ANNALS OF THE NEW YORK ACADEMY OF SCIENCES

VOLUME 168, ART. 1 PAGES 1–207

December 10, 1969

Editorial Director
PETER D. ALBERTSON

Editor-in-Chief
MARC KRAUSS

Associate Editor
HÉLÈNE RUTH BIELEFELD

RHEUMATOID FACTORS AND THEIR BIOLOGICAL SIGNIFICANCE*

Consulting Editors and Conference Cochairmen
HARRY BARTFELD AND WALLACE V. EPSTEIN

CONTENTS

Introduction. *By* HARRY BARTFELD

Introduction. *By* WALLACE V. EPSTEIN

Part I. Measurement and Distribution of Rheumatoid Factor

Methods of Measurement of Rheumatoid Factor. *By* MARION WALLER 5

Comparison of Three Serological Tests in Adult Rheumatoid Arthritis and Still's Disease (Juvenile Rheumatoid Arthritis). *By* BARBARA M. ANSELL, JOHN HOLBOROW, DEREK ZUTSHI, ARTHUR READING, AND WALLACE V. EPSTEIN 21

Distribution of Rheumatoid Factor Activity in Nonrheumatoid States. *By* HARRY BARTFELD 30

A Longitudinal Study of Rheumatoid Factors in a New England Town. *By* EDGAR S. CATHCART AND JOHN B. O'SULLIVAN 41

Part II. Structure of Rheumatoid Factors and Their Antigens

Structural and Conformational Specificity of the Antigen for Rheumatoid Factor. *By* CHRISTOPHER S. HENNEY 52

γM Rheumatoid Factors Reacting with Nitrophenyl Groups and Denatured Deoxyribonucleic Acid. *By* KRISTIAN HANNESTAD 63

Binding Properties of Monoclonal γG-Antiglobulin Factors with Human γG. *By* JEAN-CHARLES CEROTTINI AND HOWARD M. GREY 76

Rheumatoid Factors and the Structure and Function of γM Antibodies. *By* S. I. CHAVIN AND E. C. FRANKLIN 84

* This series of papers is the result of a conference entitled Rheumatoid Factors and Their Biological Significance, held by The New York Academy of Sciences on May 26 and 27, 1969.

Part III. Possible Biological Functions of Rheumatoid Factor

Interactions among Rheumatoid Factors, γG Antibodies, Lymphocytes, and Phagocytes. *By* Ronald P. Messner, Erskine M. Caperton, Jr., Richard A. King, and Ralph C. Williams, Jr. 93

The Interaction of Soluble Immune Complexes with Rheumatoid Factors. *By* Robert W. Lightfoot, Jr., Ronald E. Drusin, and Charles L. Christian 105

Relation of Rheumatoid Factor to Intracellular Inclusions. *By* John H. Vaughan, Ralph F. Jacox, George Abraham, and Richard Clark 111

The Role of Rheumatoid (Antiglobulin) Factors in Hemolytic Anemia. *By* Leonard S. Goldberg and Eugene V. Barnett 122

Histamine-Releasing Activity of Rheumatoid and Nonrheumatoid Serum and Synovial Fluid. *By* I. Broder, R. Baumal, D. Gordon, and D. Bell 126

In Vivo Interactions of Antiglobulin Factors. *By* R. T. Schultz, K. Kano, and F. Milgrom 140

Part IV. Possible Biological Functions of Rheumatoid Factor in Synovial Space

Rheumatoid Factor and the Fixation of Complement. *By* Nathan J. Zvaifler 146

Complement Components in Synovial Fluid: Activation and Fixation in Seropositive Rheumatoid Arthritis. *By* S. Ruddy, M. C. Britton, P. H. Schur, and K. F. Austen 161

Rheumatoid Factor and Kinin Generation. *By* Wallace V. Epstein, Margaret Tan, and Kenneth L. Melmon 173

Experimental Arthritis in Man and Rabbit Dependent upon Serum Anti-Immunoglobulin Factors. *By* Arnold J. Rawson, Joseph Lee Hollander, Francisco P. Quismorio, and Neva M. Abelson 188

The Joint-Fluid γG-Globulin Complexes and Their Relationship to Intraarticular Complement Diminution. *By* R. J. Winchester, V. Agnello, and H. G. Kunkel 195

Summary. *By* John H. Vaughan 204

The conference on which this monograph was based was cosponsored and supported in part by:

• THE ARTHRITIS FOUNDATION

INTRODUCTION

Harry Bartfeld, M.D.
St. Vincent's Hospital Medical Center
and New York University School of Medicine
New York, N. Y.

The first general conference on rheumatoid factors was held in New York City on January 23, 1957. It was entitled "Serological Reactions of Rheumatoid Arthritis" and was cosponsored by the National Institute of Arthritis and Metabolic Diseases and the Arthritis and Rheumatism Foundation. The presentations at that conference dealt with the various serological tests for rheumatoid factors, the fractionation of rheumatoid arthritis serum, and characterization of the factor. In its history, rheumatoid factor has been called many names: an accessory agglutinating factor, a conglutinin, a fraction of complement, a substance that upset the stabilizing properties of serum, etc. At this first conference on rheumatoid factors some workers still preferred to call it an "agglutination activating factor," as it had been named by Waaler in 1939.

Since 1957, many more investigators have further studied rheumatoid factors and they are now, courageously, considered to be antibodies to γ-globulin or anti-γ-globulins. The intent of this second general conference on rheumatoid factors, entitled "Rheumatoid Factors and Their Biological Significance," cosponsored by the New York Academy of Sciences and the Arthritis Foundation, is to bring together workers in the various scientific disciplines dealing with this subject.

In the presentations by the participants, who are from Norway, Canada, England, Switzerland, and the United States, and in the discussion periods to follow, we look forward to significant information on the following questions regarding rheumatoid factors: what they are, why and how they are formed, what they react with, and what they do in the body.

INTRODUCTION

Wallace V. Epstein, M.D.

Department of Medicine
University of California School of Medicine
San Francisco, Calif.

The occasion of a conference dealing with rheumatoid factors brings together not only a company of distinguished investigators but also those threads of research which, unassociated, seem to impart little pattern to the field, but, when assembled, suggest a current direction and a future hope. The first conference on this subject, "Serological Reactions of Rheumatoid Arthritis," was held in 1957, sponsored by The National Institute of Arthritis and Metabolic Diseases and the Arthritis and Rheumatism Foundation; it was devoted almost entirely to describing what was then the newly developed serological test system and the beginnings of our knowledge of the structure of IgM rheumatoid factor and its even less well-characterized reactant. At that time, rheumatoid factor was considered to be something between a component of the complement system and an antibody in its own right. It was at this gathering that Dr. Kunkel presented and discussed the 22S complex and its component members, an observation which proved central to the concept of rheumatoid factor as an antibody and especially to the subsequent debate concerning autospecificity.

The proliferation of information produced over the next 12 years makes categorization difficult. The present conference bears witness to the fact that exact definition of the antigen and of this very special antibody system is still beyond our reach. The fact that rheumatoid factor is not limited to the disease for which it was named may be the only fact not subject to further elaboration in our discussions; beyond that, there is little core material not still under examination.

It must be confessed at the outset that the title given this conference was an attempt to generate interest in an area we may all be attempting to avoid, namely, the biological significance of the rheumatoid factors system. It is probable that reports of clinical observations, as well as findings in the chemical, immunochemical, and serological areas, have encouraged established investigators and attracted new workers to these studies. Very likely it was Dr. Williams' observation in 1962 of the appearance of, and then the disappearance of, rheumatoid factor in the course of treated subacute bacterial endocarditis that stimulated much work dealing with the biological function and responsivity of the rheumatoid factor system. The now certain involvement of the complement system with the rheumatoid factor system opens new doors to possible biological effects.

Our 1957 conference started with a formal list of definitions and terms. Today, we share many common concepts and at least some common terms.

I should like to offer my thanks to the New York Academy of Sciences and the Arthritis Foundation for sponsoring this conference.

Part I. Measurement and Distribution of Rheumatoid Factor

METHODS OF MEASUREMENT OF RHEUMATOID FACTOR

Marion Waller, Ph.D.

Department of Medicine
Medical College of Virginia
Richmond, Va.

A survey of the recent literature has revealed a plethora of reports on rheumatoid factors in various ethnic groups and in individuals with a variety of disease states.[1] These studies often purported to demonstrate the significance of these antibodies and to imply a pathogenetic role for them. Rheumatoid factors have been demonstrated not only in the rheumatic diseases[2-41] but also in such diverse conditions as syphilis,[42-46] hypertension,[47] sarcoidosis,[48-50] infectious diseases,[51-63] myocardial infarction,[64,65] dysglobulinemia,[66-69] liver disease,[70-77] renal disease,[78] malignancy,[79] diseases of the thyroid,[80] diseases of the chest,[81-90] paroxysmal nocturnal hemoglobinuria;[91] they have been found in psychiatric populations[92] as well as in normal individuals.[93-111] Interpretation of these reports is made difficult by the variety of test systems employed, and sometimes by the conflicting results thereby obtained. Although the clinical significance of the rheumatoid factors is poorly understood, there is no doubt that these antibodies in high titer are most closely associated with the disease rheumatoid arthritis. However, there are no established changes in titer associated with therapy or duration of disease.[112,113]

A number of investigators have been concerned about the problem of standardization of these serological tests.[114,115] An excellent text has recently been published,[116] delineating in detail all of the methods that are in current use for measuring rheumatoid factors. An earlier concept[117] that these antibodies are distinctly abnormal serum factors and that a test of great sensitivity and specificity could be developed has gradually given way to the feeling that these serological responses are within the capability of almost all individuals and that the high titers observed in rheumatoid arthritis are but an exaggerated or exuberant response of what may be observed in the normal state. Thus, sensitivity is usually sacrificed for specificity and vice versa in different test systems. A comparison of this problem of standardization with that achieved for syphilis[114] is not entirely valid, since rheumatoid factors represent an antibody response of variable specificity, associated most closely with a disease of unknown etiology and ill-defined pathogenesis reflecting possibly different antigenic stimuli. Since rheumatoid arthritis is not a proven communicable disease, there are no compelling factors for the acceptance of a standardized test that is complicated, unwieldy, or exceedingly time-consuming. It has been suggested that the standardized test should achieve both specificity and sensitivity. Such a test would be capable of detecting all varieties of antiglobulin antibodies, even when present in low titers. This test could establish "diagnostic titers," which are usually not observed in the absence of rheumatoid arthritis. There are at least three test systems that could be standardized with these objectives in mind: (1) latex test, (2) FII tanned cell test, and (3) sensitized-sheep cell test. An alternate suggestion is to employ two tests: (1) a simple slide test of great sensitivity to be used as a screening test; and (2) a second test that will give a titer. The latter could be either a tube test or a slide test.

TABLE 1

TITERS OF RHEUMATOID FACTOR WITH NINE DIFFERENT TESTS

Disease*	SSC		SHC	Slide Latex		Tube Latex			FII	FII >320
	1:10	1:5		A	B	A	B	C		
Sarcoidosis (10)	—	20	—	—	—	—	—	—	320	+
	—	—	—	—	—	—	—	—	160	—
	—	—	—	—	—	—	—	—	80	—
	—	—	—	—	—	—	—	—	320	+
	—	—	—	—	—	—	—	—	80	—
	—	—	—	—	—	—	—	—	80	—
	—	20	—	+	+	40	20	160	1,280	+
	—	—	—	—	+	20	20	160	80	—
	—	—	—	—	—	—	—	—	160	—
	—	—	—	—	—	—	—	—	160	—
Rheumatoid arthritis (14)	80	320	640	+	+	1,280	1,280	1,280	20,480	+
	320	1,280	2,560	+	+	5,120	5,120	1,280	>40,960	+
	80	640	640	+	+	5,120	2,560	640	>40,960	+
	160	640	2,560	+	+	2,560	1,280	1,280	>40,960	+
	40	160	1,280	+	+	1,280	1,280	1,280	40,960	+
	640	1,280	1,280	+	+	1,280	2,560	2,560	>40,960	+
	—	40	80	+	+	40	80	320	640	+
	640	1,280	2,560	+	+	640	1,280	320	40,960	+
	80	160	80	+	—	40	40	160	80	—
	—	—	40	+	—	20	—	—	40	—
	—	—	40	+	—	40	—	—	160	—
	—	—	—	—	+	—	—	—	320	+
	—	—	—	—	—	—	—	—	40	—
	80	320	320	+	+	640	640	640	20,480	+

Degenerative arthritis (15)	—	—	40	—	—	—	—	80	40	—
	—	—	40	+	+	160	160	320	40,960	+
	—	—	40	+	+	160	80	320	640	+
	—	—	—	—	+	—	—	—	160	—
	—	—	—	—	—	—	—	—	160	—
	—	—	—	—	—	—	—	—	320	+
	—	—	—	—	—	—	—	—	80	—
	—	—	—	—	—	—	—	—	40	—
	—	—	40	+	+	20	20	160	640	+
	—	—	—	—	—	—	—	—	160	—
	—	—	—	—	—	—	—	—	160	—
	—	—	—	—	—	—	—	—	40	—
	—	—	—	—	—	—	—	—	40	—
	—	—	—	—	—	—	—	—	20	—
	—	—	—	—	—	—	—	—	160	—
Lupus (10)	—	—	40	+	+	40	640	80	2,560	+
	—	—	—	—	—	—	—	—	320	+
	—	—	—	—	—	—	—	—	320	+
	—	—	80	+	+	80	40	20	320	+
	—	—	—	+	—	20	20	—	—	—
	—	—	—	—	—	—	—	—	160	—
	—	—	—	—	—	—	—	—	40	—
	—	—	—	—	—	—	—	—	80	—
	—	—	—	—	—	—	—	—	80	—
	—	—	—	—	—	—	—	—	160	—
Normal†	160	320	1,280	+	+	2,560	2,560	2,560	>40,960	+

* Numbers in parentheses indicate number of patients whose sera were tested.
† Included for comparison.

With these problems and objectives in mind, 74 blood samples were tested with nine different serological tests. This evaluation was performed by a technician with ten years of experience in serological testing for rheumatoid factors. TABLE 1 shows the titers of rheumatoid factors in selected sera by the nine tests. The tests used in this evaluation were: the sensitized-sheep cell test (SSC),[118,119] with the sheep erythrocytes sensitized at 1:5 and 1:10 dilutions of the basic agglutinin titer of the rabbit anti-sheep cell antibody; the sensitized-human cell test (SHC);[120] two different commercially available slide test reagents; three different commercially available tube latex reagents; and the FII tanned cell test.[121]

The patients were carefully selected in order to obtain sera of specific serological activity with the test systems. All of the diagnoses were unequivocal, and some of the patients had been followed for many years. Two of the patients with rheumatoid arthritis were selected because they were known to be seronegative. Thus, this survey does not reflect the incidence of rheumatoid factors in the selected disease groups. Although the titers of rheumatoid factor tend to reflect the sensitivity of the test systems employed, the survey did not reveal spurious appearance of factor by any of the test systems. When factor was demonstrable by one of the tests, it was usually demonstrable by most of the other test systems, albeit in lower or higher titer. There was also an unexpected degree of uniformity in the pattern of results obtained with the various tests; overall, the SSC test was the most specific test, and the FII tanned cell test was the most sensitive test. It was not possible to single out any test as the most sensitive and at the same time as the most specific test. The serum from a normal young woman[122] followed for more than 11 years was included to show that from the viewpoint of serology there is no demonstrable difference between the rheumatoid factors in normal and diseased individuals, inasmuch as all of the tests used gave high titers of factor with this serum.

TABLE 2 shows the comparison of three different test systems (SSC, latex, and FII tanned cell test) for specificity and sensitivity with 64 sera. The titers from the SSC test, standardized at 1:5 and 1:10 dilutions of the basic agglutinin titer of rabbit anti-sheep cell antibody, were averaged, as were the titers performed by the three tube latex tests.

Many clinicians have been concerned about the failure of the serological tests to offer diagnostic help in juvenile rheumatoid arthritis. It has not been possible to develop a test that is very sensitive in the juvenile form of this disease and yet specific for the adult form. The nine selected sera from patients with juvenile rheumatoid arthritis were singularly negative in their serological reactions, except for one serum with the SSC test at a 1:5 dilution of the basic agglutinin titer and with the FII tanned cell test. However, the FII tanned cell test was the least specific test with sera from patients with a variety of other diseases.

TABLE 3 is used to show the observable fluctuations in titer demonstrated by the different test systems over a five-year period. Patient I.S. has had seronegative rheumatoid arthritis for 20 years, with a marked deterioration during the past five years; this deterioration was not reflected by changes in rheumatoid factor activity. Patient V.E. has also deteriorated during the past five years, but this course was reflected in her rising titer of rheumatoid factor. It was observed that all of the tests reflected these serological changes to some degree.

Since rheumatoid arthritis is not a communicable disease like syphilis, the compulsion to use a standardized test will be determined by other factors, in addition to sensitivity and specificity, especially since these two characteristics

TABLE 2

COMPARISON OF TITERS OF RHEUMATOID FACTOR OBTAINED WITH THREE DIFFERENT TEST SYSTEMS IN RELATION TO SPECIFICITY AND SENSITIVITY*

	Rheumatoid Arthritis (14)			Lupus (10)			Osteoarthritis (15)			Sarcoidosis (10)			Juvenile Arthritis (9)			Nonrheumatoids (6)		
Titer	SSC	Latex	FII	SSC	Latex	FII	SSC	Latex	FII	SSC	Latex	FII	SSC	Latex	FII	SSC	Latex	FII
> 20,000			8						1									
10,240																		
5,120																		
2,560		3				1												
1,280	1	3										1						
640	2	1	1						2						1			
320†	2	1	1			3			1			2			1			3
160	3	1	1			2		1	5			3			2			1
80	1	1	1		1	2			1			4			5		1	2
40			2			1		2	4		2							
20	1	2			2			1	1				1					
< 20	4	2		10	7	1	15	11		10	8		8	9		6	5	

* Numbers in parentheses indicate the number of patients whose sera were tested.
† The finding of titer of 320 or greater indicates a relative sensitivity of the test.

TABLE 3

OBSERVABLE FLUCTUATIONS IN TITER OF RHEUMATOID FACTOR OVER A FIVE-YEAR PERIOD

Patient*	Date of Test	SSC		SHC	Slide Latex		Tube Latex			FII
		1:10	1:5		A	B	A	B	C	
I.S.	3–16–64	–	–	–	–	–	–	–	–	40
	12–28–66	–	–	–	–	–	–	–	–	40
	11– 7–67	–	–	–	–	–	–	–	–	20
	5– 8–68	–	–	–	–	–	–	–	–	20
	2–11–69	–	–	–	–	–	–	–	–	20
V.E.	11–11–64	80	320	320	+	+	320	320	640	5,120
	11– 8–66	40	160	160	+	+	160	320	320	10,240
	9– 6–67	80	320	160	+	+	320	320	640	20,480
	7–30–68	80	320	320	+	+	640	640	640	40,960
	4– 1–69	160	640	1,280	+	+	5,120	2,560	1,280	>40,960

* I.S., a 58-year-old, white female; V.E., a 54-year-old, white female.

TABLE 4

FACTORS INVOLVED IN ACCEPTANCE OF A STANDARDIZED TEST FOR RHEUMATOID FACTOR

Test	Preparation		Time (hr)	Cost of Reagents	Skill and Cost of Labor	Apparatus*	Results		
	Inactivation	Absorption					Specificity	Sensitivity	Titer
SSC	Yes	Yes	24.0	0.25†	+++	+++	++++	+	Yes
Tube latex									
A	No	No	0.5	2.00	++	++	++	+++	Yes
B	No	No	24.0	2.00	++	++	++	+++	Yes
C	No	No	24.0	2.00	++	++	++	+++	Yes
SHC	No	No	1.5	0.10†	+	++	++	+++	Yes
Slide latex									
A	No	No	< 0.1	0.20	—	+	++	+++	No
B	No	No	< 0.1	0.20	—	+	++	+++	No
FII	Yes	Yes	24.0	0.50†	++++	+++	±	++++	Yes

* Required apparatus includes a centrifuge and waterbaths at 37° and 56°/C.

† Cost decreases with number of tests performed.

cannot be found in any single test. TABLE 4 is a simplified evaluation of those factors that will play a role in the popular acceptance of any standardized test. Both the SSC test and the FII tanned cell test require inactivation and absorption of the sera prior to testing. This is very time-consuming, and it will tend to make these two tests less popular. Some of the tube latex tests require overnight refrigeration before the final result is read, but it is quite possible that this feature could be eliminated. The cost of reagents varies considerably, and, as one might anticipate, the tests requiring the greatest technique and skill are the cheapest to perform. However, good technicians are not cheap, and thus the cost of reagents does not accurately reflect the actual cost of testing. In addition, since skilled technical help is not only expensive but also difficult to obtain, it is important to evaluate the skill required to perform an adequate test. The slide tests require practically no skill, while the FII test can only be performed by highly skilled individuals if it is to have any value at all. The clinician not directly associated with a medical complex will be concerned about the apparatus necessary to perform a test, and, of course, this physician is the least likely to have available a skilled serologist.

Conclusion

From these studies, I would conclude that neither the SSC test, with its unusually high degree of specificity, nor the FII tanned cell test, with its marked sensitivity, are suitable as standardized tests for clinicians whose chief objective in performing the test is to enjoy the diagnostic aid that it offers. The tube latex test is the most suitable titration test when time and skill are considerations. Even this test needs to be better standardized since the different reagents presently available differ in ease of performance, readability, and results obtained. The following suggestions are offered in anticipation of a standardized test that is easy to perform, whose reagent is stable, and whose test results are simple to read with accuracy: (1) use the same reagent for rapid slide and titration test; (2) color the latex particles, so that the flocculates are easy to read; (3) Standardize the test with a short incubation time, and avoid overnight tests.

There are over 200 reports in the literature since 1960 documenting the incidence of rheumatoid factors in various population groups by a variety of test procedures. It appears that further studies of this kind will only add to the confusion already existing. The most important task is the elucidation of the etiological agent or agents responsible for this interesting serological activity and the relationship of this activity to disease.

References

1. BENNETT, P. H. & P. H. N. WOOD, Eds. 1966. Population Studies of the Rheumatic Diseases. Proc. Third Int. Symp. Excerpta Medica Found. New York, N. Y.
2. ALVARO RUIZ UMAÑA, H. 1965. Serological tests in rheumatism (critical evaluation). Med. Trop. (Madrid) **41:** 251–305.
3. ANDRIOTAKIS, C., P. KAKLAMANIS & B. THOUAS. 1966. C-reactive protein, rheumatoid factor and immunoglobulin G in the serum and synovial fluid of patients with joint diseases. Rev. Rhum. **33:** 259–262.
4. BALL, J., K. J. BLACK, T. A. BURCH, J. H. KELLGREN, J. S. LAWRENCE & V. TSIGALIDOU. 1962. Comparative studies of serologic tests for rheumatoid disease. Arthritis Rheum. **5:** 61–69.
5. BERGER, H. W. & S. G. SECKLER. 1966. Pleural and pericardial effusions in rheumatoid disease. Ann. Intern. Med. **64:** 1291–1297.
6. BURCH, T. A. 1966. Epidemiological studies on rheumatic diseases. Milit. Med. **131:** 507.
7. COTTA, H. & R. LUTHER. 1964. The utility of latex tests in inflammatory, degenerative and metabolic diseases of the vertebral column and joints. Z. Orthop. **99:** 368–385.

8. Moskowitz, R. W., K. J. Bendict & R. Stauffer. 1968. *In* Population Studies in the Rheumatic Diseases. Proc. Third Int. Symp. P. H. Bennett & P. H. N. Wood, Eds. Chapt. **29:** 207–214. Excerpta Medica Found. New York, N. Y.
9. Svec, V., S. Sitaj, D. Zitnan & G. Hudakova. 1967. Laboratory tests in ankylosing spondylitis. Fysiat. Reum. Vestn. **45:** 199–203.
10. Hall, A. P., W. A. Bardawil, T. B. Bayles, A. D. Mednis & N. Galins. 1960. The relations between the antinuclear, rheumatoid and L. E. cell factors in the systemic rheumatic diseases. New Eng. J. Med. **263:** 769–775.
11. Elling, P., H. Graudal & V. Faber. 1967. Organ-specific and organ-nonspecific autoantibodies in rheumatoid arthritis. Acta Med. Scand. **182:** 707–715.
12. Gallo, G., D. Barisone & S. Accardo. 1967. Clinical use of the Singer-Plotz latex test as modified by Watson. Minerva Med. **58:** 4573—4576.
13. Rejholec, V. & M. Kralova. 1968. Therapeutic response in responsive and seronegative rheumatoid arthritis. Fysiat. Reum. Vestn. **46:** 119–122.
14. Rocha da Silva Almeida, A., M. Nahon, M. Lachtermacher & J. Houli. 1965. Comparison of the value of the Waaler-Rose test and the latex slide test for the diagnosis of rheumatoid arthritis. (A study of 134 determinations.) Rev. Brasil Med. **22:** 396–398.
15. Sato, M. 1965. Hemagglutination studies with F II-Diazo-formalinized erythrocytes and rheumatoid arthritis sera as a rheumatoid arthritis test. J. Jap. Rheum. Ass. **5:** 284–292 & 320.
16. Schöne, H. 1966. The diagnostic value of the latex fixation test. Deutsch. Gesundh. **21:** 489–491.
17. Sievers, K. 1965. The rheumatoid factor in definite rheumatoid arthritis: Analysis of 1,279 adult patients with a follow-up study. Acta Rheum. Scand. (Suppl.) **9:** 1.
18. Yuyama, H. 1967. Clinical and biochemical studies on the modified latex fixation test. J. Med. Soc. Toho Univ. **14:** 211–224.
19. Podliachouk, L., A. Eyquem & F. Jacqueline. 1964. Anti-Gm substances in rheumatoid arthritis and in cirrhosis. Transfusion **7:** 377–381.
20. Graudal, H. 1968. Distributions of the Waaler-Rose titer in rheumatoid arthritis and other types of arthritis. Ugeskr. Laeg. **130:** 1561–1565.
21. Bonomo, I., A. Samara, H. Pacheco Tavares, M. Schneider & G. Gangemi. 1967. A clinical study of the latex fixation test. Hospital (Rio) **71:** 387–394.
22. Jarløv, N. V. 1968. Seronegative rheumatoid arthritis. A reinvestigation. Ugeskr. Laeg. **130:** 1572–1574.
23. Kellgren, J. H. & W. M. O'Brien. 1962. On the natural history of rheumatoid arthritis in relation to the sheep cell agglutination test (SCAT). Arthritis Rheum. **5:** 115.
24. Dixon, A. St. J. 1960. "Rheumatoid arthritis" with negative serological reaction. Ann. Rheum. Dis. **19:** 209.
25. Hill, A. & C. C. Greenbury. 1965. Clinical interpretation of serological tests in rheumatoid arthritis. *In* Progress in Clinical Rheumatology. A. St. J. Dixon, Ed. : 42. Little, Brown & Co. Boston, Mass.
26. Sharp, J. T., E. Calkins, A. S. Cohen, A. F. Schubart & J. J. Calabro. 1964. Observations on the clinical, chemical and serological manifestations of rheumatoid arthritis, based on the course of 154 cases. Medicine **43:** 41–58.
27. Berkowitz, S. S., S. Laurian, E. Guariglia & O. Steinbrocker. 1965. Latex agglutination reaction in synovial fluid and blood serum. AIR (Arch. Interam. Rheum.) **8:** 259–267.
28. Legler, F. 1968. Serological diagnosis of rheumatoid arthritis. Med. Welt. **43:** 2354–2356.
29. Abdin, Z. H., M. S. El-Feel & M. A. M. Abul-Fadl. 1966. The differential agglutination test in Egyptian rheumatoid and rheumatic children. Egypt. Rheum. **3:** 91–97.
30. Bardfeld, R., D. Kanková & J. Duhon. 1968. Differentiation of some juvenile arthritic diseases. Fysiat. Reum. Vestn. **46:** 101–105.
31. Boni, A. & K. Fehr. 1966. Serologic aspects of juvenile rheumatoid arthritis. Z. Rheumaforsch. **25:** 81–95.
32. Cassidy, J. T. & H. A. Valkenburg. 1967. A five year prospective study of rheumatoid factor tests in juvenile rheumatoid arthritis. Arthritis Rheum. **10:** 83–90.
33. Daneo, V., A. Robecchi, Jr. & M. Viara. 1966. Serologic aspects of juvenile rheumatoid arthritis. Reumatismo **18:** 506–512.
34. Scala, M., M. Raganati & N. de Cicco. 1964. The significance of the latex fixation test in children. Pediatria (Napoli) **72:** 1252–1256.
35. Swierczynska, Z. & E. Wilkoszewski. 1966. Some serological reactions in rheumatoid arthritis. Fysiat. Reum. Vestn. **44:** 233–236.

36. Swierczynska, Z. & E. Wilkoszewski. 1967. Certain serological tests in juvenile rheumatoid arthritis. Pediat. Pol. **42:** 159–162.
37. Jansen, C. 1967. Serology in the differential diagnosis of hip joint arthritis and osteoarthritis. Deutsch. Med. J. **18:** 160–161.
38. Corcos, J. M., W. C. Robbins, B. Rogoff & R. Heimer. 1961. Some serum protein abnormalities in patients with progressive systemic sclerosis and their relatives. Arthritis Rheum. **4:** 107.
39. Vaccaro, R., R. Rossoni & P. Alestra. 1967. Antinuclear antibodies and antiperinuclear and rheumatoid factors in a series of children with collagen diseases. Minerva Pediat. **19:** 2181–2186.
40. Zachariae, E., H. Zachariae & M. S. Larsen. 1965. Psoriatic arthropathy. Nord. Med. **74:** 857–861.
41. Block, K. J., E. J. Wohl, I. I. Ship, R. B. Oglesby & J. J. Bunim. 1960. Sjögren's Syndrome. I. Serological reactions in patients with Sjögren's Syndrome with and without rheumatoid arthritis. Arthritis Rheum. **3:** 287–297.
42. Liotta, S., V. Scandariato, E. Mancini & E. Armentano. 1966. Rheumatoid factor test in syphilis. Progr. Med. (Napoli) **22:** 817–822.
43. Mustakallio, K. K., A. Lassus & O. Wager. 1967. Auto-immune phenomena in syphilitic infection: Rheumatoid factor and cryoglobulins in different stages of syphilis. Int. Arch. Allerg. **31:** 417–426.
44. Mustakallio, K. K., A. Lassus, T. Putkonen & O. Wager. 1967. Cryoglobulins and rheumatoid factor in sera from chronic false positive seroreactors for syphilis. Acta Dermatovener. **47:** 249–254.
45. Peltier, A. & C. L. Christian. 1959. The presence of the "rheumatoid factor" in sera from patients with syphilis. Arthritis Rheum. **2:** 1–7.
46. Semeraro, N., M. L. Orabona & F. La Torre. 1964. Comparison of some serological tests for determination of rheumatoid factor in syphilis patients. Progr. Med. **20:** 51–55.
47. Köröskényi, K., L. Bakos, K. Hegyi & J. Vajda. 1965. Serology in hypertension and rheumatoid arthritis. Z. Rheumaforsch. **24:** 277–279.
48. Kunkel, H. G., H. J. Simon & H. H. Fudenberg. 1958. Observations concerning positive serologic reactions for rheumatoid factor in certain patients with sarcoidosis and other hyperglobulinemic sera. Arthritis Rheum. **1:** 289–296.
49. Oreskes, I. & L. E. Siltzbach. 1968. Changes in rheumatoid factor activity during the course of sarcoidosis. Amer. J. Med. **44:** 60–67.
50. Spilberg, I., L. E. Siltzbach & C. McEwen. 1969. The arthritis of sarcoidosis. Arthritis Rheum. **12:** 126–137.
51. Cathcart, E. S., R. C. Williams, Jr., H. Ross & E. Calkins. 1961. The relationship of the latex fixation test to the clinical and serological manifestations of leprosy. Amer. J. Med. **31:** 758–765.
52. Houba, V. & A. C. Allison. 1966. M-Antiglobulins (rheumatoid factor-like globulins) and other gamma globulins in relation ot tropical parasitic infections. Lancet **i:** 848.
53. Huntley, C. C., M. C. Costas, R. C. Williams, A. D. Lyerly & R. G. Watson. 1966. Anti-gamma-globulin factors in visceral larva migrans. J.A.M.A. **197:** 552.
54. Pinto, L. & G. Barbieri. 1964. Rheumatoid factor positivity in sera from patients with leprosy. G. Mal. Infett. **16:** 456–462.
55. Bradford, D. E. 1965. R. A. latex test in infectious mononucleosis. J. Roy. Army Med. Cps. **111:** 240–243.
56. Svec, K. H. & J. H. Dingle. 1965. The occurrence of rheumatoid factor in association with antibody response to influenza A_2 (Asian) virus. Arthritis Rheum. **8:** 524–529.
57. Messner, R. P., T. Laxdal, P. G. Quie & R. C. Williams, Jr. 1968. Rheumatoid factors in subacute bacterial endocarditis—bacterium, duration of disease or genetic predisposition? Ann. Intern. Med. **68:** 746–756.
58. Williams, R. C., Jr. & H. G. Kunkel. 1962. Rheumatoid factor, complement and conglutinin aberrations in patients with subacute bacterial endocarditis. J. Clin. Invest. **41:** 666–675.
59. Bartfeld, H. 1960. Incidence and significance of seropositive tests for rheumatoid factor in non-rheumatoid diseases. Ann. Intern. Med. **52:** 1059.
60. Dalmau-Ciria, M. 1964. Latex fixation test in non-rheumatic conditions. Med. Clin. (Barc.) **42:** 148–150.
61. Dresner, E. & P. Trombly. 1959. The latex fixation reaction in non-rheumatic diseases. New Eng. J. Med. **261:** 981–988.
62. Howell, D. S., J. M. Malcolm & R. Pike. 1960. F II agglutinating factors in serums of patients with non-rheumatic diseases. Amer. J. Med. **29:** 662–671.

63. LOSPALLUTO, J., B. DORWARD & M. ZIFF. 1960. Observations on serologically positive non-rheumatoid sera. Arthritis Rheum. **3:** 277.
64. SHINA, S. & Y. YASUDA. 1965. Studies on the latex slide test in myocardial infarction. Jap. Heart J. **6:** 511–520.
65. THOMPSON, R. A. 1965. Tests for rheumatoid factor after myocardial infarction. J. Clin. Path. **18:** 808–810.
66. FUDENBERG, H., J. L. GERMAN, III & H. G. KUNKEL. 1962. The occurrence of rheumatoid factor and other abnormalities in families of patients with agammaglobulinemia. Arthritis Rheum. **5:** 565.
67. VAUGHAN, J. H. & R. A. GOOD. 1958. Relation of "agammaglobulinemia" sera to rheumatoid agglutination reactions. Arthritis Rheum. **1:** 99–111.
68. HRNČÍŘ, Z. & F. MATĚJA. 1966. Rheumatoid factor in myeloma and in Waldenstroem's macroglobulinemia. Cas. Lek. **105:** 351–354.
69. KLEIN, F. & P. MATTERN. 1965. Rheumatoid factors in primary and reactive macroglobulinemia. Ann. Rheum. Dis. **24:** 458–464.
70. BONOMO, L., J. LOSPALLUTO & M. ZIFF. 1963. Anti-gamma globulin factors in liver disease. Arthritis Rheum. **6:** 104–114.
71. COLTORI, M. C., DEL VECCHIO-BLANCO & M. CARRELLA. 1967. Serologic studies in different types of liver diseases and other diseases. Fegato **13:** 1–33.
72. SCHIRMER, A. & T. WEGMANN. 1964. The appearance and prognostic significance of the rheumatoid factor in liver diseases. Schweiz. Med. Wschr. **94:** 1751–1755.
73. TABE, K. 1967. Clinical and experimental studies on rheumatoid like factor in chronic liver disease. J. Osaka Cy. Med. Cent. **16:** 157–176.
74. VACCA, G. & G. F. FERRO. 1965. Liver disease and immunological abnormalities in the serum. Minerva Med. **56:** 2372–2374.
75. WEINREICH, J. & H. A. KUHN. 1965. The latex slide test in liver disease. Acta Hepatosplen. **12:** 44–50.
76. GRAZIANI, B., S. LIOTTA & F. BASSETTI. 1964. Positive agglutination tests for the rheumatoid factor in liver disease. Med. Clin. Sper. **14:** 380–390.
77. LANI, C. & G. P. TOMEI. 1964. The R. A. test in icteric patients. Rheumatismo **16:** 415–418.
78. WALLER, M., R. IRBY, F. MULLINAX & E. C. TOONE, JR. 1965. Connective-tissue disease and rheumatoid factors in patients with renal transplants. New Eng. J. Med. **273:** 12–18.
79. HURRI, L. & Y. PERTTALA. 1965. Observations on non-specific Waaler-Rose and latex reactions in cancer patients. Ann. Med. Intern. Fenn. **54:** 181–183.
80. OKA, M., P. SEPPÄLÄ & L. MIKKONEN. 1966. Latex slide test in thyroid diseases. Acta Med. Scand. **179:** 253–255.
81. BOD , A. 1964. Is the latex-test applicable for the assessment of tuberculous activity? Tuberk. Tudobet. **17:** 359–361.
82. BONOMO, L., U. GILLARDI & A. TURSI. 1966. Anti-γ-globulin and antinuclear factors in chronic bronchitis. Relation to disease course and hyperglobulinemia. Amer. J. Clin. Path. **45:** 313–322.
83. GOTTLIEB, A. J., H. SPIERA, A. S. TEIRSTEIN & L. E. SILTZBACH. 1965. Serologic factors in idiopathic diffuse interstitial pulmonary fibrosis. Amer. J. Med. **39:** 405–410.
84. LEVINE, H., M. SZANTO, H. G. GRIEBLE, G. L. BACH & T. O. ANDERSON. 1968. Rheumatoid factor in non-rheumatoid pleural effusions. Ann. Intern. Med. **69:** 487–492.
85. LIOTTA, S., C. OMODEI-ZORINI, B. GRAZIANI & V. SCANDARIATO. 1965. Results obtained in agglutination tests for the "rheumatoid factor" in tuberculosis. Med. Clin. Sper. **15:** 157–166.
86. PERNIS, B., E. C. VIGLIANI & I. J. SELIKOFF. 1965. Rheumatoid factor in serum of individuals exposed to asbestos. Ann. N. Y. Acad. Sci. **132:** 112.
87. SINGER, J. M., C. M. PLOTZ, F. M. PERALTA & H. C. LYONS. 1962. The presence of anti-gamma globulin factors in sera of patients with active pulmonary tuberculosis. Ann. Intern. Med. **56:** 545–552.
88. TOMASI, T. B., H. H. FUDENBERG & N. FINBY. 1962. Possible relationship of rheumatoid factors and pulmonary disease. Amer. J. Med. **33:** 243.
89. WARD, R. & R. STALKER. 1965. Sheep cell agglutination test in chronic interstitial pulmonary fibrosis. Ann. Rheum. Dis. **24:** 246–256.
90. SINGER, J. M., F. M. PERALTA, H. D. LYONS & C. M. PLOTZ. 1961. Presence of serologically active macroglobulins in sera of some patients with active pulmonary tuberculosis. Arthritis Rheum. **4:** 124.
91. KAPLAN, M. E., S. KOCHWA, L. R. WASSERMAN & R. E. ROSENFIELD. 1966. Serum anti-gamma G globulin factors in paroxysmal nocturnal hemoglobinuria. Blood **28:** 446.

92. Oreskes, I., S. Rosenblatt, H. Spiera & H. Meadow. 1968. Rheumatoid factors in an acute psychiatric population. Ann. Rheum. Dis. **27**: 60–63.
93. Aho, K. 1961. A normal series for rheumatoid serology collected by random sampling. Acta Rheum. Scand. **7**: 18.
94. Laine, V., K. Sievers, O. Wager & K. Aho. 1962. The rheumatoid factor in the personnel of a rheumatism hospital. Acta Rheum. Scand. **8**: 229.
95. Natvig, J. B. & O. Tönder. 1967. Specificity of rheumatoid factors in sera from blood donors. Acta Path. Microbiol. Scand. **69**: 437–444.
96. Valkenburg, H. A., J. Ball, T. A. Burch, P. H. Bennett & J. S. Lawrence. 1966. Rheumatoid factors in a rural population. Ann. Rheum. Dis. **26**: 497–508.
97. Waller, M., E. C. Toone, Jr. & E. Vaughan. 1964. Study of rheumatoid factor in a normal population. Arthritis Rheum. **7**: 513–520.
98. Wilson, J. A. & A. G. Steinberg. 1965. Antibodies to gamma globulin in the serum of children and adults. Transfusion **5**: 516–524.
99. Valkenburg, H. A. 1963. Rheumatoid factor in populations. *In* The Epidemiology of Chronic Rheumatism. **1**: 74–81. Blackwell Sci. Publ. Oxford, England.
100. Valkenburg, H. A. 1963. Latex fixation test (LFT). *In* The Epidemiology of Chronic Rheumatism. **1**: 337–339. Blackwell Sci. Publ. Oxford, England.
101. Holman, H. & H. R. Diecher. 1960. Appearance of hypergammaglobulinemia, positive serological reactions for rheumatoid arthritis and complement fixation reactions with tissue constituents in sera of relatives of patients with systemic lupus erythematosus. Arthritis Rheum. **3**: 244.
102. Cammarata, R. J., G. P. Rodnan, R. H. Fennell, Jr., R. J. Cestello & A. S. Creighton. 1964. Serologic reactions and serum protein concentrations in the aged. Arthritis Rheum. **7**: 297.
103. De Blécourt, J. J., F. W. Boerma & E. O. Vorenkamp. 1965. Occurrence of rheumatoid factor in serum of the aged. Ann. Rheum. Dis. **24**: 180–181.
104. De Blécourt, J. J., F. W. Boerma & E. O. Vorenkamp. 1967. Incidence of "rheumatoid factor" in aged serum. Ann. Rheum. Dis. **26**: 47–49.
105. Heimer, R., F. M. Levin & E. Rudd. 1963. Globulins resembling rheumatoid factor in serum of the aged. Amer. J. Med. **35**: 175–181.
106. Hrnčir, K., K. Dvorák & F. Matěja. 1967. Clinical importance of the rheumatoid factor in old age. Cas. Lek. Cesk. **106**: 257–263.
107. Jacqueline, F., L. Podliachouk & A. Eyquem. 1965. Rheumatoid factors and anti-Gm substances in the serum of the aged. Ann. Inst. Pasteur (Lille) Suppl. **5**: 48–57.
108. Litwin, S. D. & J. M. Singer. 1965. Studies of the incidence and significance of anti-gamma globulin factors in the aging. Arthritis Rheum. **8**: 538–550.
109. Balazs, V. & M. M. Frohlich. 1966. Anti-heavy chain activity of the monoclonal (paraprotein) cryoglobulins with rheumatoid factor effect. Amer. J. Med. Sci. **252**: 668.
110. Meltzer, M., E. C. Franklin, K. Elias, R. T. McCluskey & N. Cooper. 1966. Cryoglobulinemia: A clinical and laboratory study. II. Cryoglobulins with rheumatoid factor activity. Amer. J. Med. **40**: 837.
111. Viara, M. & M. Mellini. 1964. The latex-fixation test for rheumatoid arthritis (RA-test) in subjects of advanced age. Rheumatismo **16**: 59–64.
112. Ziff, M. 1957. The agglutination reaction in rheumatoid arthritis. J. Chronic Dis. **5**: 644–667.
113. Ziff, M. 1963. Possible clinical and pathological associations of rheumatoid factor. Arthritis Rheum. **6**: 481–489.
114. Bozsóky, S. 1963. The problem of standardization in rheumatoid arthritis serology. Arthritis Rheum. **6**: 641–649.
115. Cathcart, E. S. & J. B. O'Sullivan. 1965. Standardization of sheep cell agglutination test. Arthritis Rheum. **8**: 530–537.
116. Cohen, A. S., Ed. 1967. Laboratory Diagnostic Procedures in the Rheumatic Diseases. Little, Brown & Co. Boston, Mass.
117. Hall, A. P. 1961. Serologic tests in rheumatoid arthritis. Med. Clin. N. Amer. **45**: 1181–1196.
118. Waaler, E. 1940. On the occurrence of a factor in human serum activating the specific agglutination of sheep blood corpuscles. Acta Path. Microbiol. Scand. **17**: 172–188.
119. Rose, H. M., C. Ragan, E. Pearce & M. O. Lipman. 1948. Differential agglutination of normal and sensitized sheep erythrocytes by sera of patients with rheumatoid arthritis. Proc. Soc. Exp. Biol. Med. **68**: 1–6.
120. Waller, M. V. & J. H. Vaughan. 1956. Use of anti-Rh sera for demonstrating agglutination activating factor in rheumatoid arthritis. Proc. Soc. Exp. Biol. Med. **92**: 198.

121. HELLER, G., A. S. JACOBSON, M. H. KOLODNY & W. H. KAMMERER. 1954. The hemagglutination test for rheumatoid arthritis. II. The influence of human plasma fraction II (gamma globulin) on the reaction. J. Immunol. **72:** 66.
122. WALLER, M. & E. C. TOONE, JR. 1968. Normal individuals with positive tests for rheumatoid factor. Arthritis Rheum. **11:** 50–55.

General Discussion

DR. BARTFELD: This is a comprehensive review of the work of many years on various serological tests for rheumatoid factor by Dr. Waller. It seems appropriate that the first report of this conference concern serological tests since all of the work on rheumatoid factors began after another Waaler established a blood test for them.

E. FABRIC (*I. E. Chemical Co.*): Was there any correlation between the serological tests and the response to therapeutic agents?

DR. WALLER: With the test systems that we have used, the sensitized-human cell test and the sensitized-sheep cell test, we get no significant change of titers with any type of therapy at all. These individuals have been exposed to all types of therapy available today to rheumatologists with no marked alteration that we could note.

DR. WARREN ASH (*National Institutes of Health, Bethesda, Md.*): Does the temperature at which these tests are run have any influence upon the results?

DR. WALLER: The test procedures, particularly those in which we use commercially available reagents, follow the recommendations of the manufacturers. We have selected commercially available reagents principally because so many individuals throughout the country rely on them. We do not alter the temperature from the standard conditions established for the tests. Standard procedures were followed with the sensitized-sheep cell test and the FII tanned cell test.

DR. ASH: I ask this question because a recent paper in *Arthritis and Rheumatism* reported that tests conducted at 4° C would give a false-positive reaction compared with the same test conducted at room temperature (22° C).

DR. WALLER: In smaller hospitals and in service laboratories for clinicians in areas away from a large medical complex, tests would not be done at 4° C. Room temperature seems to be the most popular temperature at which to do the latex test. Overnight refrigeration is required in some of the tests, but I feel that these tests can be standardized so that refrigeration will not be necessary.

DR. COHEN (*Rosewell Park Memorial Institute, Buffalo, N.Y.*): We are still using aligator erythrocytes instead of sheep cells for tests, since humans lack heterophil antibodies to alligator cells and these cells are resistant to osmotic stress and mechanical trauma. The only problem, of course, is how to obtain alligator cells? We have used donors from a zoo. I feel that erythrocytes from species to which there are no human antibodies should be used in these tests There are organizations or individuals who can supply the cells of species other than the common ones that we've been using.

DR. BARTFELD: We have also performed sensitized-alligator cell tests in a large series of cases, and the results correlate well with those of the sheep cell tests; the tests are also simpler to perform.

DR. EPSTEIN: In regard to these tests, no one has attempted to advocate specificity for disease as a criterion of selection. Whether one talks about serological tests for syphilis, or almost anything else, in most areas, people have given up the idea that some number is going to significantly influence one's judgment in clinical decision making. You've made an excellent case for the fact that the most sensitive test is the best test. I don't think we can teach second- and third-year medical students that the laboratory is arbitrarily cutting off their decision-making capability. I think that unless there is some specificity beyond that which you've demonstrated, we should uniformly use the most sensitive test and then append to it those criteria which make us arbitrarily group patients into certain categories of disease.

May I add just one technical point? If one begins the tanned cell procedure at a 1:200 dilution of serum, I think it's very wise not to inactivate it for the effects it has on globulin.

DR. BARNETT: I would second Dr. Epstein's comment and add one in regard to Dr. Ash's use of the words "false positive." We should, I think, avoid the use of terms like false positive and false negative. We have a variety of tests with a wide range of sensitivities. These different tests also have a wide range of specificities – not necessarily specific for disease, but specific immunochemically, that is, antibody to different terminants or species of γ-globulin. If we keep those two terms in mind, we can then interpret the data on a particular serum.

I would like to ask a question regarding the occasional patient that has classical rheumatoid arthritis with the destruction of cartilage and bone and rheumatoid nodules. Statistically, we can make the generalization that such patients should have positive serology and a high-titer of antiglobulins in one or another test. However, we occasionally find patients who are seronegative in whole panel of tests. Would you comment on such sera and would you advise fractionating sera in such situations?

DR. WALLER: I think any process, fractionation, or immunochemical test that elucidates these basic mechanisms would be important I would like to point out that we seem to be oriented in terms of a large medical complex. Whether we like it or not, these tests do offer a diagnostic aid; they should not be the determining factor in diagnosis, but they are an aid to clinicians throughout the country. I think that they would all like to have a test that is relatively easy to do and offers them this diagnostic aid with caution.

DR. MALTZ (*San Jose, Calif.*): Your implication that a slide test is simpler to perform and often the only one that's available bears some consideration in these studies. Do you think there is some way that we might improve the specificity of the slide test without a loss of sensitivity? Do you think that use of euglobulin instead of serum might provide this? On that same topic, would you comment about the use of euglobulin in the other methods and also something about inhibition tests.

DR. WALLER: In this survey, I purposely avoided using serum fractions such as the euglobulin fraction or modifications which are employed in large research laboratories in their efforts to achieve specificity and sensitivity. I tried to make a survey of the most popular systems in use today by the majority of people. I do think that with isolated euglobulins you can demonstrate factor in many instances where you might not with whole serum.

This is not, however, a practical test for very small hospitals. We must get this test into a form that is relatively simple to perform. Most technicians perform many other types of tests, and do this test only once or twice a week. Thus, we want a test that clinicians can use as a diagnostic aid, not as the diagnosis itself. It was with this idea in mind that I performed this series of tests rather than approach the problem from the point of view of the research laboratory. I am not really able to answer all of these questions on the basis of my results, because I did not do euglobulin fractions in the entire series of tests.

DR. JANOFF (*Princeton Laboratories*): In connection with this paper, I would like to comment on some sera that were examined in parallel with the sensitized-sheep cell tube tests and with the latex FII slide test (Hyland) and a sensitized-sheep cell slide test (Rheumaton). The data affirm the general consensus that the sensitized-sheep cell test is very specific and the FII latex test is less specific and more sensitive. The sensitized-sheep cell slide test was almost as specific as the Waller-Rose test, and had increased sensitivity, as well.

DR. WALLER: Dr. Maltz asked if I had any recommendations for making a slide test more specific and a better test. I do not, and I think that most clinicians would like to have a titer: we should, however, bear in mind the problem that the obstretician has had for years in getting anti-Rh antibody titers, which are not at all uniform in the various hospital laboratories. He is very disconcerted if you say that a patient does not have anti-Rh antibody when indeed the patient does. But whether you give him a titer of 600 or 1,000 probably doesn't alter the pattern he is going to follow. Such tests are important in his handling of the patient and the projected handling of the child by the pediatrician. The tests have not been standardized to a great degree in the various hospitals, except that the hospitals have adhered to certain guidelines set down by the American Association of Blood Banks. I believe if one were to send out a sample of serum to various hospitals throughout the country, the difference in titers of specific anti-Rh antibodies would be shocking. We find ourselves in a similar situation today as far as rheumatoid factor is concerned.

DR. E. ORESKES (*Mount Sinai Hospital School of Medicine, New York, N.Y.*): It has been thirteen years since Drs. Singer and Plotz reported the latex fixation test. In all that time, we have still not achieved adequate standardization of this most commonly used procedure, and we should give this matter some thought. This test is the one most widely used, and its variations are innumerable. At least two points in the procedure which are critical to me are the standardization of the size and number of latex particles employed and, perhaps even more important, the standardization of the concentration of the γ-globulin, since some is not absorbed to the surface of these particles.

I agree with Dr. Epstein that for many purposes the most sensitive test is the most useful. We use the FII tanned sheep cell test: it is quite valuable in our own work. I agree that we ought to obtain data and evaluate it rather than censor it in a technical sense. The FII tanned sheep cell test, by virtue of its greater sensitivity, is, in our opinion, one of the most useful.

DR. WALLER: Actually, I much prefer the sensitized-human cell test, but I am a realist too. The man who donates the sensitizing antiserum (Ripley) is a single individual, and the use of this test will not appreciably add to or help the problem of standardization throughout the country. This man will not live forever, and the chances of finding another such serum in the near future is rather slim. I would like to help the average internist in the country and to think of a test that would be the best for him and the most practical at this time. In the very near future, we might develop a much better test than the latex test, but at the moment it seems to be the most practical test we can offer.

DR. SINGER (*Montefiore Hospital and Medical Center, The Bronx, N.Y*): In the performance of serological tests, we should realize their intrinsic technical limitations on a qualitative and semiquantitative measurement. This is true in regard to the varibility of the commercial production of latex from batch to batch; the content and nature of detergents used for stabilization of particles; differing degrees of aggregation of γ-globulin (on standing at room temperature or under refrigeration); buffers other than glycine buffer at pH 8.2; freezing of the latex particles; instability of any precoated particle standing at room or refrigeration temperatures; and reading results by lens or overreading.

The efforts of the Arthritis Foundation as well as those of Dr. Waller, for the standardization of rheumatoid arthritis sera are of considerable significance in the confidence of laboratories employing this technique. In spite of limitations, the latex test is used world-wide, and I fully agree with Dr. Waller that this test performs qualitatively in either the physician's office or in a small remote laboratory. The importance of confirmation of the slide test by tube cannot be overemphasized, however. We have recently developed three new techniques in our laboratory which I hope may make this procedure a quantitative one: (1) utilization of a detergent that will stabilize latex particles coated with γ-globulin for a period of a year; (2) chemical binding of γ-globulin on latex particles: and (3) an automated technique for direct recording to the patient's chart.

COMPARISON OF THREE SEROLOGICAL TESTS IN ADULT RHEUMATOID ARTHRITIS AND STILL'S DISEASE (JUVENILE RHEUMATOID ARTHRITIS)

Barbara M. Ansell, F.R.C.P., John Holborow, M.D., Derek Zutshi, M.B., and Arthur Reading, F.I.M.L.T.

Rheumatism Research Unit
Canadian Red Cross Memorial Hospital
Taplow, Maidenhead, England

and

Wallace V. Epstein, M.D.

Department of Medicine
University of California School of Medicine
San Francisco, Calif.

This study on the FII test[1] was undertaken to investigate whether serum antiglobulin factors could be detected in arthritis usually considered seronegative, and particularly in Still's disease.

Materials and Methods

From May of 1966 to August of 1967, all sera sent from the wards and outpatient departments for differential-agglutination tests (DAT)* and latex tests which are performed by the methods described by Bywaters and Scott,[2] were also tested by the FII technique. Control sera for the adults were obtained from 23 healthy subjects, 71 outpatients with no signs of rheumatic diseases, and 65 patients admitted to the hospital with diseases of the respiratory system. For the children, control sera were obtained from 203 patients who had recovered from rheumatic fever, and 70 sick children not suffering from any rheumatic diseases.

For the FII test, sera were titrated over a range of doubling dilutions from 1:25 to 1:12,800. To obtain mean titers for comparison of different groups of subjects, the tubes in this dilution range were numbered consecutively from 1 to 10, and the titers of individual sera were scored as tube numbers (0 = > 1:25, 1 = 1:25, 2 = 1:50, etc.). The geometric mean FII titers and their variances were calculated on this basis.

Results

The distribution of anti-γ-globulin activity in a mixed population, consisting of patients with rheumatic diseases of varying types as well as controls, form a continuing gradent from nil to high levels (FIGURE 1). There was good correlation between the latex test and FII hemagglutination test, particularly at high and low titers (FIGURE 1). If we take a dilution of 1:16 or more as positive, the correlation between the FII test and the DAT titer of Rose-Waaler was not as good (FIGURE 2) as that between the latex and FII tests; more than 50% of sera showing FII titers at any level gave negative DAT results.

When only cases of classical and definite rheumatoid arthritis were considered out of the group as a whole, there was an upward gradation of the FII titer (FIGURE 3), but a small group, 42 of 435 cases, remained negative. In definite Still's disease, 142 out of 286 showed no demonstrable FII titer, and there was not the same tendency to a rising gradation.[3] A comparison of the three

* A modification of the sensitized-sheep cell test.

tests in those patients who fulfilled the criteria for classical and definite rheumatoid arthritis showed that 42% had positive DAT results, 75% positive latex tests, and 87% an FII titer of 1:200 or more (TABLE 1). Of the nine patients who showed no FII titer, three had positive DAT results. The percentage of controls with FII titers of 1:200 or more was considerably higher than the percentage of those showing positive DAT or latex tests. The mean tube titer was 7.4 in rheumatoid arthritis, compared with 1.4 in healthy controls, 1.2 in the sick-adult controls, and 1.8 in the respiratory-disease controls. Thus, on tube titers there was a significant difference in the results found in rheumatoid arthritis patients and the various control groups. There was no significant difference in the results of the control groups, so it was decided to combine all three for purposes of comparison with other rheumatic diseases, giving a mean tube titer of 1.5. The mean tube titer in degenerative joint disease, ankylosing spondylitis, arthritis associated with gastrointestinal disorders, Reiter's syndrome, and gout showed no statistical difference from that of the control group.[4]

In definite Still's disease, however, there was a similar increase in the percentage with positive results according to the tests (TABLE 2); thus, 7% had positive DAT results, 15% latex tests, and 26% an FII titer of 1:200 or more. The mean FII titer in Still's disease was 2.3, which was significantly greater ($p = 0.001$) than

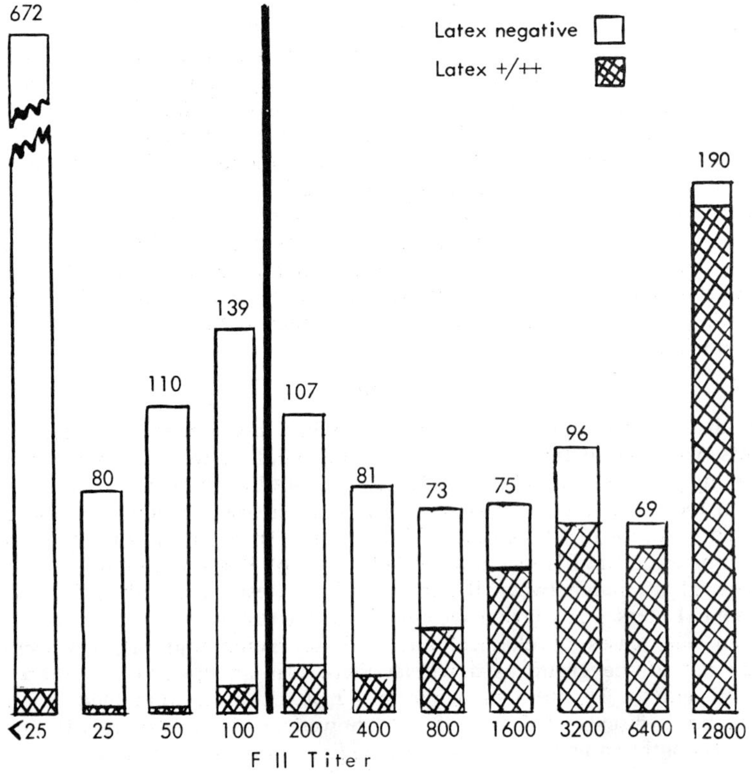

FIGURE 1. Comparison of FII and latex results in 1,692 patients.

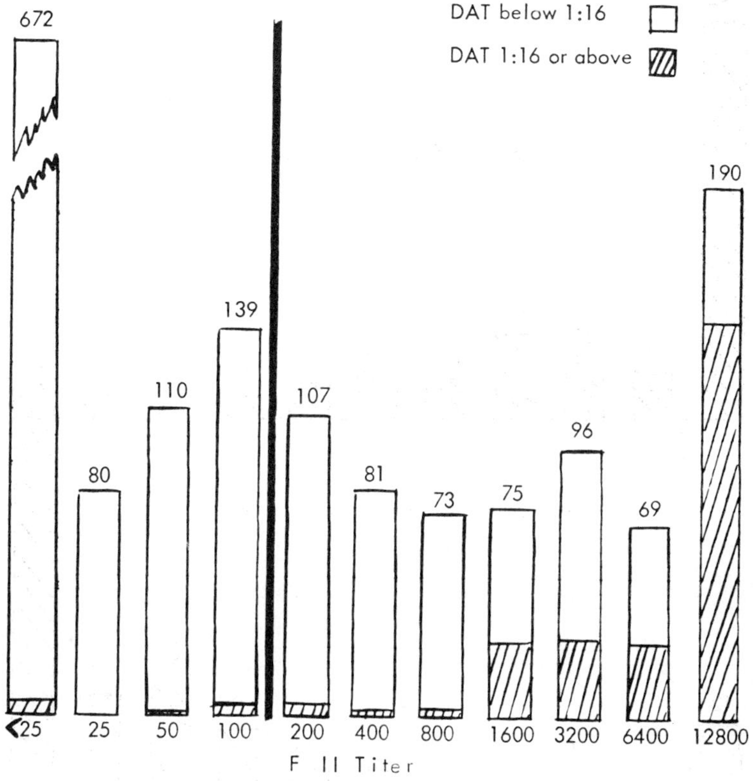

FIGURE 2. Comparison of FII and DAT results in 1,692 patients.

the 1.6 for controls of the same age distribution, but does not approach the 7.4 of the rheumatoid arthritis subjects.

The material was analyzed with regard to the activity of the disease. By active disease we mean tenderness or pain on movement of one or more joints, with soft tissue swelling, with or without a raised sedimentation rate.[3] Active disease is associated with a significantly higher ($p = 0.001$) mean titer than is inactive disease, the latter being the same as the control group (TABLE 3). When the cases are subdivided for sex, the mean tube titer is considerably higher in females with active disease than it is in males. The mean titer in active males is not significantly greater than that of the controls. In both females and males the inactive cases showed the same tube titer as the controls did. In active Still's disease, the mean FII titer increases with age in both sexes (TABLE 4) but it rises earlier in the females than in the males; a similar increase was not seen in inactive cases. This rise in tube titer correlates with the age of onset of disease, rather than with the age at the time of testing, and is irrespective of the duration of the disease. The mean tube titer in those whose illness commenced between the ages of 10 and 14 years was 3.4 compared with 1.8 in the youngest group, where the duration of follow-up was longer.

The mean tube titer in those patients who had a monarticular onset was 1.6, i.e., not significantly different from that of the controls; similarly, at no time was

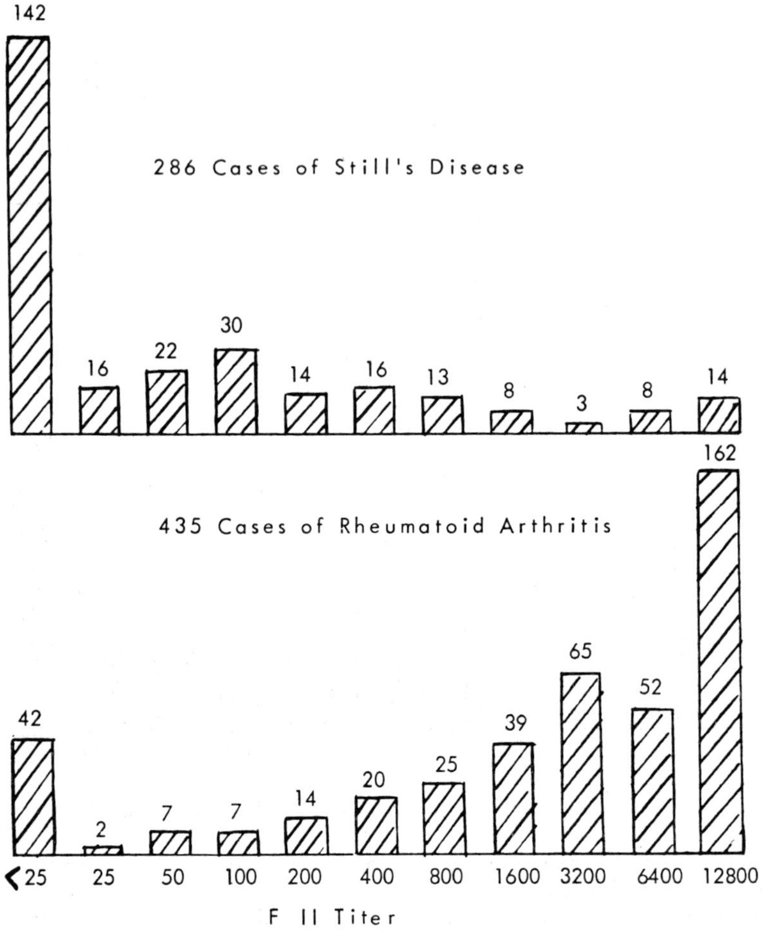

FIGURE 3. Distribution of FII titer in 286 cases of definite Still's disease and 435 cases of classical and definite rheumatoid arthritis.

iridocyclitis associated with any rise in FII titer, nor was the development of psoriasis, ankylosing spondylitis, or amyloidosis. The only close correlation between a rise in titer and some other factor was found in the presence of nodules in the active cases: Patients with nodules were found to have a mean tube titer of 8.6, i.e., similar to that of adult rheumatoid arthritis patients; two of these patients had associated vascular lesions. Radiographs of the hands, feet, and cervical spine were available in all except one patient. In active cases, there was a significantly higher ($p = 0.001$) mean FII titer (3.9) in those cases with erosions than in those who showed no radiological change or who had healed or degenerative lesions. In the 12 cases with severe residual deformity leading to a chair or crutch existence, there was a significantly higher FII titer, irrespective of the activity of the Still's disease.[5]

In 211 cases of Still's disease, an antinuclear factor test was carried out on the

TABLE 1

COMPARISON OF DAT, LATEX, AND FII RESULTS IN RHEUMATOID ARTHRITIS AND CONTROL SUBJECTS

Experimental Group	No.	DAT of 1:16 or more (%)	Latex +/++ (%)	FII Hemagglutination Titer %			Mean FII Titer
				1:200 or more	1:25–1:100	1:25	
Rheumatoid arthritis							
Classical and definite	435	42	75	87	4	9	7.4
Probable and possible	69	5	30	50	17	33	3.8
Controls							
Healthy	70	0	0	11	34	55	1.4
Sick (adult)	71	0	4	16	20	46	1.2
Chest disease	65	1.5	11	26	14	60	1.8

TABLE 2

COMPARISON OF DAT, LATEX AND FII RESULTS IN STILL'S DISEASE AND JUVENILE CONTROLS

Experimental Group	No.	DAT of 1:16 or more (%)	Latex +/++ (%)	FII Hemagglutination Titer %			Mean FII Titer
				1:200 or more	1:25–1:100	1:25	
Definite Still's disease	286	7	15	26	24	50	2.3
Juvenile Controls	273	0.4	2	18	30	52	1.6

TABLE 3

MEAN FII TITER IN ACTIVE AND INACTIVE CASES OF STILL'S DISEASE

Experimental Group	Both Sexes		Male		Female	
	No.	Mean Titer	No.	Mean Titer	No.	Mean Titer
Active Still's disease	169	2.8*	48	1.9	121	3.2†
Inactive Still's disease	117	1.6	48	1.4	69	1.7
Controls	273	1.6	129	1.4	144	1.7

* $p = < 0.001$.
† $p = < 0.001$.

TABLE 4

EFFECT OF AGE ON FII TITER IN ACTIVE STILL'S DISEASE

Age at Time of Test (years)	Mean Titer	
	Male	Female
0–4	1.0	0
5–9	1.8	1.3
10–14	0.7	3.0
15–24	1.9	4.1
25–34	4.3	3.3
35–44	5.0	6.0

TABLE 5

EFFECT OF AGE OF ONSET ON MEAN FII TUBE TITER IN ACTIVE STILL'S DISEASE

Age at Onset (years)	No.	Mean Titer	Duration (years)
0–4	45	1.8	10.5
5–9	58	2.7	9.7
10–14	62	3.4	7.4
15	4	6.0	11.8

same sera.[6] There was no overall correlation: Of the 92 cases with negative FII titers, 25 were positive for antinuclear factors. However, six of the 11 patients with an FII titer of 1:12,800 or more were positive for antinuclear factor. In adult rheumatoid arthritis, there was a close correlation between the high-titer FII tests and postive antinuclear factor findings.

Discussion

As might be expected, many sera negative by the DAT and/or latex test in classical and definite rheumatoid arthritis were shown to possess anti-γ-globulin activity. Despite this finding, there is no fundamental alteration in the serological state, since a small group (10%) of patents satisfying the criteria for classical and definite rheumatoid arthritis remained persistently seronegative, as did patients with ankylosing spondylitis, Reiter's syndrome, gout, and arthritis associated with gastrointestinal disorders. In Still's disease, only 26% of cases had FII titers of more than 1:200, compared with 87% in adult rheumatoid arthritis. The excess anti-γ-globulin activity in Still's disease compared with the controls is accounted for very largely by female patients with active disease. The mean age of onset in these patients tends to be higher than in the group as a whole. The correlation of a higher anti-γ-globulin activity with the presence of nodules and joint erosions suggests that these patients may represent a subgroup within the main group with an early onset of adult rheumatoid arthritis. Even in these females with active disease, the antiglobulin levels are still below those seen in adult rheumatoid arthritis. There is no clue as to whether this is due to a difference in the mechanism of onset of the disease in juvenile patients compared with adults, or whether similar etiological factors cause different degrees of autoimmune response in the two populations.

Summary

The distribution of anti-γ-globulin activity in a mixed population of rheumatic and nonrheumatic subjects formed a gradient from high levels to zero. In classical and definite rheumatoid arthritis, the FII titer was significantly raised, showing a downward gradation from 1:12,800 to 1:100. Low titers were found in patients with rheumatic diseases usually regarded as seronegative. In Still's disease, the mean tube titer was significantly higher than in juvenile controls; this was particularly evident in females with active disease and a late age of onset, and also correlated with the presence of nodules and erosions.

References

1. HELLER, G., A. S. JACOBSON, M. H. KOLODNY & W. H. KAMMER. 1954. J. Immunol. **72:** 66.
2. BYWATERS, E. G. L. & F. E. T. SCOTT. 1960. *In* Recent Advances in Clinical Pathology. S. C. Dyke, Ed. : 278–302. J. & A. Churchill, Ltd. London, England.

3. BYWATERS, E. G. L. & B. M. ANSELL. 1959. Bull. Rheum. Dis. **9:** 189.
4. ZUTSHI, D. W., C. A. READING, W. V. EPSTEIN, B. M. ANSELL & E. J. HOLBOROW. 1969. Ann. Rheum. Dis. **28:** 289.
5. ZUTSHI, D W., B. M. ANSELL, E. G. L. BYWATERS, W. V. EPSTEIN, E. J. HOLBOROW & C. A. READING. 1969. Ann. Rheum. Dis. In press.
6. HOLBOROW, E. J. & G. D. JOHNSON. 1969. Association of Clinical Pathologists, Broadsheet 65. J. Clin. Path.

Discussion of the Paper

DR. VAUGHAN: I would like to know whether you are willing to suggest that the juvenile patients who are seropositive and have nodules and erosions are actually cases of rheumatoid arthritis of the adult variety and have a different disease from the remainder of the children studied.

DR. ANSELL: Yes, I am. Over the last ten years, most of my clinical work has involved a long-term follow-up of our juvenile cases. On the basis of a 15-year follow-up, there is no doubt that there is a small subgroup within a group of some 200 children who are behaving just like adults; even their nodules sometimes resemble those of adults. I think we have demonstrated that within the group as defined by serological terms, there is this small subgroup.

In addition, we are finding a higher incidence of ankylosing spondylitis in the 20-year follow-ups: 10% of the boys we followed for 20 years have ankylosing spondylitis. We don't really know what this means, and that is why I think the disease should not be called juvenile rheumatoid arthritis, but rather juvenile chronic polyarthritis; only a small subgroup of these patients have true juvenile rheumatoid arthritis.

DR. BARNETT: What is your experience with the result of therapy and changes in serum titers in this group? Also, you indicated that among your patients with gout or ankylosing spondylitis as a group there was no statistically significant difference in serum titer from that of your controls; however, do some of the individuals with higher titers have certain characteristics pointing to peripheral joint involvement and activity of disease, progression, and longer attacks of gout?

DR. ANSELL: In respect to your first question, 23 of our juvenile patients were treated with gold out of a total of 70 that we followed sequentially with the FII test over a one-year period. We compared them with 50 other cases of Still's disease studied monthly during that period, and there was a significant fall in the serum titer from 3.2 to 2.3 in the treated cases over the six months of therapy, with our usual, standard course of gold treatment. We have noted similar reductions in rheumatoid factors measured by the DAT test in juvenile patients treated with gold over a six-month period. The disappointing thing is that one or two patients who originally did extremely well on gold started to deteriorate when put on maintenance gold treatment, and their DAT titers have gone up again.

In answer to your second question on ankylosing spondylitis, we investigated these cases thoroughly, but we could find nothing to account for the one or two cases with higher titers. The finding of high titer did not correlate with the presence of peripheral arthritis in the ankylosing spondylitis cases. There were two interesting ankylosing spondylitis patients with high FII titers, whose serum electrophoresis showed a single band which Arthur Howard feels is indistinguishable from what he believes to be myeloma globulin in their γ-globulins. These two patients are currently under study, but neither of them has myeloma disease. I do not have enough data on gout to be able to make any definitive statements.

DR. G. J. FRIOU (*University of Southern California School of Medicine, Los*

Angeles, Calif.): In terms of the nature of the antigen that might be responsible for either the FII factor or the DAT factor, I think some of the most interesting patients are the few who have positive DAT tests that are out of proportion to the FII titer; I wonder if there's anything unusual or characteristic about those patients from a clinical point of view.

DR. ANSELL: One of them has amyloid disease now, but did not have it at the time that he was tested. Another is one of those very rare cases of Still's disease who, right at the beginning of his illness, within three months of the onset, showed a strongly positive DAT test (1:256) and a negative latex and a negative FII test. I can't remember anything else particular about them, although we examined their sera carefully.

DR. COHEN: On the basis of all your experience, would you subscribe to the statement that a patient who is seropositive at the onset of disease has a stormier course, whether he is an adult or juvenile patient?

DR. ANSELL: Among the juvenile patients, yes. I personally follow up the juvenile cases, and I have no doubt that they remain with active disease longer, have more destructive lesions, and are much more likely to be left with severe residua. Among the adults, I personally have not undertaken a major study.

In regard to male and female patients aged 16–21 years at the onset of their disease, the females who are seropositive within a few weeks of the onset have all done extraordinarily badly. The boys in this age group, irrespective of their serology, seem to have done better.

DR. O'SULLIVAN: I was interested in your comments on the decreased titers for these rheumatoid factors with treatment of your rheumatoid patients. I wondered whether you had any controls. As you know, these factors are continuously distributed in the population, and there is no phenomenon of a regression toward the mean; if you select people who are positive to any test under these circumstances and then retest them, you will find that a higher proportion is negative on retesting. The same results are found in tests for high cholesterol and high blood sugars, and high titers of serological factors would tend to come down partly due to the technical variation of the test itself.

DR. ANSELL: I obviously didn't make myself clear. In the juvenile patients, we selected those patients with active disease who were currently attending the clinics regularly and performed monthly DAT, latex, and FII tests on them over a one-year period. After six months, I selected about 50 who had never received gold or chloroquine therapy and compared them with the 22 that had received gold treatment. The 22 who were to receive gold treatment started with a higher titer, which fell and approached that of the others at the end of the six-month treatment.

DR. MONTAN (*New York University, New York, N. Y.*): I would like to know what percentage or how many of the patients originally used as controls and thought to have rheumatic fever turned out to have juvenile chronic polyarthritis after they were followed.

DR. ANSELL: We did not use acute rheumatic fever patients as controls. We used patients who had recovered from the disease for at least one year. We are in the process of a 20-year follow-up study of them, and no one was included in this long-term study who had not been followed for at least one year without any sign of active disease in the rheumatic fever category. To date, none of these patients has subsequently progressed to persistent arthritis.

The acute rheumatic fever cases form a small but interesting group in that we found a certain number with raised titers on DAT, latex, and FII tests. From an investigational point of view, it's unfortunate that rheumatic fever is such a declining disease; the group in our study numbers only about 20.

Dr. Williams: Have you any data on the serum complement levels in these same patients.

Dr. Ansell: No.

Dr. Williams: Do you have those sera frozen? It would be interesting to find out if the presence of anti-γ-globulin factors in these patients was inversely proportional to the mean level of complement. Also, do you know of any data by others who have studied this particular question in a longitudinal fashion? I ask this because John Davis has said that rheumatoid factors protect patients from complement.

Dr. Ansell: I have no data on this. The sera seem to be scattering themselves to the four winds; they constitute a rather valuable collection, and everyone wants them. Currently, most of them are in Birmingham for immunoglobulin studies. Perhaps the most interesting work that's being done on them at the moment is at the Middlesex Hospital, where Roitt is testing these sera for antibodies to IgG and IgM. He has found that some of these children had antibodies to IgG, correlated with activity of the disease. Antibodies to IgM were found in a few sera in which rheumatoid factor could not be detected by any other of the techniques we have used.

DISTRIBUTION OF RHEUMATOID FACTOR ACTIVITY IN NONRHEUMATOID STATES*

Harry Bartfeld, M.D.

St. Vincent's Hospital Medical Center
and New York University School of Medicine
New York, N. Y.

In 1940, Waaler[1] reported the presence of a factor in human serum which caused the agglutination of amboceptor-sensitized sheep erythrocytes. He named this factor the agglutinating activating factor and found it in the sera of 35% of 50 rheumatoid arthritis patients and 9% of 202 controls (patients with cancer, peptic ulcer, pneumonia, neurasthenia, etc). This factor was discovered in 1922, as Waaler pointed out, by Meyer,[2] who, in the examination of 100,000 sera for the Wasserman reaction, found ten sera that agglutinated sensitized sheep erythrocytes. The first serum was from a patient with liver cirrhosis, and the second was from a patient with chronic bronchitis. Thus, rheumatoid factors were really first discovered in nonrheumatoid diseases.

In this survey of the work of our laboratories and others, patients having possible as well as definite connective tissue diseases were omitted. The sensitized-sheep cell agglutination tests (SSC) used were either the differential-agglutination test[3] or the heterophile absorbed test serum modification,[35] usually the latter. The human fraction II (Hu FII) studies were mainly latex FII precipitation tests,[4] although some were FII tanned sheep cell tests.[5]

TABLE 1 shows that the incidence of seropositive tests increases with age. Although the positive titers were generally low, some of the SSC titers in healthy donors were as high as 1:256. One such patient had a 22S component in the serum and did not develop rheumatoid arthritis over a two-year follow-up.[6]

In a study done in the United States, there was a higher incidence of seropositive individuals among women and Negroes.[10] It was also found that there were more seropositive individuals in Africa in those tribes that had poor nutrition.[11] Rheumatoid factor is present in significant numbers of older individuals having degenerative diseases: 30% of 235 patients with an average age of 71 years (excluding those with tuberculosis, syphilis, lung disease, and sarcoidosis) were Hu FII positive; among these, 64% of those with Parkinsonism, 47% of those with diabetes mellitus, and 17% of those with arteriosclerotic cardiovascular disease were seropositive.[12]

TABLE 2 shows that patients may have rheumatoid factors in their sera in the course of infectious diseases. In fact, tests for rheumatoid factors have been used to help confirm the diagnosis of subacute bacterial endocarditis (SBE). Following remission of SBE in one to two months, the titers fall to zero, and it has been suggested that this is due to absence of the antigenic stimulus.[24] The viral diseases studied showed 14–17% seropositivity and include viral pneumonia, influenza, and herpes zoster; as in SBE with remission the tests became negative.[13] In six cases of rubella synovitis, the Hu FII tests were positive in two, and one of these was SSC positive. [14a&b,39] The incidence of seropositive individuals is higher in infectious hepatitis than in any other viral disease except infectious mononucleosis.

Parasitic diseases, especially when accompanied by involvement of the liver

* This work was aided by grants from the New York chapter of the Arthritis Foundation and the Commonwealth Foundation.

TABLE 1

INCIDENCE OF RHEUMATOID FACTORS WITH AGE

Age (years)	Hu FII Tests		Reference	SSC Tests		Reference
	Total No.	% Positive		Total No.	% Positive	
0–29	2,828	2	7	2,828	0.7	7
30–59	2,536	4	7	2,536	0.2	7
60–93	413	24	7–9	375	6.0	7–9

TABLE 2

INCIDENCE OF RHEUMATOID FACTOR IN INFECTIOUS DISEASES

Diagnosis	Hu FII Tests		Reference	SSC Tests		Reference
	Total No.	% Positive		Total No.	% Positive	
Bacterial disease	51	20	13–15	77	11	16–21
Subacute bacterial endocarditis	58	48	14a & b, 22–24	76	22	17, 22–27
Syphilis	215	13	13, 28–30	198	5	17–19, 29, 31, 32
Viral disease*	60	17	13, 30, 33	42	14	17, 19, 20, 27
Infectious hepatitis	12	24	13, 14a & b, 23	47	21	14, 20, 21, 34, 35
Leishmaniasis	10	100	36	10	90	36
Schistosomiasis	24	4	37			
Larvae migrans	59	44	37			
Trypanosomiasis	104	27	36, 38	104	44	36, 38

* Including viral pneumonia, influenza, and herpes zoster.

and reticuloendothelial system, produce a significant incidence of seropositivity. This was seen in a study of visceral larvae migrans in children ranging from one to five years in age, in which 44% of the children were seropositive; the titers decreased with remission. In a concurrent study of 33 juvenile rheumatoid arthritis patients, only 15% were seropositive; the authors suggested that the stimulus for rheumatoid factor production was greater in helminth infections.[37]

In view of the striking reticuloendothelial hypertrophy and hyperplasia of lymph nodes in leishmaniasis and trypanomiasis, it is not surprising that there is a very high incidence of rheumatoid factors in each condition, both by the Hu FII and SSC tests, approaching or surpassing the incidence in rheumatoid arthritis. In trypanosomiasis, the percentage of seropositivity was increased, especially in those patients with increased IgM levels; positive reactions became negative after treatment of sera with mercaptoethanol. Two cases with an acute onset had SSC titers of 1:16 and 1:128 five weeks after the infecting sting.[38]

Lung diseases are associated with a high number of seropositive tests (TABLE 3). Bronchitis, due mainly to bacterial infections, showed an incidence of rheumatoid factors almost double that of bacterial infections in general. In 50 bronchitis patients treated with antibiotics and followed for two to eight weeks, the titers became lower or negative.[40]

In a study of coal miners[1] pneumoconiosis, 42% of patients without associated arthritis showed a positive SSC test, but 89% with associated rheumatoid arthritis were seropositive. This incidence was higher than that found for rheumatoid arthritis alone.[41] Although pneumoconiosis is associated with rheumatoid arthritis, other industrial dust diseases are not. In asbestosis and

TABLE 3

INCIDENCE OF RHEUMATOID FACTORS IN LUNG DISEASES

Diagnosis	Hu FII Tests		Reference	SSC Tests		Reference
	Total No.	% Positive		Total No.	% Positive	
Bronchitis	105	62	40	71	18	40
Asthma	23	17	40	18	0	40
Coal miners' disease						
Simple pneumoconiosis	23	0	41	23	4	41
Massive fibrosis	56	25	41, 42	63	23	41, 42
Asbestosis	315	21	43			
Silicosis	212	15	43			
Idiopathic pulmonary fibrosis	66	32	44–46	66	46	44–46

silicosis, seropositivity increases after long exposure, usually 15 years, but the highest titers are not always found in the most serious cases. It has been suggested that there is an increase of immunologically competent cells in the lungs in chronic granulomatous diseases of the lungs.[43]

Isolated perfused lungs of rabbits produce antibodies,[47] and some patients with lung diseases associated with pleurisy (tuberculosis, cancer, pneumonia) demonstrate rheumatoid factor present in the pleural fluid but not in the serum.[15] In idiopathic pulmonary fibrosis, the incidence of seropositivity was found to be higher with the SSC test than with the Hu FII test. It was suggested that since the lungs are the first large capillary bed after synthesis of rheumatoid factor in lymph nodes, local precipitation of antigen-antibody complexes could initiate disease processes. Thus, in a study of 14 rheumatoid arthritis patients with high titers of rheumatoid factor, 64% had radiographic signs of lung disease, but there was no lung disease present in 14 rheumatoid arthritis patients with low titers of rheumatoid factor. Intermediate complexes were present in the sera of these rheumatoid arthritis and idiopathic pulmonary fibrosis patients. There was no evidence of arthritis in the idiopathic pulmonary fibrosis patients.[44]

TABLE 4 shows the incidence of seropositivity in sarcoidosis, tuberculosis, and leprosy. The cases of sarcoidosis reported did not have joint involvement. The incidence of seropositive individuals was twice as great when arthritis was present.[51] In a series of sarcoidosis patients, there were more seropositive cases among those in whom the disease had been present for two yars or more. In this series, 38 seropositive patients were followed for two years. When retested, 19 of 26 who were clinically well had Hu FII titers that were negative or had dropped by three tube dilutions. In the 12 whose clinical activity was worse or stationary, the titers of rheumatoid factors were unchanged or increased.[50]

In active chronic pulmonary tuberculosis and leprosy, there was no correla-

TABLE 4

INCIDENCE OF RHEUMATOID FACTORS IN SARCOIDOSIS, TUBERCULOSIS, AND LEPROSY

Diagnosis	Hu FII Tests		Reference	SSC Tests		Reference
	Total No.	% Positive		Total No.	% Positive	
Sarcoidosis	231	17	14a & b, 48–51	157	5	14, 22, 26, 32, 48–51
Tuberculosis	377	11	13, 23, 28, 52	289	6	17, 52
Leprosy	101	24	53	101	15	53

TABLE 5

INCIDENCE OF PHEUMATOID FACTORS IN DYSPROTEINEMIAS AND PARAPROTEINEMIAS

Diagnosis	Hu FII Tests		Reference	SSC Tests		Reference
	Total No.	% Positive		Total No.	% Positive	
Hypergamma-globulinemia	207	19	13, 14a & b, 30, 54–56	61	32	32, 55
Purpura hyperglobulinemia	5	100	58	16	62	57, 58
Multiple myeloma	88	18	13, 14a & b, 23, 30, 55, 57	122	4	14a & b, 17, 35, 55, 57–59
Liver cirrhosis	115	36	13, 14a & b, 23, 30	206	16	17, 19, 21, 27, 55
Macroglobulinemia						
Secondary	48	35	13, 14a & b, 38	36	16	38
Primary	76	30	13, 14a & b, 34, 38, 55, 57	77	22	38, 55, 57
Leukemia and lymphoma	54	19	13, 14a & b, 56	23	4	17, 22, 26, 34, 60
Cancer	151	22	13, 14a & b, 15, 22, 23, 30	75	11	14a & b, 16, 19, 20, 22, 26, 32, 34, 58, 60

tion between activity or duration of the disease and level of titer of rheumatoid factors.[52,53] In the serum of 17 of 20 seropositive leprosy patients, prior absorption with lepromin or tuberculin removed the agglutinating factors, and ultracentrifuge studies showed similar, if not identical, agglutinating factors in leprosy and rheumatoid arthritis.[53]

TABLE 5 shows the incidence of seropositivity in patients with hypergammaglobulinemia, secondary or reactive macroglobulinemia not associated with known infectious causes, noninfectious diseases of the lymphoreticular system, and primary macroglobulinemia. In the overall or reactive synthesis of macroglobulins under these conditions, some are produced that have rheumatoid factor properties.[61] In primary macroglobulinemia, it is possible that malignant clones of cells arise and synthesize macroglobulins having rheumatoid factor properties.[58] Serum of a patient with liver disease, seropositive with the Hu FII test and the SSC test, contained a 22S complex similar to that found in rheumatoid arthritis.[62]

TABLE 6 lists the incidence of seropositivity in a group of patients having

TABLE 6

INCIDENCE OF RHEUMATOID FACTOR IN CRYOGLOBULINEMIA AND INFECTIOUS MONONUCLEOSIS

Diagnosis	Hu FII Tests		Reference	SSC Tests		Reference
	Total No.	% Positive		Total No.	% Positive	
Purpura cryoglobulinemia	13	90	63, 64	13	30	63, 64
Infectious mononucleosis	70	4 (22° C)	65			
	50	72 (4° C)	65			
Infectious mononucleosis cryoprecipitates	20	100	66			

cryoglobulinemia unassociated with multiple myeloma or primary macroglobulinemia. These patients had a complex symptomatology, consisting of purpura, weakness, and arthritis.[63] The cryoglobulins could be separated into 19S IgM and 7S IgG components. The cryoglobulinemic sera, isolated cryoglobulins, and the 19S IgM isolates also agglutinated cells coated with aggregated heavy chains but not those sensitized with light chains.[64]

It was demonstrated that cold-reactive rheumatoid factors were present in the sera of infectious mononucleosis and reticulum cell sarcoma patients. Hu FII tests done at 4° C with sera from infections mononucleosis patients were 18 times more positive than when done at room temperature; similarly, there was a sevenfold increase of positive reactions with sera of reticulum cell sarcoma patients. This difference was not found with sera from rheumatoid arthritis or sick hospital patients.[65]

TABLE 7 shows the incidence of seropositive tests in a group of syndromes with possible autoimmune mechanisms, such as Sjörgren's syndromes and Behcet's syndrome, both of which are characterized by multiple autoantibodies. In both syndromes, polyarthritis may be present. The Sjörgren's syndrome cases summarized in TABLE 7 did not have any associated connective tissue disease; however the incidence of rheumatoid factors, both by the Hu FII test and SSC test; was much higher than that found in definite rheumatoid arthritis.[67] Biopsies of lymph glands in these patients showed infiltration with lymphocytes and plasma cells; malignant lymphoma was reported to have developed in some.[67]

A group of investigators followed 132 patients with Behcet's syndrome. They performed Hu FII tests in 30 cases and found 66% positive.[68] In a previous study, they had found 64% of 85 patients of this group with articular symptoms.[73] These results contrast with another study of 25 patients with this syndrome, 76% of whom had polyarthritis although all 25 were seronegative for rheumatoid factor.[69]

Two groups of investigators have reported positive tests for rheumatoid factor in recipients of renal homografts. These patients had received immunosuppressive and corticosteroid therapy. In one series of 21 recipients, the factors appeared in approximately eight weeks. Seven patients developed musculoskeletal complaints, with periarthritis of knees and ankles; three developed erythematous nodular skin lesions, and nine developed peripheral neuritis. A total of 12 of the 21 had some symptom. In most cases, the musculoskeletal complaints developed when the steroid dose was decreased. Only one of the 14 recipients demonstrating positive rheumatoid factor tests rejected the transplant, while two of the seven who were seronegative rejected their transplants.[70] In another series of 60 recipients, 38% developed musculoskeletal complaints of synovitis

TABLE 7

INCIDENCE OF RHEUMATOID FACTORS IN SJÖRGREN'S SYNDROME, RENAL HOMOGRAFTS, AND MYOCARDIAL INFARCTIONS

Diagnosis	Hu FII Tests		Reference	SSC Tests		Reference
	Total No.	% Positive		Total No.	% Positive	
Sjörgren's Syndrome	23	96	67	19	74	67
Behcet's syndrome	55	36	68, 69			
Renal homograft	81	74	70, 71	75	8	70, 71
Myocardial infarction	55	12	72	55	20	72

TABLE 8
INCIDENCE OF RHEUMATOID FACTORS IN PSYCHIATRIC DISEASES

Diagnosis	Hu FII Tests		Reference
	Total No.	% Positive	
Endogenous depression	27	63	74
Schizophrenia	45	38	74
Psychoneuroses	14	57	74

or arthalgia and pain. Rheumatoid factors appeared between the second and 28th week following the transplant in 93% of the patients, with no relation to the musculoskeletal complaints.[71]

Positive tests for rheumatoid factors have also been found following myocardial infarction. Factors were present more often in those patients for whom there was a history of previous infarction or who had suffered a more serious infarct. Titers were not very high, and tests were negative in most patients by the time they were discharged.[72]

TABLE 8 shows the incidence of rheumatoid factors in psychiatric diseases. When schizophrenia and psychoneuroses were associated with depression, the incidence of positive tests were even higher.[74] The reason for these seropositive tests is unknown. It has been reported, however, that stimulation of the rat hypothalmus increased γ-globulins levels.[75] It is known, also, that symptoms of schizophrenia and reactive depression, as well as rheumatic factors, can be present in systemic lupus erythematosus. The psychiatric patients were not tested for antinuclear factor.[74]

Immunization and Rheumatoid Factor

A study of 27 postepidemic influenza patients showed that four produced Hu FII- and SSC-positive rheumatoid factors in association with the influenza antibody response. Two of these patients had active influenza, and the other two had been vaccinated.[33]

It has also been reported that the injection of brucella antigens into normal individuals caused induction of rheumatoid factors that reacted with Hu FII. However, if red cells were coated with antibrucella 7S γ-globulin produced by the patient, the cells were not agglutinated by the individual's own rheumatoid factor.[76] In another study, brucella vaccine was injected into rheumatoid arthritis patients, healthy relatives of these patients, and matched controls. Following vaccination, seven (33%) of 21 rheumatoid arthritis patients initially negative became SSC positive, 14 (16%) of 90 seronegative relatives became SSC positive, and three (3%) of 106 matched controls became SSC positive. All individuals, rheumatoid and nonrheumatoid, showed an equal degree of brucella antibody response.[77]

Repeated transfusions have been shown to cause the production of rheumatoid factors, and there was correlation between the number of transfusions and the incidence of Hu FII-positive tests. Following 50 transfusions, the incidence was 15%; following 100, it was 50%; and following 200, it was 71%.[78]

Similar Immunological Reactions or Positive Sera

Ouchterlony double-agar gel-diffusion studies with seropositive sera of rheumatoid arthritis and nonrheumatoid patients showed similar macroglobulin precipitin lines of identity when reacted against aggregated Hu FII, antirheumatoid euglobulin serum, and antimacroglobulin serum. These precipitin lines did not form following prior absorption of the test sera with Hu FII.[79]

Discussion and Summary

Rheumatoid factors that are reactive with both human IgG and rabbit IgG are present to a significant degree in nonrheumatoid states. While on the whole they react more often with human IgG, as does the classical rheumatoid factor of rheumatoid arthritis, they do not react as often with rabbit IgG. There are many exceptions, including trypanosomiasis, leishmaniasis, idiopathic pulmonary fibrosis, Sjörgren's syndrome, and purpura hypergammaglobulinemia.

The finding of rheumatoid factor in nonrheumatoid states may explain its connection with rheumatoid arthritis:

1. Its presence in infectious diseases and following vaccination, repeated transfusions, renal homografts, and in the aged established that humans produce rheumatoid factor in response to immunization.

2. It can be produced in a short time, in infections within two to five weeks and following homografts in two to eight weeks.

3. When the stimulus for its production is removed in acute infections, it disappears. Its presence in chronic infectious disease is associated with tissue breakdown and the presence of autologous and foreign antigen with sustained immunogenic stimulus; this supports the hypothesis that IgG complexed with antigen may be a stimulus for production of rheumatoid factors (anti-γ-globulins). The antigenic stimulus for rheumatoid factor in the aged could follow a series of repeated infections or modification of autologous IgG, since aging is a series of nonlethal somatic mutations. It has been shown that prior absorption of seropositive leprosy sera with lepromin or tuberculin removed the rheumatoid factors.

4. Diseases affecting the lymphoreticuloendothelial system, whether primary or secondary (reactive), and whether due to infectious or noninfectious causes, are associated with hypergammaglobulinemia and macroglobulinemia. Some of the polyclonal or monoclonal macroglobulins produced in such states are rheumatoid factors.

5. The presence of a high incidence of rheumatoid factors in nonrheumatoid states when organs such as the lung, liver, and the lymphoreticuloendothelial system are involved is noteworthy and points to local production of rheumatoid factor in these organs.

6. The presence of high-titer rheumatoid factors (that react with both human and rabbit IgG), 22S, and intermediate complexes for long periods of time in nonrheumatoid individuals without producing rheumatoid arthritis points to a nonpathogenic role of this factor in the latter disease.

7. Alternately, these rheumatoid factors and complexes may be needed to express or reinforce pathogenic phenomena present in those individuals with diathesis for rheumatiod arthritis.

8. Grabar has suggested that antibodies against endogenous substances may be only the pathological expression of a normal physiological process: the formation of immunoglobulins, whose function is to fix and carry products of metabolism or degradation.[80]

References

1. Waaler, E. 1940. Acta Path. Microbiol. Scand. **17**: 172.
2. Meyer, K. 1922. Immunitatsforsch. Exp. Ther. **34**: 229.

3. Rose, H. M., C. Ragan, E. Pearce & M. O. Lipman. 1948. Proc. Soc. Exp. Biol. Med. **68:** 1.
4. Singer, J. M. & C. M. Plotz. 1956. Amer. J. Med. **21:** 888.
5. Heller, F., A. S. Jacobson, M. H. Kolodny & W. H. Kammerer. 1954. J. Immunol. **72:** 66.
6. Waller, M. V., B. Decker, E. C. Toone & R. Irby. 1961. Arthritis Rheum. **4:** 579.
7. Waller, M. V., E. C. Toone & E. Vaughan. 1964. Arthritis Rheum. **7:** 513.
8. Heimer, R., F. M. Levin & E. Rudd. 1963. Amer. J. Med. **35:** 175.
9. de Belecourt, J. J., S. W. Boerma & E. O. Vorenkamp. 1965. Ann. Rheum. Dis. **24:** 180.
10. Lichtman, M. A., J. H. Vaughan & C. G. Hames. 1967. Arthritis Rheum. **10:** 204.
11. Valkenberg, H. A. 1963. *In* The Epidemology of Chronic Rheumatism. J. H. Kellgren, M. R. Jeffery & J. Ball, Eds. : 74. Blackwell Sci. Publ. Oxford, England.
12. Litwin, S. D. & J. Singer. 1965. Arthritis Rheum. **8:** 538.
13. Dresner, E., P. Trombly & G .F. O'Brien. 1959. Clin. Res. **7:** 49.
14a. Bartfeld, H., E. Mahood & E. F. Hartung. 1958. Ann. Rheum. Dis. **17:** 83.
14b. Bartfeld, H. & E. F. Hartung. Unpublished data.
15. Levine, H., Szanto, H. G. Grieble, F. L. Bach & T. O. Anderson. 1968. Ann. Intern. Med. **69:** 587.
16. Scott, F. E. T. 1952. Lancet **i:** 392.
17. Harter, F. & F. Dickgiesser. 1953. Deutsch Arch. Klin. Med. **200:** 202–235.
18. Ball, J. 1952. Ann. Rheum. Dis. **11:** 97.
19. Wager, O. 1950. Ann. Med. Exp. Fenn. **28** (Suppl. 8): 154.
20. Svartz, N. & K. Schlossmann. 1952. Acta Med. Scand. **142:** 420.
21. Tawil, G. S. & E. M. Abd El Dahab. 1955. Amer. J. Clin. Path. **25:** 166.
22. Jacobson, A. S., W. H. Kammerer, J. Wolf, W. V. Epstein & G. Heller. 1956. Amer. J. Med. **20:** 490.
23. Rothermich, N. O. & V. K. Phillips. 1957. J.A.M.A. **164:** 1999.
24. Williams, R. C. & H. G. Kunkel. 1963. J. Clin. Invest. **41:** 666.
25. Brown, R., J. J. Bunim & C. McEwen. 1949. Ann. Rheum. Dis. **8:** 299.
26. Winbald, S. 1952. Acta Med. Scand. **142:** 458.
27. De Forest, G. K., M. B. Mucci & P. Boisvert. 1956. Amer. J. Med. **21:** 897.
28. Rheins, M. S., F. W. McCoy, R. G. Burrell & E. V. Buehler. 1957. J. Lab. Clin. Med. **50:** 113.
29. Peltier, A. & C. L. Christian. 1959. Arthritis Rheum. **2:** 1.
30. Block, K. J. & J. J. Bunim. 1959. J.A.M.A. **169:** 307.
31. Miller, J. E., E. R. Lynch & J. Lansbury. 1949. J. Lab. Clin. Med. **34:** 1218.
32. Craig, H. W., G. P. Kerby & E. L. Persons. 1957. J. Lab. Clin. Med. **49:** 635.
33. Svec, K. & J. Dingle. 1965. Arthritis Rheum. **8:** 524.
34. Jawetz, E. & E. V. Hook. 1949. Proc. Soc. Exp. Biol. Med. **70:** 650.
35. Heller, G., A. S. Jacobson & M. H. Kolodny. 1949. Proc. Soc. Exp. Biol. Med. **72:** 316.
36. Houba, V. & A. C. Alison. 1966. Lancet **i:** 848.
37. Huntley, C. C., M. G. Costas, R. C. Williams, A. D. Lyerly & R. G. Watson. 1966. J.A.M.A. **197:** 552.
38. Klein, F. & P. Mattern. 1965. Ann. Rheum. Dis. **24:** 458.
39. Chambers, R. J. & E. G. L. Bywaters. 1963. Ann. Rheum. Dis. **22:** 269.
40. Bonomo, L., U. Gillardi & A. Tuisi. 1966. Amer. J. Path. **45:** 313.
41. Caplan, A., R. B. Payne & J. L. Withy. 1962. Thorax **17:** 205.
42. Schroeder, W., E. C. Franklin & C. McEwen. 1962. Arthritis Rheum. **5:** 673.
43. Pernis, B. & E. C. Vigliani. 1965. Ann. N. Y. Acad. Sci. **132:** 112.
44. Tomasi, Jr., T. B., H. H. Fudenberg & N. Finby. 1962. Amer. J. Med. **33:** 243.
45. Turner-Warwick, M. & D. Donich. 1965. Brit. Med. J. **I:** 886.
46. Ward, R. & R. Stalker. 1965. Ann. Rheum. Dis. **24:** 246.
47. Askonas, B. A. & J. H. Humphrey. 1958. Biochem. J. **70:** 212.
48. Kunkel, H. G., H. J. Simon & H. Fudenberg. 1958. Arthritis Rheum. **1:** 289.
49. Puticonen, T., M. Virkkunen & O. Wager. 1965. Acta Rheum. Scand. **11:** 53.
50. Oreskes, I. & L. E. Siltzbach. 1968. Amer. J. Med. **44:** 60.
51. Spilberg, I., L. E. Siltzbach & C. McEwen. 1969. Arthritis Rheum. **12:** 126.
52. Singer, J. M., C. M. Plotz, M. Peralta & H. C. Lyons. 1962. Ann. Intern. Med. **56:** 545.
53. Cathcart, E. S., R. C. Williams, Jr., H. Ross & E. Calkins. 1960. Arthritis Rheum. **3:** 436.
54. Plotz, C. M. & J. M. Singer. Amer. J. Med. **21:** 893.

55. WALDENSTRÖM, J., S. WINBALD & S. LUINGMA. 1964. Acta Med. Scand. **176:** 629.
56. FINKEL, H. E., M. J. BRAUER, R. N. TAUB & W. DAMESHEK. 1968. Blood **28:** 634.
57. HAMMACK, W. J. & H. HOLLEY. 1965. J. Lab. Clin. Med. **58:** 366.
58. WALDENSTRÖM, J. & S. WINBLAD. 1958. Acta Rheum. Scand. **4:** 3.
59. SVARTZ, N. 1965. J.A.M.A. **194:** 516.
60. SULKIN, S. E., R. M. PIKE & H. C. COGGESHALL. 1949. Proc. Soc. Exp. Biol. Med. **70:** 475.
61. BARTFELD, H. 1960. Ann. Intern. Med. **52:** 1059.
62. KUNKEL, H. G., H. J. MÜLLER-EBERHARD, H. H. FUDENBERG & T. B. TOMASI. 1965. J. Clin. Invest. **40:** 117.
63. MELTZER, M., E. C. FRANKLIN, K. ELIAS, R. T. MCCLUSKEY & N. COOPER. 1966. Amer. J. Med. **40:** 837.
64. BALAZS, V. & M. M. FROHLICH. 1966. Amer. J. Med. Sci. **251:** 80; **252:** 668.
65. CAPRA, J. D., R. J. WINCHESTER & H. C. KUNKEL. 1969. Arthritis Rheum. **12:** 67.
66. KAPLAN, M. E. 1968. J. Lab. Clin. Med. **71:** 754.
67. BLOCH, K. J., W. W. BUCHANAN, M. J. WOLFE & J. J. BUNIM. 1965. Medicine (Balt.) **44:** 187.
68. SHIMIZU, T., Y. KATSUTA & Y. OSHIMA. 1965. Ann. Rheum. Dis. **24:** 494.
69. STRACHAN, R. W. & F. W. WIGZELL. 1963. Ann. Rheum. Dis. **22:** 26.
70. WALLER, M., R. IRBY, F. MULLINAX & E. C. TOONE. New Eng. Med. **273:** 12.
71. BROWN, J. F., J. H. HERMAN & C. J. SMYTH. 1967. Ann. Intern. Med. **66:** 87.
72. THOMPSON, R. A. 1965. J. Clin. Path. **18:** 808.
73. OSHIMA, Y., T. SHIMZU, R. YOKOHARI, T. MATSUMOTO, K. KANO, T. KAGAMI & H. NAGAYA. 1963. Ann. Rheum. Dis. **22:** 36.
74. ORESKES, I., S. ROSENBLATT, H. SPIERA & H. MEADOW. 1968. Ann. Rheum. Dis. **27:** 60.
75. FESSEL, W. J. 1963. Arthritis Rheum. **6:** 771.
76. MCDUFFIE, F. 1965. (See reference to Pitts, N.) Southern Med. J. **58:** 1126.
77. RHODES, K., A. SCOTT, R. L. MARKHAM & M. E. MONK-JONES. 1969. Ann. Rheum. Dis. **28:** 104.
78. ALLEN, J. C. & H. G. KUNKEL. 1966. J. Clin. Invest. **45:** 29.
79. BARTFELD, H. 1960. J. Lab. Clin. Med. **56:** 303.
80. GRABER, P. 1957. Texas Rep. Biol. Med. **15:** 1.

General Discussion

DR. ORESKES: Some years ago we published a report on six hundred consecutive sera received in our laboratory for routine rheumatoid factor tests. We found that the vast majority of sera came from individuals who had diseases other than rheumatoid arthritis, and most of the sera demonstrating positive rheumatoid factor tests also came from patients with diseases other than rheumatoid arthritis; the spectrum of diseases was very wide. Our series was admittedly biased in favor of rheumatoid arthritis, and yet it was clear that most of the seropositive patients did not have this disease.

We also found that the people who have rheumatoid factors are generally sicker than the people who do not have them. Dr. Bartfeld alluded to our work in sarcoidosis, and we have found this also in other diseases. In general, increased titers or the perpetuation of rheumatoid factor in a patient was associated with continuing disease of a more chronic or more fulminating nature than in those who did not have rheumatoid factor or in those whose titers tended to decrease or disappear. This brings us to the question whether rheumatoid factor is good or bad. Dr. Davis argues that rheumatoid factor is good, but if you look at all kinds of diseases, you might suppose that rheumatoid factor is bad.

DR. ZVAIFLER: An interesting study is being conducted by Drs. Bilonti and Leppet at our institution which directs itself to one of the questions Dr. Bartfeld raised, the local production of rheumatoid factor. There are some children with an idiopathic form of parotiditis which comes and goes; to date, the etiological agent has not been determined. In these children, the parotid secretions draining from the affected parotid gland contains both rheumatoid factors and antinuclear factors, while the opposite, uninvolved parotid does not. In the majority of these children, the rheumatoid factors and antinuclear factors either are not demonstrated in the bloodstream at all, or, when they are present, appear in much lower titers. I think this finding not only supports the concept of local production, but also is in keeping with the hypothesis that these factors may simply relate to the body's response to chronic inflammation of any kind.

DR. FRIOU: A clinical study of gold therapy is being carried out by Dr. Arthur Logger, a member of our rheumatology group at the University of Southern California. We don't have enough data to comment at this point about the clinical response of the patients, but I think the study itself is of interest in terms of the data that we are recording on changes of rheumatoid factor titers. The project is an attempt to evaluate crysotherapy, with atomic absorption spectrophotometry used as a guide to gold levels. The patients under study are all seropositive definite rheumatoids who have completed conventional gold therapy trials without favorable response. The levels are maintained at 400 μ/100 ml by adjusting the dose; this requires, in some patients, several times the conventional dosage schedule. Fifteen patients have been included in the study to date. Holding the dose level at this has not yet produced toxicity, but we have observed a striking fall in rheumatoid factor titers in all of the patients that have been observed for a reasonably adequate length of time. It would be premature to comment on these clinical data; the patient group is small, but we hope to report our findings when more patients have been followed. Although the patients are not being studied "blind" insofar as the physicians are concerned, an independent evaluation of the range of joint motion and other clinical aspects of the patients is being conducted without knowledge of the therapy; we shall report data on this aspect in the future.

DR. ANSELL: Some years ago we studied a number of cases of rubella arthritis, all of whom were adolescent or young women. We found only one with a high latex titer. Recently, we've seen some other cases, including some cases of rubella without arthritis as well as some with it. It seems that the older patient, between 15 and 25 years old, is the one who shows a positive latex test; we've only seen one positive sheep cell test, and these positive reactions seem to be of fairly short duration. In our experience, they've disappeared in three to four weeks. What is the duration of rheumatoid factor in rubella?

DR. BARTFELD: Generally, rubella synovitis occurs mainly in the older age group. One patient that we followed had synovitis and was positive by both the human FII test and the sensitized-sheep cell test for about three months.

DR. EPSTEIN: In general, the pathology of seronegative synovitis is almost indistinguishable from seropositive synovitis. I believe what you are saying about nonrheumatic conditions is that there is either an infectious agent or an antigenic stimulus present, and therefore we would conclude that the persistence of rheumatoid factor in the rheumatoid arthritic means the persistence of the antigenic stimulus or the infectious agent, or both. We can't really see anything in the tissue response of seronegative disease. It seems to me that many people have been commenting around the question whether rheumatoid factor can be demonstrated in seronegative synovitis. Do you know of anyone who really feels, as was once claimed with reference to the euglobulin inhibition test and other modifications, that all inflammatory rheumatoid synovitis can be shown to be associated with greater than normal concentration of the rheumatoid factor by some technical procedure?

DR. BARTFELD: Morris Ziff and Martin Tanner are not here, but I was trained at New York University, and we believe strongly in the euglobulin inhibition test. It's true that with this test you find more positive reactions in nonrheumatoid arthritis patients, but you also find more in the rheumatoid patients. Rheumatoid arthritis patients may have some predisposing factors, such as x, y, and z, but they also need rheumatoid factor to express this diathesis. Everyone has rheumatoid factor in minimal amounts, but a minimal amount may be quite potent in a predisposed rheumatoid. No one knows how much Ig is needed to cause an autoimmune reaction; if it is high-affinity Ig, minimal amounts may suffice. There is no real answer to that question at this time.

DR. VAUGHAN: I'd like to comment on Dr. Ansell's observations on rubella arthritis; two things were not clear to me. One was the incidence with which the seropositivity is seen in the older individuals who get rubella arthritis; the other is the incidence of seropositivity found in individuals with rubella without arthritis.

DR. ANSELL: I can't quote our actual incidence, but we have seen positive latex tests in patients with rubella without arthritis, and they have tended to be older patients. Let us remember one thing about rubella: Not every epidemic is associated with polyarthritis. There was a big epidemic in our area about two years ago, in which we saw practically no polyarthritis; last year, however, we saw quite a lot of polyarthritis, but we found only a small incidence of positive latex tests in these cases. One of these patients had a remission after two or three months and has just recently developed arthritis again; she is one of the cases that demonstrated a very positive latex test. Seven years ago, when we conducted our first study, we only found one positive case out of seven; in the more recent study, four out of eleven were positive.

DR. MALTZ: A comment was made regarding the production of rheumatoid factor locally in certain tissues. How significant is a positive test for rheumatoid factor on synovial fluid?

DR. BARTFELD: While significant when present in synovial fluid, since in some such cases it may be absent in the serum, it has also been shown in the cells of synovial fluid. A means of demonstrating rheumatoid factors in patients who were not seropositive was reported by Braunsteiner: He took bone marrow of seronegative rheumatoid arthritis patients, smeared the bone marrow on glass slides, and incubated them with fluorescent fraction II; he found cytoplasmic fluorescence in significant numbers of lymphocytes and plasma cells. In other words, rheumatoid factor can be produced at low levels within tissues, by local lymphocytes and plasma cells—perhaps not enough to get into the blood, but maybe enough to do damage, if we believe rheumatoid factor does damage, and I'm not taking either side.

A LONGITUDINAL STUDY OF RHEUMATOID FACTORS IN A NEW ENGLAND TOWN

Edgar S. Cathcart, M.D.* and John B. O'Sullivan, M.D.

Diabetes and Arthritis Field Research Station
Division of Chronic Diseases, Public Health Service
United States Department of Health, Education, and Welfare
Boston, Mass.

The Sudbury study of chronic disease has been used to determine the point prevalence of rheumatoid factors in a normal population and to test initial assumptions on the biological significance of these factors by prolonged and repeated observations. The present paper describes the measurement and distribution of rheumatoid factors in persons between 15 and 75 years of age and presents certain preliminary observations based on a three-year follow-up of persons who initially demonstrated a positive sheep cell agglutination test (SCAT) and bentonite flocculation test (BFT).

Design on the Sudbury Study

In 1964, the total adult population of Sudbury, Mass. was invited to participate in an ongoing study of arthritis, diabetes, and other conditions. Following completion of a questionnaire, each respondent was examined by a physician and subjected to special blood tests, including the SCAT and BFT. In 1965 (FIGURE 1), a preselected, age-stratified random sample, comprising 21% of the total population, and 330 persons (representing all those individuals with initial SCAT titers $\geqq$1:4 or with initial BFT titers $\geqq$1:8) were invited back for a second physical examination and another series of blood tests. During this phase of the study, hand x-rays were obtained on all respondents. A third phase of the study was completed in 1967 with the same random sample in addition to the original seropositive individuals. During this third examination, foot x-rays were obtained.

Methods and Materials

Each respondent was rated according to criteria for rheumatoid arthritis proposed at the New York Symposium on Population Studies of the Rheumatic Diseases (New York criteria).[1] A positive history refers to an episode of joint pain, past or present, involving three or more limb joints. Each joint group, e.g., the proximal interphalangeal joints, counts as one joint, and each side of the body is rated separately. A positive examination for rheumatoid arthritis is largely dependent on involvement of three or more joint groups by soft-tissue swelling, limitation of motion, or characteristic rheumatoid deformity. Of the three joints affected, at least one must be a hand, wrist, or foot; there must also be symmetry of one joint pair. Joints such as the first carpal-metacarpal or the distal interphalangeals are excluded from consideration since they are frequently associated with degenerative joint disease.

The SCAT and BFT were performed on serum according to methods previously described.[2] Aliquots of serum from pools of varying titer of rheumatoid factors were repeatedly introduced to measure the technical variation, and an exchange of sera with several other centers with ongoing population studies was

* Present address: Department of Medicine, Boston University School of Medicine, Boston, Mass.

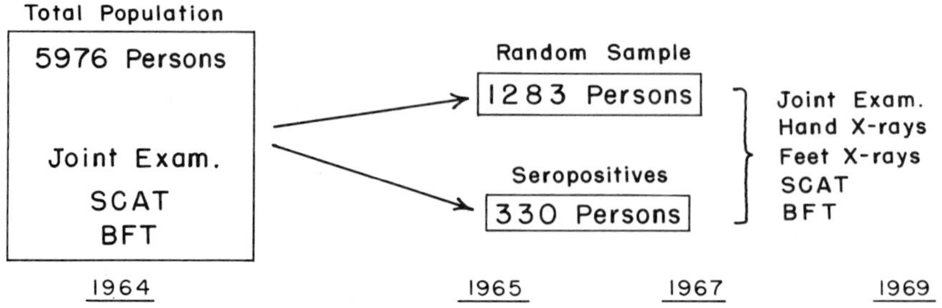

FIGURE 1. Design of the Sudbury health study.

initiated.[3] The SCAT, in particular, was calibrated against results obtained by Dr. J. Ball of Manchester, England, so that comparisons could be made with previous European population studies.[4] Results obtained on positive-reacting sera were consistently within one titer of those obtained by Dr. Ball on the same sera.

Results

Of 5,820 persons between 15 and 75 years of age, 78% (2,188 males, 2,364 females) responded in 1964. Of these, 64 persons (1.4%) had a BFT titer ≧1:32, and 40 persons (0.9%) had a SCAT titer ≧1:32. A marked rise in the percentage of positive reactions according to age was noted for both tests when a titer of 1:4 was arbitrarily chosen as the cutoff between positive and negative

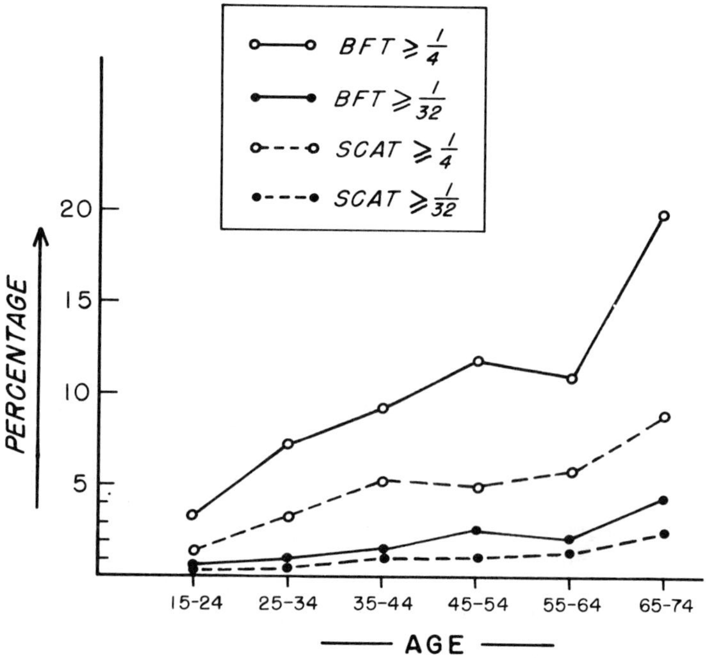

FIGURE 2. Age distribution of seropositive individuals of both sexes in 1964.

TABLE 1

BFT TITER DISTRIBUTION BY AGE AND SEX

Sex	Age (years)	No. Tested	Reciprocal of Titer									No. Not Tested	Percent ≥32
			<4	4	8	16	32	64	128	256	512+		
Male	15–24	371	362	5	3				1				0.27
	25–34	531	491	19	9	5	3	1		2		1	1.13
	35–44	749	674	30	18	9	5	2	3	2	2	4	1.88
	45–54	323	277	25	6	7	4	1	3				2.48
	55–64	137	122	9	2	3					1		0.07
	65–74	79	63	3	5	4	1	2		1			5.06
Total		2,190	1,989	91	43	28	13	6	7	5	3	5	1.55
Female	15–24	391	374	10	2	1	1		1	1		1	0.77
	25–34	708	661	25	12	3	4	1				2	0.71
	35–44	703	641	21	16	15	4		2	1		3	1.00
	45–54	302	274	14	3	3	3	3	1			1	2.33
	55–64	171	153	5	4	4	2	1	1	1			2.92
	65–74	91	73	8	2	5	1		2				3.30
Total		2,366	2,176	83	39	31	15	5	7	3		7	1.27
Both sexes		4,556	4,165	174	82	59	28	11	14	8	3	12	1.40

TABLE 2

SCAT TITER DISTRIBUTION BY AGE AND SEX

Sex	Age (years)	No. Tested	Reciprocal of Titer									No. Not Tested	Percent ≥32
			<4	4	8	16	32	64	128	256	512+		
Male	15–24	371	368	1	1					1			0.27
	25–34	531	519	4	2	2		1	1	1		1	0.57
	35–44	749	704	14	10	7	4	2	1		2	5	1.08
	45–54	323	309	5	5	1		3					0.93
	55–64	137	129	3	2	2					1		0.73
	65–74	79	72	4	1	1		1					1.27
Total		2,190	2,101	31	21	13	4	7	2	2	3	6	0.82
Female	15–24	391	383	3	2		2					1	0.51
	25–34	708	679	15	6	3	1		2			2	0.42
	35–44	703	670	13	7	3	3	2	2			3	1.00
	45–54	302	285	7	4	1	1		2			2	1.00
	55–64	171	161	2	2	2	1	1	1	1			2.34
	65–74	91	85			3		2	1				3.30
Total		2,366	2,263	40	21	12	8	5	8	1		8	0.93
Both Sexes		4,556	4,364	71	42	25	12	12	10	3	3	14	0.88

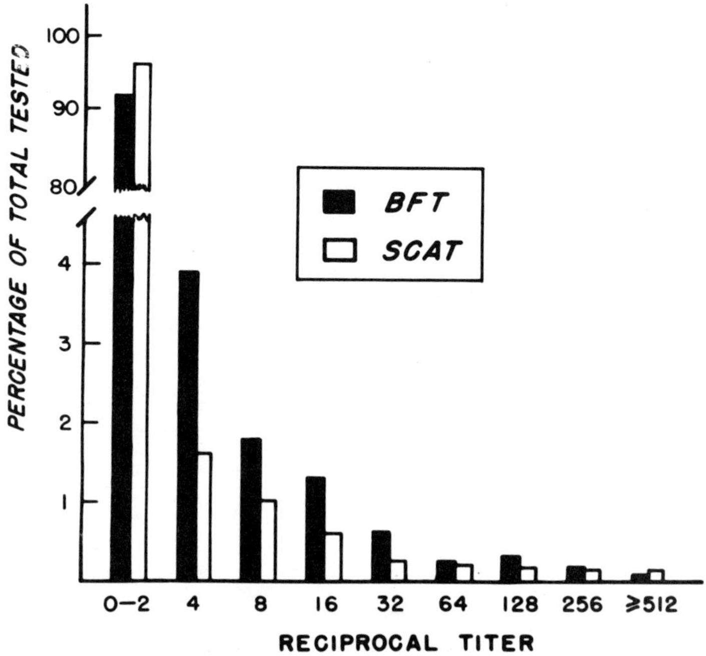

FIGURE 3. Distribution of BFT and SCAT titers in both sexes in 1964.

reactions. On the other hand, the influence of increasing age on the frequency of positive reactions for both tests was less pronounced when a titer of 1:32 was arbitrarily chosen as the cutoff between positive and negative reactions (FIGURE 2). The distribution of positive reactions according to age and sex was also determined for the BFT (TABLE 1) and the SCAT (TABLE 2). A continuous distribution of positive reactions at various titers by BFT and SCAT was noted (FIGURE 3), although the sensitivity of the former appeared to be approximately twice that of the latter, particularly in the lower range of positive titers.

The relationship of the BFT to the SCAT was explored for those sera with titers ≥ 1:32 (positive reactions), those with titers between 1:4 and 1:16 (borderline reactions), and those with titers less than 1:4 (negative reactions). In persons with negative reactions, the agreement between the two methods was 90%, but for those with positive and borderline reactions the agreement was only 14% (TABLE 3). Thus, the majority of persons with borderline or positive reactions by the BFT were negative by the SCAT, and vice versa.

A follow-up was obtained on 58 persons with BFT titers ≥ 1:32 in 1964 and whose sera was available for testing in 1965 (TABLE 4). It was found that 36 persons (62%) differed by no more than one titer, whereas seven persons (12%) were completely negative in 1965. Similar results were obtained on the 1965 follow-up of 40 persons with SCAT titers ≥ 1:32 in 1964 (TABLE 5). Twenty-eight persons (70%) demonstrated no more than one titer difference over a one-year period, and seven persons (18%) had a negative test in 1965. Data on persons first positive by SCAT in 1964 and retested in 1967 indicated a remarkable degree of constancy over a prolonged period of time. Those individuals whose tests were negative by SCAT in 1965 following a positive test in 1964 remained negative in 1967; 91% of those positive in 1964 and 1965 remained positive when retested in 1967.

Relationship of the BFT and SCAT to Rheumatoid Arthritis

In Sudbury, 16 persons demonstrated a positive history and examination for rheumatoid arthritis; of these five persons (31%) had a positive BFT and a positive SCAT. On the other hand, of 64 persons with BFT titers ≧1:32 in 1964, 16 gave a positive history of rheumatoid arthritis, and five of these demonstrated a positive examination for rheumatoid arthritis. In 1967, 54 of those originally positive in 1964 were again available for examination. Two additional persons

TABLE 3

RELATIONSHIP OF BFT TO SCAT IN 1964

Reciprocal of BFT Titer	Reciprocal of SCAT Titer		
	<4	4–16	≧32
<4	4,067	96	1
4–16	265	35	14
≧32	32	7	25

TABLE 4

BFT POSITIVES IN 1964 RETESTED IN 1965

Reciprocal of 1965 Titer	Reciprocal of 1964 Titer				
	32	64	128	256	512
<4	4	0	2	1	0
4	1	1	0	0	0
8	5	0	0	1	0
16	5	0	0	0	0
32	9	3	2	1	0
64	0	6	4	3	0
128	0	0	3	0	0
256	0	0	1	2	1
≧512	0	0	1	0	2

TABLE 5

SCAT POSITIVES IN 1964 RETESTED IN 1965

Reciprocal of 1965 Titer	Reciprocal of 1964 Titer				
	32	64	128	256	512
<4	4	1	1	0	1
4	0	0	0	0	0
8	0	0	0	0	0
16	3	0	0	0	0
32	3	1	0	0	0
64	0	1	1	0	0
128	2	7	4	1	0
256	0	2	3	0	0
≧512	0	0	1	2	2

TABLE 6

THREE-YEAR FOLLOW-UP OF RHEUMATOID ARTHRITIS AMONG 1964 SEROPOSITIVES

	No. Tested	1964 Results		1967 Results		
		Positive History	Positive Examination	Positive History	Positive Examination	No Follow-Up
BFT-positive	64	16	5	20	7	10*
SCAT-positive	40	10	5	13	7	2

* Four dead.

now satisfied the criteria for rheumatoid arthritis by examination, and another two persons gave a positive history for polyarthritis (TABLE 6). Based on the emergence of new cases over a three-year period, the annual incidence of rheumatoid arthritis in BFT-positive individuals without previous evidence of arthritis was calculated to be 1.1% according to examination and history, and 2.8% according to history alone.

Of the 40 persons with SCAT titer ≧1:32, ten gave a positive history of rheumatoid arthritis, and five of these demonstrated a positive examination for rheumatoid arthritis. In 1967, 38 from this group were again available for examination. Three additional persons then gave a positive history for rheumatoid arthritis, and two of these also showed a positive examination (TABLE 6). From these data, the annual incidence of rheumatoid arthritis in SCAT-positive individuals without arthritis was calculated to be 1.9% according to examination and history and 3.3% by history alone.

When the incidence of rheumatoid arthritis by the New York criteria in BFT-positive individuals who had been followed for three years was analyzed according to age and sex, it was found that all persons who were positive, both by history and by examination, were over the age of 45 years (FIGURE 4). Furthermore, in the

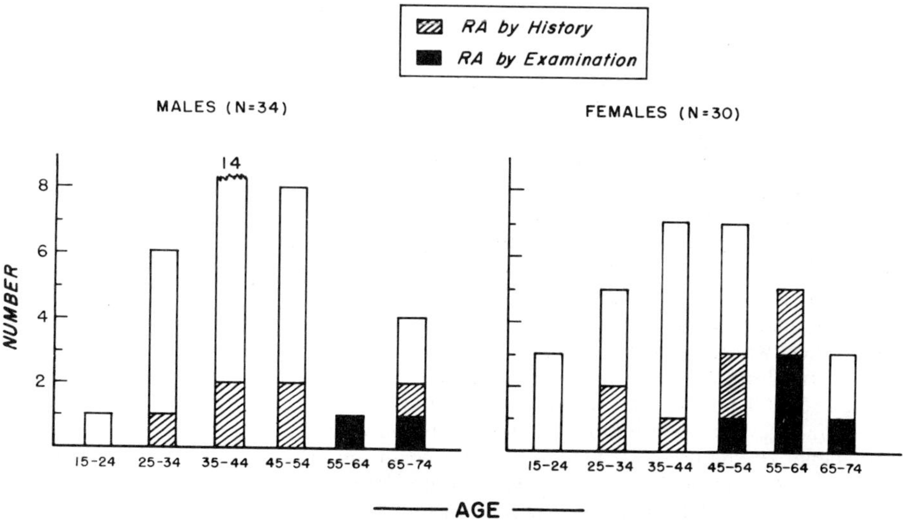

FIGURE 4. Rheumatoid arthritis among BFT-positive individuals by age (three-year follow-up).

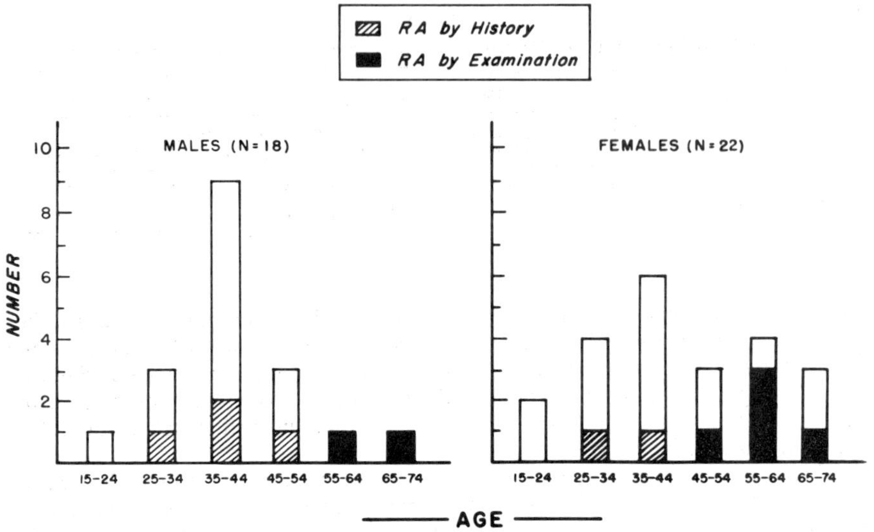

FIGURE 5. Rheumatoid arthritis among SCAT-positive individuals by age (three-year follow-up).

total Sudbury population, only eight persons (two males, six females) over the age of 45 years had a positive BFT and no evidence of rheumatoid arthritis. Similar results were obtained by analysis of SCAT-positive individuals (FIGURE 5), in that only seven persons (two males, five females) over the 45 years of age demonstrated a SCAT titer $\geqq$1:32 with negative findings for rheumatoid arthritis.

Discussion

In Sudbury, Mass., the incidence of BFT-positive individuals was 1.3% and the incidence of SCAT-positive individuals was 0.9%. On the other hand, if a titer by either test of 1:4 was considered positive, then the prevalence of positive reactions by BFT and SCAT rose to 8.6% and 4.2%, respectively. Little can be gained by comparing the BFT results with those obtained in other populations, since interlaboratory standardization for this test was not attempted. However, comparisons can be made with certain results obtained by Ball and Lawrence, who measured the prevalance of positive SCAT results in different European populations in 55-to-64-year-old individuals.[4] For this age group, the prevalence of positive SCAT results (titer $\geqq$1:32) in Sudbury was 1.6%, as compared with 1.6% in Heinola, Finland, 3.5% in Glamorgan, Wales, 4.8% in Rotterdam, The Netherlands, and 5.4% in Leigh, England. In this regard, therefore, the Sudbury population would appear to resemble a rural rather than an urban community in that rural communities are alleged to have a significantly lower prevalence of positive SCAT results than are urban communities.

As in previous population studies,[4-7] no noteworthy sex differences in the prevalence of rheumatoid factors were found in this study. At low titer, positive reactions by both SCAT and BFT were more common among older than among younger persons. Nevertheless, the relationship of increasing age to positive reactions was less marked at the higher titer of 1:32. The latter finding is in keeping with results obtained in the populations of Wenslydale, where no positive results were obtained for persons over the age of 55 years,[4] and in Jerusalem, where the presence of rheumatoid factors, as measured by their reactivity with rabbit amboceptor, was less common among older than among younger persons.[7] It was observed in Sudbury that positive reactors by BFT were frequently negative by SCAT, and vice versa. Even when adjusted to comparable sensitivity, the two tests, particularly at low titer, usually identified different persons. As noted by others,[8] these results suggest that the two tests are of different biological significance.

Positive reactors by both SCAT and BFT at titers $\geqq$1:32 tended to be positive when their serum was tested one and three years later. This finding is in keeping with that of Waller and co-workers, who found that of 125 "normal" individuals with a positive sensitized human red cell test, 78% still showed positive reactions one to three years later.[6] It differs from that of Adler and co-workers, who found that 65% of 55 persons with a positive latex fixation test had dropped to negative values when tested less than one year later.[7] Studies are now in progress, based on the Sudbury data, to determine the incidence of newly positive reactors, i.e., persons whose tests were originally negative but later turned positive.

Finally, mention should be made of the relationship between positive BFT and SCAT results and rheumatoid arthritis as measured by the New York criteria. Of 16 persons with a past history of polyarthritis and involvement by swelling, limitation of motion, or deformity of three or more joints, five persons (31%) had a positive BFT and a positive SCAT. Although this figure is somewhat lower than that percentage of seropositive rheumatoid arthritis observed in a hospital or clinic, the discrepancy is probably due to the larger number of subclinical or mild forms of polyarthritis that prevail in the normal population. The finding that 25% of those persons in Sudbury with a positive SCAT or BFT gave a positive history of polyarthritis affirms the clinical importance of these serological reactions when read at high titers. The association between positive tests for rheumatoid factors and rheumatoid arthritis was most marked in older individuals, whereas the majority of younger persons with positive BFT and SCAT results appeared to be in good health. One of the most intriguing findings in the present study was the evidence that among persons without rheumatoid arthritis, a positive BFT or SCAT appeared to increase the probability of developing polyarthritis in the future. Whereas the annual incidence of new cases of rheumatoid arthritis in a random sample of the Sudbury population which included seropositive as well as seronegative persons had previously been estimated to be $0.29 \pm 0.16\%$[10] the incidence of new cases among SCAT-positive individuals appeared to be between 1.9 and 3.3%. These results, albeit based on different clinical criteria, support the previous findings of Ball and Lawrence[11] but contradict those of Ako and co-workers[12] and Waller and Toone.[13] Follow-up of the Sudbury population over a longer period of time will be necessary, however, before the accuracy and validity of these preliminary observations can be verified.

Summary and Conclusions

1. Sixty-four persons (1.4%) were positive by BFT at titer $\geqq$1:32, and 40 persons (0.9%) were positive by SCAT at titer $\geqq$1:32.

2. The percentage of positive reactions by BFT and SCAT, particularly when low titers were considered positive, increased with age.

3. The sex distributions for positive reactors by BFT and SCAT were approximately equal.

4. Positive and borderline reactors by BFT were frequently negative by SCAT, and vice versa.

5. Positive reactors by BFT and SCAT tended to be positive one and three years later.

6. Of persons with BFT and/or SCAT titers ≥1:32, 25% appeared to have rheumatoid arthritis by history or physical examination (New York criteria).

7. The annual incidence of rheumatoid arthritis in positive reactors without previous history of polyarthritis was 1.9–3.3%.

Acknowledgment

We are indebted to Miss Grace Lincoln for expert technical assistance.

References

1. BENNETT, P. H. & T. A. BURCH. 1967. N. Y. Symp. Population Studies Rheum. Dis. Bull. Rheum. Dis. **17**: 453.
2. CATHCART, E. S. 1967. Rheumatoid factors. *In* Laboratory Diagnostic Procedures in the Rheumatic Diseases. A. S. Cohen, Ed. : 96–113. Little, Brown & Co. Boston, Mass.
3. O'SULLIVAN, J. B. & G. W. MCDONALD. 1966. Decisive factors in designing the Sudbury Study of Chronic Disease. Public Health Rep. **81**: 891.
4. BALL, J. & J. S. LAWRENCE. 1961. The epidemiology of the sheep cell agglutination test. Ann. Rheum. Dis. **20**: 235.
5. MIKKELSEN, W. M., H. J. DODGE, I. F. DUFF, F. H. EPSTEIN & J. A. NAPIER. 1963. Clinical and serological estimates of the prevalence of rheumatoid arthritis in the population of Tecumseh, Michigan, 1959–60. *In* The Epidemiology of Chronic Rheumatism. J. H. Kellgren, M. R. Jeffry and J. Ball, Eds. **1**: 239–248. Blackwell, Sci. Publ. Oxford, England.
6. WALLER, M., E. C. TOONE & E. VAUGHAN. 1964. Study of rheumatoid factor in a normal population. Arthritis Rheum. **7**: 513.
7. ADLER, E., J. H. ABRAMSON, R. GOLDBERG, Z. ELKAN & S. BEN HADOR. 1966. Rheumatoid arthritis in a Jerusalem population. 2. Epidemiology of rheumatoid factors. Amer. J. Epidemiol. **85**: 378.
8. BENNETT, P. H. & T. A. BURCH. 1968. Rheumatoid factor in the Blackfeet and Pima Indians. *In* Population Studies of the Rheumatic Diseases. P. H. Bennett & P. H. N. Wood, Eds. : 192–199. Excerpta Med. Found. Amsterdam, The Netherlands.
9. ROPES, M. W., G. A. BENNETT, S. COBB, R. JACOX & R. A. JESSAR. 1959. Diagnostic criteria for rheumatoid arthritis: 1958 Revision. Ann. Rheum. Dis. **18**: 49.
10. O'SULLIVAN, J. B., E. S. CATHCART & J. A. BOLZAN. 1968. Diagnostic criteria and the incidence of rheumatoid arthritis in Sudbury, Massachusetts. *In* Population Studies of the Rheumatic Diseases. P. H. Bennett & P. H. N. Wood, Eds. : 109–113. Excerpta Med. Found. Amsterdam, The Netherlands.
11. BALL, J. & J. S. LAWRENCE. 1963. The relationship of rheumatoid serum factor to rheumatoid arthritis. A 5-year follow up of a population sample. Ann. Rheum. Dis. **22**: 311.
12. AKO, K., J. KIRPILA & O. WAGER. 1959. The persistance of the agglutination activating factor in the circulation. A nine-year study of 27 patients. Ann. Med. Exp. Fenn. **37**: 377.
13. WALLER, M. & E. C. TOONE. 1968. Normal individuals with positive tests for rheumatoid factor. Arthritis Rheum. **11**: 50.

Discussion of the Paper

DR. J. L. ABBRUZZO (*Jefferson Medical College, Philadelphia, Pa.*): Have you had an opportunity to do any antinuclear antibody tests on this group of patients? I am particularly referring to the group with a history of arthragia and arthritis but no evidence of joint disease on examination.

DR. CATHCART: No, we haven't performed such tests.

DR. ABBRUZZO: I noted that the incidence of seropositive arthritis in your group, five out of 16, is rather low, but I presume that the list of exclusions in the American Rheumatism Association (ARA) criteria for diagnosing rheumatoid arthritis does not apply to this group. Is that correct?

DR. CATHCART: That's true.

DR. BARNETT: It's obvious that insurance companies, for instance, and the Federal Government, and third parties that are responsible for the payment of patient care are very interested in the data from this type of study. It would appear from your report of a prospective study in a closed community, as well as from hospital studies, that rheumatoid serology is a poor method of case screening for rheumatoid arthritis. In a normal population, as you pointed out, seropositivity at random in the population is more likely to be from nonrheumatoid individuals than from rheumatoid individuals.

You also noted, with particular relevance to the insurance companies, that an asymptomatic person who submits his serum for multiphasic testing and is found to have positive rheumatoid serology apparently is ten to twenty times as likely to develop the clinical polyarthritis that we call rheumatoid arthritis than is an individual who is found to be seronegative. However, this likelihood still only increases the incidence of the disease by 1% or less than 2% of the seropositive group per annum. Is that correct?

DR. CATHCART: Dr. Barnett, you raise a very crucial question, and that is the prevalence of rheumatoid arthritis. I refrain from using ARA criteria because with them we find that perhaps 2–4% of the Sudbury population have probable rheumatoid arthritis. But for anyone who's involved in a study such as this, it becomes obvious that this is a totally inaccurate and very false impression of rheumatoid arthritis. As shown in the Tecumseh study, most people who have rheumatoid arthritis by the ARA criteria on initial examination no longer show evidence of the disease when examined one year later. And if one looks at these people during the ongoing study, it is quite obvious that most of them do not have rheumatoid arthritis but other diseases, or that the criteria were used inaccurately. For example, the ARA criteria require that joint swelling be observed for six weeks or longer. No population study that I know of to date has really applied this criterion properly.

DR. FRIOU: In order to evaluate the significance of your figure of 1–1.7% of new cases per year in the seropositive group, one would need to know what the increment of new seropositive normal individuals was during your sequence of studies.

DR. CATHCART: We don't have that data at this time; obviously, we're working on it. There are factors involved in the variability of our test, and one must know how much a test, when applied to thousands of reactions, is going to vary from year to year before one can adequately say that a given person is seronegative and not seropositive.

Part II. Structure of Rheumatoid Factors and Their Antigens

STRUCTURAL AND CONFORMATIONAL SPECIFICITY OF THE ANTIGEN FOR RHEUMATOID FACTOR

Christopher S. Henney, Ph.D.

World Health Organization
Immunology Research and Training Center
Lausanne, Switzerland

The classification of rheumatoid factor as an antibody is inextricably related to the identification of the antigen that elicits its formation. It seems paradoxical, therefore, that although the antibody nature of rheumatoid factor is widely accepted, its antigen is still the subject of much conjecture. The findings of Waaler[1] and Rose and co-workers,[2] that rheumatoid arthritic sera specifically caused the agglutination of red cells coated with γG-globulins, early established the likelihood that the antigen was some form of γG-globulin. This concept found support with the finding[3] that some γG-globulin preparations caused direct precipitation on addition to rheumatoid arthritic serum. Further investigations[4-6] have emphasized the importance of the configuration of the γG-globulin in this system, since it has become apparent that only aggregated γG-globulins will effect precipitation.

The present paper reports a detailed investigation into the configurational and antigenic requirements for combination with rheumatoid factor and its direct precipitation. Following establishment of the basic requirements for combination with rheumatoid factor, the immunogenicity of proteins possessing these antigenic and configurational requirements was studied under autologous, homologous, and heterologous situations. In this way, the feasibility that these molecules are possible antigens for rheumatoid factor production was assessed. It should be emphasized, however, that although the term rheumatoid factor is used in its singular form in this text, it is a collective term, representing a heterogeneous group of antibodies with a wide range of specificities. Similarly, it would be misleading to think of the "antigen" eliciting rheumatoid factor production as a number of well-defined determinants represented on a single antigen molecule. The antigens, like their corresponding antibodies, are undoubtedly a very heterogeneous group, and the approach used here, of necessity, limits this population to a number of antigenic determinants which are capable of explaining some, but not all, of the reported rheumatoid factor specificities.

Human γG-globulin preparations isolated by DEAE-cellulose chromatography were subjected to controlled denaturation by incubation of the protein (at a concentration of 10 mg/ml) for 20 minutes at temperatures ranging between 20° C and 65° C. Following incubation, the samples were cooled rapidly to room temperature and subjected to analytical ultracentrifugation at both 29,500 rpm and 59,780 rpm in a Spinco model E centrifuge. The specific optical rotation (α) of each sample was measured at six wavelengths (λ) between 350 mμ and 600 mμ, and the rotatory dispersion constant (λ_c) was calculated by the method of Yang and Doty[7] by plotting $(\alpha)_\lambda \lambda^2$ against $(\alpha)_\lambda$. Native γG-globulin preparations were found to have λ_c values in the range of 198–202 mμ; after heating at 63° C for ten minutes, this value rose to approximately 220 mμ, a value characteristic of fully denatured globular proteins[8] and indicative of gross conformational unfolding.

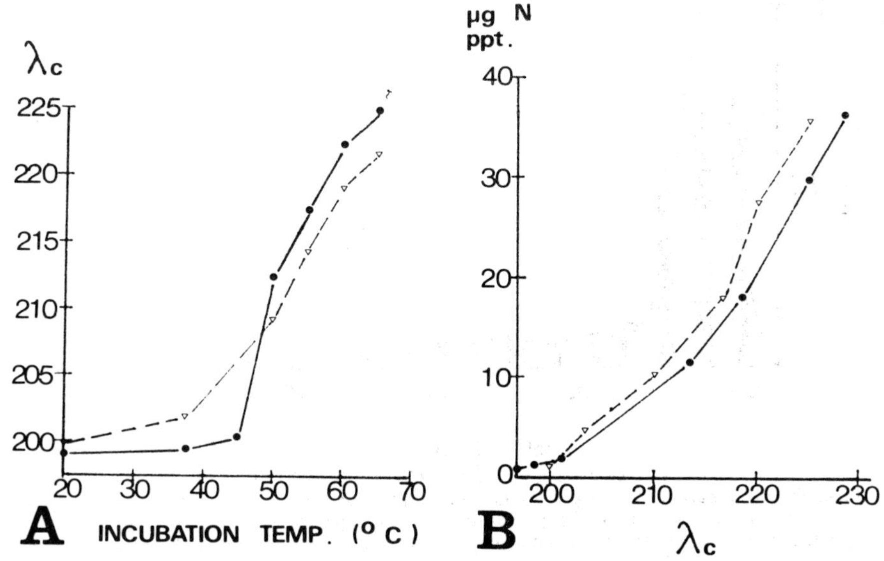

FIGURE 1. (A) The effect of temperature on the rotatory dispersion constant (λ_c) of two γG-globulin preparations. (B) The relationship between the λ_c values of these two γG-globulin preparations and their ability to precipitate rheumatoid factor.

Aliquots (5 mg) of each of the denatured samples were added to 0.5 ml of rheumatoid arthritic serum or to 1 mg of isolated rheumatoid factor preparations. The amount of precipitate formed in each case was measured. The structural alteration observed on denaturation was associated with increased rheumatoid factor precipitability, a linear relationship being observed between the λ_c values of the heat-denatured γG-globulins and thc amounts of rheumatoid factor precipitated (FIGURE 1).

Essentially similar findings were made following denaturation by other means (e.g., with NaOH or sodium dodecyl sulfate). In each case, the ability to precipitate rheumatoid factor was observed only after optical rotatory dispersion measurements had shown evidence of structural unfolding. Maximum precipitating properties were always associated with λ_c values characteristic of fully denatured γG-globulin preparations.[6]

Analytical ultracentrifugation of the variously denatured preparations invariably showed the presence of polydisperse, high-molecular-weight aggregates sedimenting between 20S and 40S. In our hands, denaturation (as evidenced by optical rotation measurements) was invariably accompanied by aggregate formation. Thus, the question was raised whether the structural unfolding was necessary for the precipitation of rheumatoid factors, because it revealed new antigenic determinants against which the rheumatoid factor is directed, or whether it was necessary simply because the aggregates thus formed, owing to decreased solubility, render visible a reaction that is essentially one of monomer γG-rheumatoid factor interaction. Thus, do monomer γG-globulin molecules themselves have antigenic determinants capable of reacting with rheumatoid factor?

In order to attempt to answer this question, a preparation of pooled normal human γG-globulin was heat-aggregated (at 63° C for 20 minutes) and then

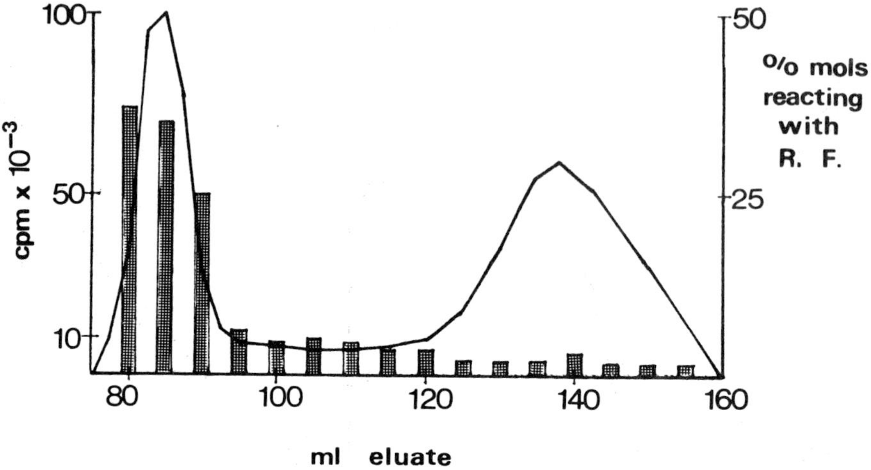

FIGURE 2. Separation of a heat-aggregated (63° C for 20 minutes), ^{131}I-labeled, human γG-globulin preparation on Sephadex G-200. Aliquots of each fraction eluted were incubated with a rheumatoid factor (R.F.) preparation, and the percentage of γG-globulin molecules specifically bound in each case was calculated. These values are plotted in the vertical columns.

labeled with ^{131}I.[9] The resulting mixture, containing both monomeric and polymeric forms of γG labeled with ^{131}I, was resolved on Sephadex G-200 (FIGURE 2). Aliquots (10 μg) of each fraction eluted were added to 0.2 ml of rheumatoid arthritic sera and to 1 mg of an isolated rheumatoid factor preparation, a situation of gross antibody excess in each case. Following incubation at 37° C for four hours, an excess of a rabbit antiserum specific for human μ chains was added, sufficient to cause total precipitation of rheumatoid factor. The amount of antigen bound to rheumatoid factor was thus evaluated by counting the radioactivity in the immune precipitate. The results are shown in FIGURE 2. Note that only polymers of γG-globulin (eluted with the void volume from Sephadex G-200) showed significant binding to rheumatoid factor, monomeric γG being essentially negative. Even among the γG polymers, however, only a portion of the molecules (25–40%) apparently possess antigenic determinants capable of

TABLE 1

REACTIVITY OF γG SUBCLASSES WITH RHEUMATOID FACTOR

	Molecules Reacting with Rheumatoid Arthritic Sera (%)		Inhibition by 20-Fold Monomer Excess (%)	Molecules Reacting with Rheumatoid Factor Preparation (%)		Inhibition by 20-Fold Monomer Excess (%)
	Monomer	Aggregate		Monomer	Aggregate	
Normal γG	<1	29	4.2	<1	28	3.0
Myeloma proteins						
γG_1	<1	21	3.1	<1	20	2.2
γG_2	<1	23	4.0	<1	18	0.9
γG_3	<1	10	4.3	<1	8	1.0
γG_4	<1	35	2.5	<1	32	2.0
Normal Fc fragment	<1	35	4.0	<1	39	3.4

reacting with rheumatoid factor. In order to ensure that these results did not simply reflect a difference in avidity for the rheumatoid factor between aggregated and monomeric γG, and to confirm that γG-globulin in its native form did not combine with rheumatoid factor, the binding of ^{131}I-aggregated γG to rheumatoid factor was repeated in the presence of a 20-fold weight excess of γG monomer. As shown in TABLE 1, no significant inhibition of the combination occurred, indicating that the γG monomer apparently lacks the antigenic (rheumatoid factor-reactive) determinants present on aggregates.

Since only a portion of aggregated γG-globulin molecules apparently possess rheumatoid factor-reactive determinants, it seemed possible that this reactivity might be confined to one or more of the γG-globulin subclasses. Consequently, the previously described experiments were repeated with γG myeloma proteins representative of each of the four known subclasses (i.e., γG_1, γG_2, γG_3, γG_4). Aggregation was carried out either by heating the proteins at a concentration of 10 mg/ml of 63° C for 20 minutes or by treatment with bisdiazotized benzidine (BDB).[10] The proteins were then labeled with ^{131}I and separated into monomer and polymer fractions by filtration on Sephadex G-200.

As noted previously, 10 μg of ^{131}I-labeled protein was added to 0.2 ml of pooled rheumatoid arthritic sera, and, following incubation, rheumatoid factor was precipitated by an excess of an antiserum specific for μ chains. As shown in TABLE 1, all four γG-globulin subclasses form, on aggregation, antigenic determinants capable of reacting with rheumatoid factor. In no case was binding of the γG-globulin monomer to rheumatoid factor demonstrable, nor did the presence of excess monomer affect the polymer-rheumatoid factor interaction.

Earlier studies had revealed, both by direct precipitation and by hemagglutination techniques, that rheumatoid factor-reactive sites were located within the Fc region of the aggregated γG-globulin molecule. Antigen-binding experiments, similar to those outlined above, performed with ^{131}I-labeled BDB-aggregated Fc fragments, again demonstrated that reactivity occurred only with aggregated fragments;[11] Fc monomer preparations neither combined with rheumatoid factor nor affected the ability of Fc aggregates to combine with this antibody (TABLE 1).

Thus, it appears that the γG-globulin monomer does not possess rheumatoid factor-reactive determinants. Moreover, the close correlation that exists between rheumatoid factor reactivity and a structural unfolding of the γG-globulin molecule (FIGURE 1), together with the fact that it has proved impossible to obtain either denatured γG-globulin in a monomeric form or aggregated γG-globulin preparations which are native by optical rotatory dispersion criteria, makes it unlikely that the presence of rheumatoid factor-reactive determinants on γG-globulin aggregates merely results from the conglomeration of "subdeterminants" contributed by several γG-globulin monomers. It appears more likely that rheumatoid factor has a specificity directed against antigenic determinants revealed in a portion of γG-globulin molecules as a result of the structural unfolding which accompanies denaturation.

The gross nature of the conditions used to effect nonspecific denaturation of γG-globulin, although producing aggregates with a high specific reactivity for rheumatoid factor, precludes their consideration as possible *in vivo* mechanisms for the revelation of autoantigenic determinants. Accumulated evidence[12-14] now suggests that the most likely manner for *in vivo* denaturation of γG-globulin results from antigen-antibody combination. The changes in optical rotation which occur when antigen and antibody combine, as originally demonstrated by Ishizaka and Campbell,[13] have been repeated in this laboratory with a number of anti-

TABLE 2

SPECIFIC OPTICAL ACTIVITY, SULFHYDRYL CONTENT, AND RHEUMATOID FACTOR REACTIVITY OF SOME ANTIGEN-ANTIBODY COMPLEXES

Soluble Complex	Antigen-Antibody Weight Ratio	Specific Optical Rotation* (degrees)			Sulfhydryl Groups Revealed† (mol/mol Ab)	Rheumatoid Factor Reactivity
		Immune Complexes	Antigen-Non-Ab γG Mixture	Difference		
BSA-rabbit anti-BSA	1.9:1	−64.6	−58.8	+5.8	0.66	+++
	2.4:1	−61.0	−59.3	+1.7	0.52	+++
	3.2:1	−60.4	−59.8	+0.6	0.20	++
	4.5:1	−60.6	−60.3	−0.3	NDI	(±)
	9.1:1	−61.0	−61.1	−0.1	NDI	−
Ovalbumin-rabbit anti-ovalbumin	4.2:1	−36.6	−33.5	+3.1		+++
	6.7:1	−33.5	−32.7	+0.8		+
	10.7:1	−32.4	−31.7	+0.7		+
	14.3:1	−31.2	−31.3	−0.1		−
Ferritin-rabbit anti-ferritin	2.7:1	−40.2	−31.9	+8.3		+++
	4.1:1	−35.2	−30.9	+4.3		+++
	5.4:1	−33.8	−30.3	+3.5		++
	6.8:1	−30.2	−29.9	+0.3		+
	13.6:1	−28.3	−29.0	−0.7		−
	19.0:1	−28.6	−28.7	−0.1		−

* At 589.5 mμ (α^D). Heat-denatured (at 56° C for ten minutes) human γG-globulin produced a rise in α^D of 12.2°.

† Calculated as sulfhydryl in immune complex minus that present in antigen-nonantibody γG mixtures. NDI = no demonstrable increase.

gens.[14,15] Typical results obtained following combination of bovine serum albumin (BSA) and ferritin with their respective rabbit antibodies are shown in TABLE 2. As shown, antigen-antibody combination in certain proportions, particularly in the region of low antigen excess, results in a marked increase in levorotation, indicative of structural alteration. Supporting evidence of such alteration is the finding that there is also an increase in the amount of titratable sulfydryl groups in these complexes.[12] Furthermore, the increase in levorotation and thus of structural alteration in γG-globulin antibody, induced specifically by combination with antigen, in some cases approaches that demonstrable by nonspecific denaturation procedures such as heating (TABLE 2). In keeping with the earlier findings of Edelman and co-workers,[4] it was found that these complexes, which by optical rotation studies contained structurally altered antibody, were capable of reacting with rheumatoid factor, while both free antibody and complexes formed in gross antigen excess, in which structurally altered antibody was not demonstrable, were not rheumatoid factor-reactive.

Although these denatured γG-globulins react with rheumatoid factor *in vitro,* their classification as antigens necessitates that they are capable of directly inducing antibodies with rheumatoid factor specificities. The following experiments were thus devised: Rabbits of known allotype (As-3, 4, and 6) were immunized with a variety of antigens, and the γG-globulin fraction from the immune sera was isolated. Homologous antigen was added in predetermined amounts so that soluble complexes, containing structurally altered antibody, were formed. These complexes were than used to immunize rabbits of the same As-3, 4, or 6 allotype as the antibody donor. The animals were bled at weekly intervals and examined for the presence of anti-antibodies by hemagglutination and gel-diffusion precipitin analysis. By the third week following immunization with 5 mg of BSA-anti-BSA complexes, antibody was formed which agglutinated sheep red cells passively coated with rabbit γG-globulin. The hemagglutination

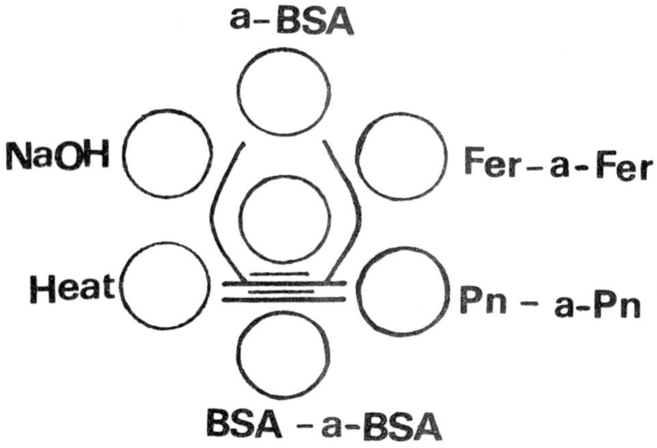

FIGURE 3. Diagrammatic representation of gel-diffusion precipitin analysis of a rabbit antiserum (center well) obtained following immunization with soluble immune complexes of bovine serum albumin (BSA) and rabbit antibody. The antigens placed in the peripheral wells were: a-BSA, rabbit antibody used in immunizing complex; BSA-a-BSA, soluble complex used for immunization; Fer-a-Fer, soluble complexes of ferritin and rabbit antibody; Pn-a-Pn, soluble complexes of pneumococcal polysaccharide type III and rabbit antibody; NaOH, NaOH-denatured rabbit γG-globulin; and Heat, heat-denatured rabbit γG-globulin.

TABLE 3

COMPARISON BETWEEN THE SPECIFICITIES OF HUMAN RHEUMATOID FACTORS AND RABBIT ANTI-ANTIBODIES

	Antigen	Principal Immunoglobulin Class	Precipitability							
			Monomeric γG	Aggregated γG		Antigen-Antibody Complexes	Aggregated Homologous γG			
							Chains		Fragments	
				Homologous	Heterologous		Heavy	Light	Fab	Fc
Human rheumatoid factor	?	γM	−	+	+	+	+	−	−	+
Rabbit anti-antibody	BSA-a-BSA	γG	−	+	−	+	+	−	+	+
	Ferritin-a-Ferritin	γG	−	+	+	+	+	−	+	+

titer of this antibody rose until the end of the second month following sensitization and remained at this level for several months thereafter. Gel-diffusion precipitin analysis (FIGURE 3) showed that antibodies reacting with the immunizing complex, but not with free antibody, were formed. This anti-antibody reacted with heat- or NaOH-denatured rabbit γG-globulin but not with the undenatured protein. Moreover, a reactivity was demonstrable with heterologous antigen-antibody complexes consisting of rabbit antibody complexed to antigens unrelated to that contained in the immunizing complex (FIGURE 3).

Anti-antibodies raised in an identical manner to soluble complexes of ferritin and rabbit γG antibody showed many similar specificites. Thus, in both cases the anti-antibodies were of the γG class and reacted only with γG-globulin molecules following denaturation. However, while the anti-antibodies raised against BSA-anti-BSA complexes reacted only with denatured rabbit γG-globulin, those raised against ferritin-anti-ferritin complexes showed a wide species cross-reactivity.[15] Although this study has to date only been performed with a limited range of antigens, there is some indication that the presence of large antigens in the immunizing complex evokes the best anti-antibody responses. The results indicate, moreover, that immunogenic determinants are revealed following antigen-antibody combinations, and that at least a portion of these autoantigenic determinants are formed consistently, irrespective of the nature of the antigen involved. A recent detailed antigenic analysis of the determinants formed following both specific (antigen-antibody) combination and nonspecific (heat, NaOH, etc.) denaturation of human γG-globulin has indicated that at least a portion of these determinants are a consistent feature of the molecule in its denatured state.[16]

While it is dangerous to draw too closely analogies that cross the species barrier, it is perhaps of some interest to compare the similarities and differences in specificity between rabbit anti-antibodies and human rheumatoid factors. A summary is therefore given in TABLE 3. Despite the differences that exist between these anti-antibodies and rheumatoid factors, there are enough similarities to suggest that an antigen-antibody complex comprising γG antibody and a large (viral?) antigen fulfills both the structural and immunogenic requirements of the "antigen" for rheumatoid factor.

Acknowledgment

I would like to thank Drs. D. R. Stanworth and K. Ishizaka for collaboration in many aspects of this work.

References

1. WAALER, E. 1940. Acta Path. Microbiol. Scand. **17:** 172.
2. ROSE, H. M., C. RAGAN, E. PEARCE & M. O. LIPMAN. 1948. Proc. Soc. Exp. Biol. Med. **68:** 1.
3. EPSTEIN, W. V., E. P. ENGLEMAN & M. ROSS. 1957. J. Immunol. **79:** 441.
4. EDELMAN, G. M., H. G. KUNKEL & E. C. FRANKLIN. 1958. J. Exp. Med. **108:** 105.
5. CHRISTIAN, C. L. 1958. J. Exp. Med. **108:** 139.
6. HENNEY, C. S. & D. R. STANWORTH. 1965. Immunology **9:** 139.
7. YANG, J. T. & P. DOTY. 1957. J. Amer. Chem. Soc. **79:** 761.
8. URNES, P. & P. DOTY. 1961. Adv. Protein Chem. **16:** 401.
9. MCCONAHEY, P. J. & F. J. DIXON. 1966. Int. Arch. Allerg. **29:** 185.
10. ISHIZAKA, K. & T. ISHIZAKA. 1960. J. Immunol. **85:** 163.
11. HENNEY, C. S. & K. ISHIZAKA. 1968. J. Immunol. **101:** 79.
12. ROBERT, B. & P. GRABAR. 1957. Ann. Inst. Pasteur (Paris) **92:** 56.
13. ISHIZAKA, K. & D. H. CAMPBELL. 1959. J. Immunol. **83:** 318.
14. HENNEY, C. S., D. R. STANWORTH & P. G. H. GELL. 1965. Nature **205:** 1079.
15. HENNEY, C. S. & D. R. STANWORTH. 1966. Nature **210:** 1071.
16. HENNEY, C. S. & K. ISHIZAKA. 1968. J. Immunol. **100:** 718.

General Discussion

DR. KUNKEL: I am sure somebody would like to express the other point of view, that these rheumatoid factors are directed against native sites of the γ-globulin molecule. I would like to ask Dr. Henney to clarify one point: What percentage of the rheumatoid factors in a given serum are directed against sites that are only revealed by denaturation?

DR. HENNEY: I don't think I can give quantitative figures. I think there is perhaps some limitation in the system that we are using. Isolated rheumatoid factor preparations from a number of sera were shown in these test systems to combine only with aggregated γ-globulin molecules. We could never show any specificity for monomeric γG, although that does not mean that it cannot happen.

DR. SCHUR: At the 1965 annual meeting of the American Rheumatism Association in Philadelphia, Dr. Kunkel and I presented results of studies in which it was demonstrated that almost all of 19S γM rheumatoid factor reacted with monomeric (or aggregate-free) preparations of 7S γ-globulins. Greatly purified rheumatoid factors were isolated from the sera of four individuals with rheumatoid arthritis by the method of Schrohenloher and his colleagues. The 19S rheumatoid factors were then reacted in the Spinco model E analytical ultracentrifuge with aggregate-free preparations of normal 7S γ-globulins and isolated 7S γG

TABLE 1

REACTIONS OF 19S RHEUMATOID FACTORS

Protein	Percent 19S Anti-γG-Globulins Reacting to Form a Soluble 22S Complex
Normal human 7S γG-globulins	
Preparation 1	$\leqq$ 100
Preparation 2	$\leqq$ 100
Autologous 7S γG-globulin	$\leqq$ 100
7S myeloma (γG) proteins	
Ke (γG_1)	$\leqq$ 100
Le (γG_1)	95
Ku (γG_1)	$\leqq$ 100
Go (γG_1)	95
Ne (γG_2)	$\leqq$ 100
Ma (γG_2)	95
Ka (γG_2)	95
Ge (γG_4)	95
Vi (γG_3)	40–50
Do (γG_3)	40–50
B Jo (γG_3)	40
Animal 7S γ-globulins	
Baboon	75
Rabbit, chimpanzee	40–60
Sheep, horse, pig	5–10
Dog, bovine, chicken	0
γA 7S myeloma protein	0
γM 19S Waldenström macroglobulin	0

myeloma globulins. When the reaction was performed in antigen (7S γ-globulin) excess, close to 100% of the 19S combined to form a soluble 22S complex. All the 19S rheumatoid factor reacted with isologous and autologous 7S γG globulins and myeloma globulins of the γG_1, γG_2, and γG_4 subgroups (TABLE 1). Only about one-half of individual 19S rheumatoid factor preparations reacted with nonhuman primate and rabbit γ-globulin, but there was little reaction with other animal γ-globulins tested (see TABLE 1), nor with a 7S γA myeloma protein and a 19S γM Waldenström macroglobulin. Close to 100% of the 19S rheumatoid factor also reacted with an Fc fragment of a γG1 myeloma globulin (to form a 215 complex), but not with its Fab of $F(ab')_2$ fragments. The valence of this reaction was 5.

The results of these studies indicate that nearly 100% of 19S anti-γ-globulins, or rheumatoid factors, isolated from different sera, complex with aggregate-free preparations of human 7S γ-globulins. This reaction is highly specific, and differential patterns of reactivity appear with proteins of different human γ-globulin subgroups, and with animal γ-globulins.

The findings are compatible with the concept that the rheumatoid factors represent antibodies to native 7S γ-globulins, which are nonprecipitating in character because of the limited valence of the antigen. Rather than revealing new antigenic sites, aggregation might simply represent a method of increasing the valence of the antigen in order to bring about a better lattice formation and precipitation.

DR. HENNEY: I'm not at all happy with the lack of correlation between the 22S complex, which certainly does occur and which one can see in the centrifuge, and the fact that one is not able in this test system to show reactivity with monomeric γ-globulin. There are, however, several things that I find it difficult to reconcile with the reactivity of rheumatoid factor with 7S γ-globulin in the centrifuge. If you add aggregated γ-globulin to a mixture of 19S and 22S rheumatoid factors, there seems to be no preferential precipitation of the 19S. Moreover, the precipitation of 22S that is produced with aggregated γG-globulins apparently does not take place by liberation of the 7S which is bound to it. In other words, this evidence seems to suggest that the aggregated γG-globulin, when binding to the rheumatoid factor, does not bind on the same sites as the 7S monomers.

DR. HANNESTAD: I seem to remember from your paper in Immunology that when you did quantitative precipitation between heat-aggregated γG and rheumatoid factor serum you found inhibition in antigen excess when you had not separated the aggregates from native γG. At that time, you suggested that the explanation for this was inhibition of the reaction by native γG. How do you reconciliate this observation with your present findings?

DR. HENNEY: I find it very difficult to do so. I think that we are dealing with two different systems.

DR. EPSTEIN: One of the questions that we are faced with is whether monomeric 7S γG is active in terms of its capacity to react with rheumatoid factor. I would particularly question whether it is possible to produce configurational changes in γ-globulin by heat and yet see no difference by optical rotation or ultracentrifugation? Thus, I wonder if we ought to use a better term now than "native" for γ-globulin; we should talk about the presence or absence of the configuration that gives reactivity with rheumatoid factor.

DR. FRIOU: Did you exclude the possibility of the involvement of complement components as an antigen, both in your immunizations and also in your test system? Also have you excluded the possibility of allotypic differences between rabbits that produce the anti-BSA serum and those with which you did the test?

I presume that you did, but I'd like to know whether the animals that produce the anti-BSA serum also develop this type of rheumatoid factor activity.

DR. HENNEY: I think we can definitely exclude any effect of allotypic factors in this series. The animals were typed by Dr. Kelus in Birmingham. I think we can also exclude any effect of complement in this system.

γM RHEUMATOID FACTORS REACTING WITH NITROPHENYL GROUPS AND DENATURED DEOXYRIBONUCLEIC ACID

Kristian Hannestad, M.D.

Institute for Experimental Medical Research
University of Oslo, Ullevål Hospital
Oslo, Norway

Introduction

Several Waldenström macroglobulins have been reported that combine with human γG.[1] In one instance, it has been shown that the binding activity was located on the Fab fragment of the macroglobulin.[2] Thus, the specificity and location of binding activity on the γM molecule support the contention that these are true antigen-antibody reactions.

A human γG myeloma protein with anti-hapten activity was first described in 1967.[3] Subsequently, γA mouse myeloma proteins were found with activity against hapten nucleic acid bases and/or nitrophenyl derivatives,[4] and a Waldenström macroglobulin was described which possessed both anti-protein activity (against the Fc fragment of human γG) and anti-hapten activity.[1] Evidence was obtained that polyclonal γM rheumatoid factors from rheumatoid arthritis sera also possessed anti-hapten activity.[1]

In the present experiments, the reactions between the trinitrophenyl (TNP) group and polyclonal γM rheumatoid factor of serum from a patient with classical rheumatoid arthritis were studied further. In addition, this paper reports a Waldenström macroglobulin with anti-γG and anti-hapten activity which precipitates denatured deoxyribonucleic acid (DNA).

Materials and Methods

Reagents. 2,4,6-Trinitrobenzenesulfonic acid (TNBS) was obtained from Nutritional Biochemical Corporation, and 2,4-dinitrophenol (DNP) sodium salt from British Drug Houses Ltd. Highly polymerized calf thymus DNA (sodium salt) Type 1 was supplied by Sigma Chemical Co. From Kock Light Laboratories Ltd. were obtained: yeast ribonucleic acid (RNA); DNase from bovine pancreas, with an approximate activity of 450 units/mg; and RNase from bovine pancreas, crystallized four times. Human Cohn fraction II was a product of Kabi A.S., and rabbit γ-globulin was purchased from Mann Research Laboratories. Hemocyanin (HCy) was obtained from the gastropod *Buccinum undatum.*

Human Sera. Serum J. M. with a γM type M-component was obtained from Dr. O. Wager of Helsinki, Finland; this M-component, which has activity against human γG and nitrophenyl derivatives, has been characterized previously.[1] It was found by Dr. M. Harboe to contain only κ (light) chains. Serum Öh. with large amounts of polyclonal γM rheumatoid factor was from a patient with classical rheumatoid arthritis. Anti-CD Ripley was obtained from Dr. Marion Waller.

Antisera. Rabbit antisera specific for human γG and γM were given by Dr. M. Harboe, and had been tested for specificity according to criteria outlined previously.[5] Rabbit antiserum against whole human serum was obtained from Behringwerke AG.

Isolation of Proteins from Serum Öh. Euglobulin was obtained by diluting serum 1:20 in cold distilled water and incubating overnight in the cold. The precipitate was collected by centrifugation, washed once in cold distilled water, and dissolved in phosphate-buffered (0.01 M) saline at pH 7.4. γM rheumatoid factors were isolated from euglobulin by specific precipitation with heat-aggregated human γG according to the method of Edelman and co-workers,[6] as previously described.[1] By immunoelectrophoresis against anti-human serum antiserum, the isolated γM rheumatoid factor preparation contain only γM; by double diffusion, a very weak reaction with anti-γG antiserum was found, and was either due to contamination by trace amounts of γG or to the precipitation by γM rheumatoid factor of soluble immune complexes present in the absorbed antiserum.

Macroglobulin. Macroglobulin was obtained by sucrose-density-gradient ultracentrifugation of 0.1 ml of euglobulin; the fraction was collected from the macroglobulin zone with peak protein concentration. Immunoelectrophoresis showed that it contained only γM.

Aggregation of γG. Human γG was heat-aggregated and concentrated according to previously described methods.[1] Aggregation of rabbit γG was achieved by heating to 69°–70° C for 25 minutes, and the aggregates were concentrated as as noted previously for human γG.[1]

Trinitrophenyl-Hemocyanin Conjugates. Trinitrophenyl-hemocyanin conjugates were prepared by modification of a procedure described by Rittenberg and Amkraut.[7] The main advantage of this procedure compared to the method used previously[1] is that the reaction takes place at neutral pH when the HCy molecule remains associated. Thus, a much larger protein carrier for the TNP-groups results at pH 7.4 than at alkaline pH, thereby rendering the precipitating system that detects anti-TNP activity more sensitive.

A 64-mg sample of HCy was dissolved in 8 ml of 0.1 M phosphate buffer (pH 7.4) and dialyzed overnight against this buffer. Then, 14.3 mg of TNBS were dissolved in 0.5 ml of 0.15 M Tris buffer (pH 7.4) and added dropwise, with stirring, to the HCy solution. The solution was stirred at room temperature in the dark for 15 hours. Unreacted TNBS was removed by dialysis for six days against phosphate-buffered saline, and small amounts of precipitate were removed by centrifugation. The conjugates were tested by double diffusion in 1% agarose made in phosphate-buffered saline.

Nucleic Acid Antigens. DNA and RNA were dissolved in 0.015 M NaCl made 0.001 M with phosphate buffer (pH 7.4). DNA was denatured at a concentration of 2 mg/ml by boiling for ten minutes at 100° C, followed by cooling in iced water. Digestion with DNase was performed by incubating denatured DNA at 37° C for one hour with DNase in the presence of 0.003 M $MgCl_2$; the enzyme-to-substrate ratio was 1:20 by weight. Denatured DNA was treated with RNase in the same manner. The digestion products were not dialyzed, and were tested against serum J.M. by double diffusion in 1% agarose in 0.06 M veronal buffer (pH 8.6).

Hemagglutination Inhibition. Details of this procedure have been described previously.[1]

Results

The Reaction of Polyclonal γM Öh. with Trinitrophenyl-Hemocyanin

The protein concentration of fractions from a sucrose density gradient containing ultracentrifuged dissolved precipitate between euglobulin Öh.-aggregated human γG is shown in FIGURE 1. Fractions number 13 and 14 precipitated strongly with heat-aggregated γG, and with TNP-HCy (FIGURE 2). The other fractions had none of these activities. Unconjugated HCy was not precipi-

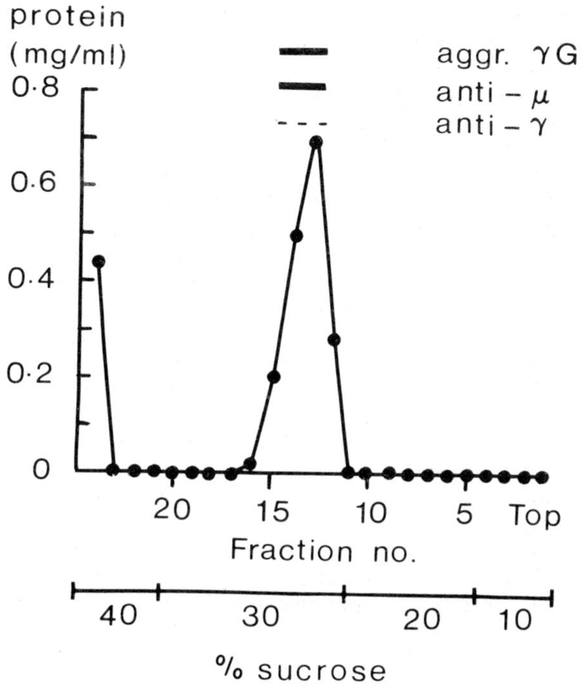

FIGURE 1. Sucrose-density-gradient ultracentrifugation (at pH 3.6) of dissolved precipitate between euglobulin Oh. and aggregated human γG. Fractions were collected from the top; γG aggregates were pelleted at the bottom. A distinct protein peak containing γM (precipitation with anti-μ) and rheumatoid factor activity (precipitation with heat-aggregated γG) were obtained. The very weak reaction with anti-γ may be due to slight contamination by γG or to precipitation of soluble immune complexes in the anti-γ antiserum. Direction of sedimentation is to the left.

tated. The finding that fractions 13 and 14 contained γM and essentially no γG shows that γM, which precipitates with aggregated γG, also reacts with TNP-groups. The reaction with TNP-HCy, although distinct in 1% agarose made in phosphate-buffered saline, was barely visible in 1% agarose made in 0.06 M veronal buffer (pH 8.6), indicating that pH and/or ionic strength have a marked effect on the precipitation of the reactants.

To test whether all or only a fraction of the γM rheumatoid factor isolated in this manner percipitated with TNP-HCy, the following experiment was performed: γM rheumatoid factor and TNP-HCy which had been dialyzed against phosphate-buffered saline were mixed in amounts of 0.5 mg each. Instantaneous turbidity resulted. After incubation at 37° C for 30 minutes, the resulting precipitate was spun down. The supernatant, which did not precipitate with TNP-HCy by double diffusion, still precipitated strongly with aggregated γG. This shows that only a fraction of the γM rheumatoid factor had sufficient affinity for the TNP-group to precipitate with TNP-HCy.

To be confident that TNP-HCy precipitated with γM rheumatoid factor in the isolated rheumatoid factor preparation, and not with an undetected contaminant, recovery of rheumatoid factor activity from the precipitate was attempted.

The precipitate between TNP-HCy and γM rheumatoid factor obtained as noted previously, was washed three times in cold phosphate-buffered saline. To the washed precipitate was added 0.2 ml of 0.1 M DNP, and, after incubation for 60 seconds at 37° C, the precipitate had dissolved completely. The large TNP-HCy molecules (molecular weight, approximately 8 million) were then separated from the lighter γM rheumatoid factor by sucrose-density-gradient ultracentrifugation (the sucrose had previously been dissolved in phosphate-buffered saline containing 0.1 M DNP). Fractions were collected from the top to avoid contamination of γM rheumatoid factor with the faster-sedimenting TNP-HCy, and were dialyzed for 24 hours against phosphate-buffered saline to remove sucrose and DNP. The protein concentration of the fractions is shown in the lower part of FIGURE 3, and the rheumatoid factor activity (Ripley) in the upper part. There was distinct rheumatoid factor activity corresponding to the peak protein concentration. No rheumatoid factor activity was detected in the phosphate-buffered saline used for the last washing of precipitate. To exclude the possibility that the agglutinating activity against the anti-CD Ripley sensitized cells was due to complement components, the fractions were heated to 56° C for 30 minutes. No decrease in agglutination resulted from this treatment. The results demonstrated that the rheumatoid factor was bound to TNP-HCy in the precipitate.

The γM rheumatoid factor used in the previous experiments had been isolated by precipitation with human γG. It was of interest to examine whether γM rheumatoid factor isolated by precipitation with rabbit γG would also precipitate with TNP-HCy. The results of experiments with γM rheumatoid factor from

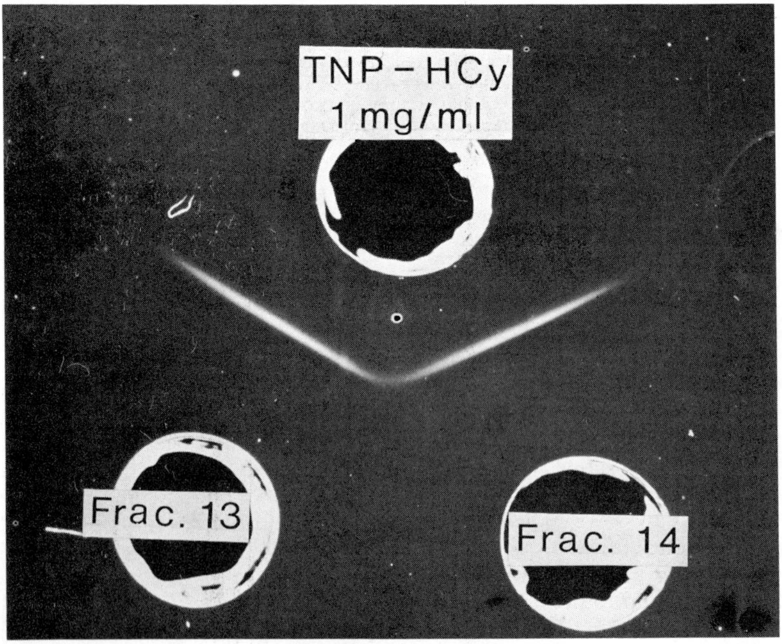

FIGURE 2. Fractions nos. 13 and 14 of FIGURE 1 precipitate with TNP-HCy. (1 mg/ml) by double diffusion in 1% agarose made in phosphate-buffered saline.

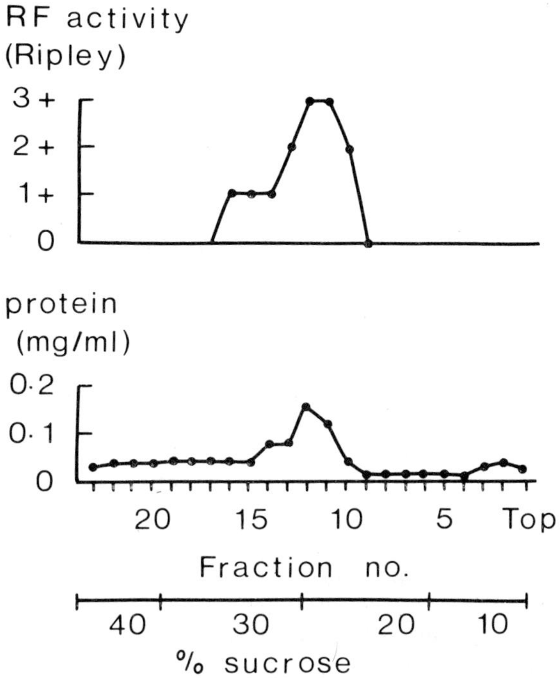

FIGURE 3. Sucrose-density-gradient ultracentrifugation in 0.1 M DNP of dissolved precipitate between γM rheumatoid factor and TNP-HCy. The γM rheumatoid factor was obtained as in FIGURE 1, and the precipitate was dissolved by adding 0.1 M DNP. Fractions were collected from the top. Distinct rheumatoid factor activity (Ripley) was found in fractions with peak protein concentration.

serum Öh. isolated from aggregated rabbit γG are shown in FIGURES 4 and 5. Pure γM rheumatoid factor thus obtained agglutinated red cells sensitized with both human (anti-CD Ripley) and rabbit γG (FIGURE 4), precipitated aggregated γG from both species (FIGURE 5), and precipitated TNP-HCy (FIGURE 5). Since a population of rheumatoid factor molecules reacting exclusively with rabbit γG was not obtained, the question still remains whether such a population has specificity for the TNP-group.

To test whether there is γM which precipitates TNP-HCy but not aggregated human γG, the following experiment was performed: 0.9 mg/ml of γM, isolated from euglobulin Öh., was subjected to intrabasin absorption with heat-aggregated γG after it had been established that 2 mg/ml of human aggregated γG did not precipitate TNP-HCy by double diffusion in 1% agarose made in phosphate-buffered saline. The well was first filled with 2 mg/ml of γG aggregates, and after three hours, when the well was empty, it was refilled with γM Öh. A dense precipitate formed around the well. The molecules that diffused into the agarose from this well did not precipitate with aggregated γG in a neighbor well, but formed a faint but definite precipitate with 2 mg/ml of TNP-HCy. This indicated that precipitation of TNP-HCy is not limited to γM molecules that precipitate heat-aggregated γG.

The Reaction of Monoclonal γM Rheumatoid Factor with Denatured DNA

Previously, the M-component of serum J.M. has been shown to have anti-γG and anti-nitrophenyl activity.[1] When serum J.M. was diffused against denatured DNA in 1% agarose made in 0.06 M barbital buffer (pH 8.6), distinct precipitation resulted. Treatment of denatured DNA with DNase abolished precipitation, while RNase had no effect (FIGURE 6). γM in serum J.M. was separated from γG by sucrose-density-gradient ultracentrifugation; only fractions from the macroglobulin zone precipitated denatured DNA, demonstrating that the reaction proceeded independent of γG. In immunoelectrophoresis of serum J.M., the slow segment of the γM-anti-γM precipitin arc corresponded exactly to the arc that developed with denatured DNA (FIGURE 7). Denatured DNA in a concentration of as little as 0.1 mg/ml was sufficient to produce a distinct arc. This showed that the denatured DNA reacted with the M-component of serum. The precipitin reaction was not visible in 1% agarose made in phosphate-buffered saline, and established precipitates disappeared when the agarose was soaked in phosphate-buffered saline. Precipitation was visible in 1% agarose made in 0.10 M phosphate buffer (pH 7.4) or phosphate-buffered saline diluted 1:2 in distilled water, and precipitation became stronger in 0.05 M phosphate buffer (pH 7.4) or 0.06 M barbital buffer (pH 8.6), indicating that the concentration of salt in the system had marked effect on precipitation. No precipitation was observed with native DNA in 0.6% agarose or RNA in concentrations of 2 mg/ml. Inactivation of serum J.M. at 56° C for 30 minutes had no effect on the precipitin reaction with denatured DNA. No precipitation occurred between isolated polyclonal γM rheumatoid factor Öh. (1.0 mg/ml) and denatured DNA.

Several aggregated human γG preparations were tested in double diffusion against a serum (E.H.) containing a γM M-component with strong precipitating activity against denatured DNA, but no anti-γG activity. No precipitation was

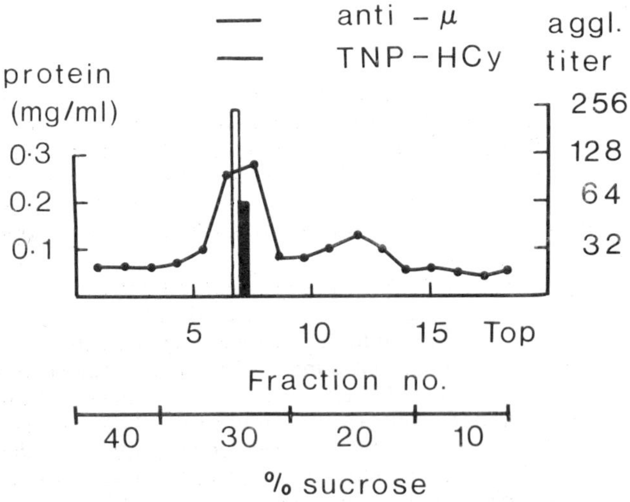

FIGURE 4. Sucrose-density-gradient ultracentrifugation (at pH 3.6) of dissolved precipitate between euglobulin Oh. and aggregated rabbit γG. Fractions were collected from the bottom. A protein peak was obtained containing γM with rheumatoid factor activity, as evidenced by agglutination of red cells coated with human (open bar) and rabbit (solid bar) γG.

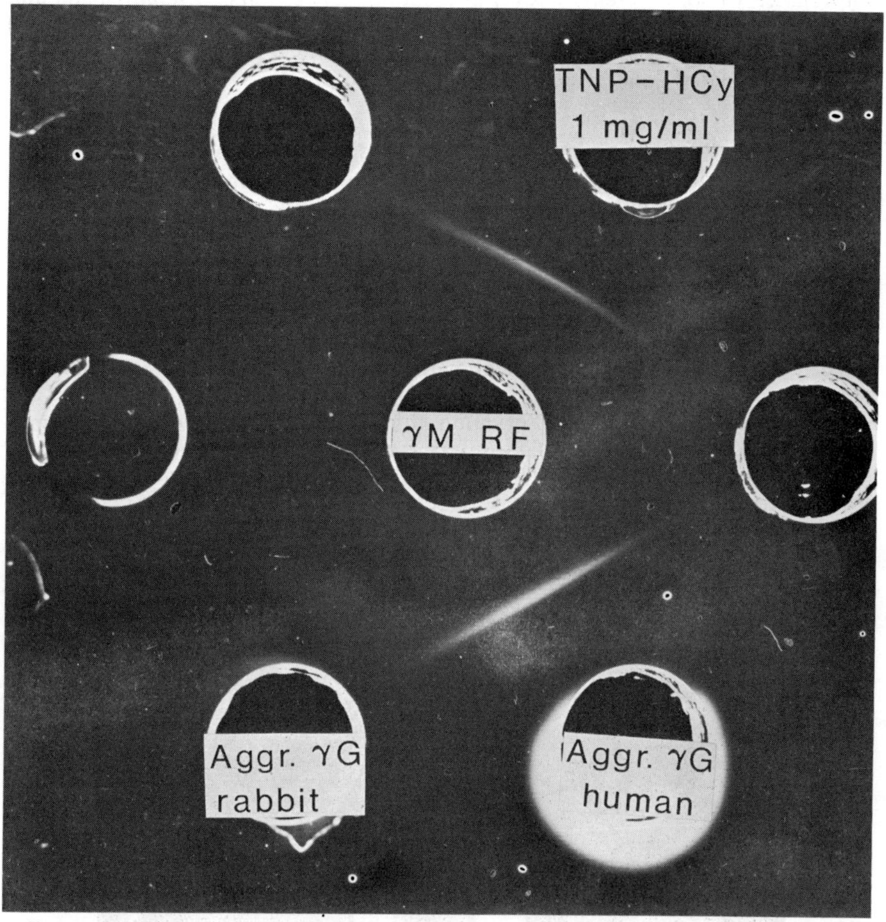

FIGURE 5. Pooled fractions nos. 6 and 7 of FIGURE 4 precipitate with aggregated human γG, rabbit γG (the latter precipitate was very diffuse), and TNP-HCy.

observed, demonstrating that aggregated γG was not contaminated by significant amounts of denatured DNA.

It was of interest to test whether DNA would inhibit the anti-γG activity of the γM M-component J.M. To this end, a fixed dilution of macroglobulin J.M., obtained by sucrose-density-gradient ultracentrifugation of serum J.M., was employed together with human red cells (CDe/CDe) sensitized with anti-CD Ripley antibodies, giving a 2+ agglutination (score from 0 to 4+) on glass plates. Denatured DNA (2 mg/ml) dissolved in 0.015 M NaCl inhibited the agglutination completely* when the plate was examined after a ten-minute incubation of the reactants. When denatured DNA (2 mg/ml) was dissolved in 0.15 M NaCl,† no inhibition of the agglutination reaction was observed, again demonstrating the

* Final molarity of NaCl, 0.10 M.
† Final molarity of NaCl, 0.15 M.

importance of ionic strength for the reaction between the M-component and denatured DNA. No inhibition was found with native DNA, whether dissolved in 0.015 M or 0.15 M NaCl, also showing that in this test system the M-component discriminated between native and denatured DNA.

Discussion

The conjugation of large numbers of TNP molecules on associated HCy afforded a very sensitive precipitating system whereby γM rheumatoid factor with anti-TNP activity could be isolated. It was thus possible to confirm, in a more unequivocal fashion, previous observations[1] that polyclonal γM rheumatoid factor reacts with the TNP group. Three additional observations are noteworthy: Only a fraction of the polyclonal γM rheumatoid factor precipitated with TNP-HCy; the precipitation of TNP-HCy by γM was not limited to γM that precipitated γG; and a γM M-component with anti-γG and anti-TNP activity also reacted with denatured DNA.

It follows from the first observation that a subpopulation of γM rheumatoid factor can be isolated which differs from the remaining population by its specificity for the TNP-group. This heterogeneity with regard to anti-TNP activity was expected,[1] and indicates that the reaction with the TNP-group involves the Fab part of the γM molecules. It will be important to find out whether this "anti-

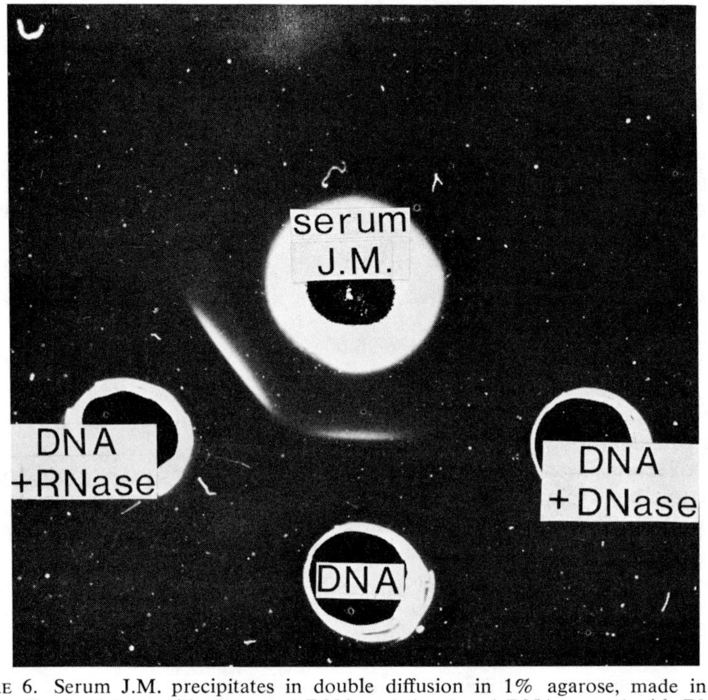

FIGURE 6. Serum J.M. precipitates in double diffusion in 1% agarose, made in 0.06 M barbital buffer (pH 8.6), with denatured DNA and denatured DNA treated with RNase, but does not precipitate with denatured DNA treated with DNase. Plate incubated overnight at 4° C.

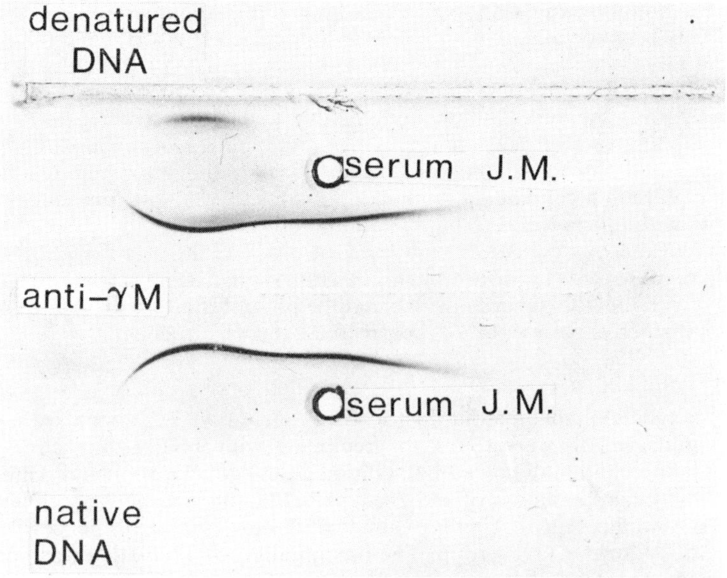

FIGURE 7. Immunoelectrophoresis of serum J.M. in agarose. The slow convex segment of the γM-anti-γM arc corresponds exactly to the precipitin arc which formed with denatured DNA. No precipitate formed with 2 mg/ml of native DNA. The cathode is on the left side.

TNP" fraction of polyclonal γM rheumatoid factor contains a population of molecules with specificity for denatured DNA.

The precipitation of TNP-HCγ was not unique for γM which precipitated aggregated γG, suggesting that antibodies with specificities other than anti-γG also cross-react with the TNP-group. The basis for the reactivity of γM rheumatoid factor with the TNP-group is not known. The affinity of γM rheumatoid factor for the TNP-group is probably low, since the precipitin reaction (a) is sensitive to changes in pH and ionic strength, which usually do not affect reactions of induced antibodies to homologous hapten; (b) requires a high degree of conjugation of the protein carrier with TNP-groups; and (c) a high concentration of hapten is necessary to dissolve the precipitates. It is therefore unlikely that the nitrophenyl group represents the homologous antigenic determinant for the γM rheumatoid factor.

Another possibility is that there may be TNP-like conformations on the Fc fragment of human γG, and that a small portion of γM rheumatoid factor has its specificity directed toward such conformations, causing them to cross-react with TNP-groups. However, one cathodically migrating γM M-component (E.H.) is being studied which reacts with DNP-TNP structures and denatured DNA, but has no detectable anti-γG activity. A hypothetical resemblance between TNP and Fc fragment structures might, therefore, be due not only to conformation, since one would then expect that every M-component which reacts with TNP should also react with γG; the resemblance may, therefore, rather be based on electrical charge or hydrophobic groups, more difficult to define.

A third possibility is that the reactivity by γM rheumatoid factor with nitrophenyl groups and denatured DNA may reflect the fact that γM rheumatoid factor can be produced in response to several antigenic stimuli, and not exclusively by immunization with γG. According to this hypothesis, the Fc fragment of γG may function as a cross-reacting antigen. Such hypothetical cross-reactions with the Fcγ fragment would probably be of low avidity, requiring very sensitive systems to be detected.

Finally, the observed reactions may be due to salt-like binding between molecules of opposite electrical charge, a negatively charged antigen (TNP-groups and denatured DNA) and positively charged γM, and where the reaction does not take place in a genuine antibody-combining site of γM. If this is the case, the reaction with nitrophenyl groups should not be correlated to any particular specificity (anti-γG, cold agglutinin, etc.) of γM, and the reacting γM population would be expected to discriminate minimally between different polyanions. Clearly, with the information available at the present time, the described reactions require further experimentation before they can be explained.

Summary

Polyclonal γM rheumatoid factor from serum of a patient with classical rheumatoid arthritis were found to precipitate with TNP groups conjugated to HCy. The precipitate dissolved by addition of 0.1 M dinitrophenol. Only a fraction of the total population of γM rheumatoid factor molecules precipitated with TNP-HCy, indicating that γM rheumatoid factor is heterogenous with regard to specificity for the TNP-group. The precipitation of TNP-HCy was not limited exclusively to γM which precipitated aggregated γG, indicating that γM with specificities other than anti-γG reacts with the TNP group.

A Waldenström macroglobulin with anti-γG and anti-nitrophenyl activity was found to precipitate with denatured DNA, but not with native DNA or RNA. The precipitin reaction with denatured DNA was visible only when the ionic strength was decreased below the physiological level. Inactivation of the Waldenström serum had no effect on the reaction, while incubation of denatured DNA with DNase abolished it. Possible explanations for the reactions of γM rheumatoid factor with structures other than γG were also discussed.

References

1. Hannestad, K. 1969. Monoclonal and polyclonal γM rheumatoid factors with anti-di- and anti-trinitrophenyl activity. Clin. Exp. Immunol. **4:** 555.
2. Metzger, H. 1967. Characterization of a human macroglobulin. V. A. Waldenström macroglobulin with antibody activity. Proc. Nat. Acad. Sci. **57:** 1490.
3. Eisen, H. N., J. R. Little, C. K. Osterland & E. S. Simms. 1967. A myeloma protein with antibody activity. Cold Spring Harbor Symp. Quant. Biol. **32:** 75.
4. Schubert, D., A. Jobe & M. Cohn. 1968. Mouse myelomas producing precipitating antibody to nucleic acid bases and/or nitrophenyl derivatives. Nature **220:** 882.
5. Hannestad, K. 1968. Rheumatoid factors reacting with autologous native γG globulin and joint fluid γG aggregates. Clin. Exp. Immunol. **3:** 671.
6. Edelman, G. M., H. G. Kunkel & E. C. Franklin. 1958. Interaction of rheumatoid factor with antigen-antibody complexes and aggregated gamma globulin. J. Exp. Med. **108:** 105.
7. Rittenberg, M. B. & A. A. Amkraut. 1966. Immunogenicity of trinitrophenyl-hemocyanin: Production of primary and secondary anti-hapten precipitins. J. Exp. Med. **97:** 421.

General Discussion

Dr. Williams: When you absorbed your monoclonal serum with the denatured DNA, did you lose the lines? Did you have any evidence that you were dealing with exactly the same antibody molecules in the two reactions?

DR. HANNESTAD: I have not conducted such an experiment yet. These are very recent observations. I have performed one experiment, i.e., I have taken serum and mixed it with red cells that were coated with anti-Rh antibodies. When I added native γG to this system, I observed no inhibition; when I added denatured DNA, distinct inhibition resulted. I have shown previously that all the rheumatoid factor activity of this serum resides in the M-component. Thus, I definitely think that it is the M-component that reacts.

DR. GOLDBERG: This work may relate to some work which Dr. Barnett and I have recently completed. We found that in mixed γG-γM cryoglobulins, there was a significant amount of DNA-like material that was detected by either a diphenylamine reagent test or by antisera which was monospecific for DNA. Interestingly, the DNA found in these mixed cryoglobulins appeared to be associated with the γM component; however, despite the fact that we could apparently disassociate the DNA from the γM component, we could never show anti-DNA activity in this γM. All of these γM components had rheumatoid factor activity.

DR. HENNEY: This seems to contradict, superficially at least, many of the preconceived notions about antibody. Would you comment on the binding constants of these different antigens for your sera. You did mention briefly that they were very low. Can you give us some values?

DR. HANNESTAD: No, I have not performed the equilibrium dialysis, so I cannot give you precise equilibrium constants. The reason why I think the affinities are very low is that the reactions are easily influenced by changes in ionic strength. If you increase ionic strength, then the visible reaction, the precipitation, decreases. I think this indicates low affinity, although it doesn't prove it. Another reason is that very high concentrations of free antigen are required to dissolve the precipitates. This also indicates that the affinity is low. Finally, the specificity is very different from that usually encountered in animals.

DR. HENNEY: Have you proved that these are, in fact, binding to the Fab analogue of the γM molecules?

DR. HANNESTAD: No, I haven't, and this is obviously something that must be done. However, the inhibition of the reactions with aggregated γG indicates that the same region of the molecule reacting with γG reacts with the haptens. And with one monoclonal protein it has been shown that the reaction of monoclonal rheumatoid factor with γG is in the Fab fragments.

DR. AGNELLO: In the gel experiment showing the reaction of serum with denatured DNA, was the serum heated?

DR. HANNESTAD: No, it was not heated.

DR. AGNELLO: Recently we have found that C′1q in normal serum will react with heat-denatured DNA, and this could very well be the case in your experiment.

DR. HANNESTAD: I don't think so, because the location of the precipitin arc in the agarose is distinctly different from the location of C′1q, which has a faster mobility; my precipitin arc had a slow mobility in the γ-region.

DR. AGNELLO: Actually, C′1q does have a very slow mobility, and it would be difficult to distinguish it from γ-globulin by immunoelectrophoresis.

DR. BARNETT: This is a very provocative and obviously very controversial area. I believe it is more than ten years ago that Gray, in a paper in the *Journal of Immunology*, suggested that rheumatoid factors were anti-DNA antibodies. Have you other macroglobulins besides the one from patient J.M. that do not react with the TNP-group or with DNA as controls?

DR. HANNESTAD: Of 70 macroglobulins, there was only one that reacted with both aggregated γG and TNP. Of these 70, however, there were about four that reacted by precipitation with DNP hemocyanin. Thus, the reaction with a DNP-group is more frequent than the combined reaction with DNP and aggregated γG.

DR. VAUGHAN: Dr. Hannestad, the number of myeloma proteins that have been found to react with DNP is rather large, and now you present these. Is it possible that DNP is reacting with the invariant part of Fab fragment if, indeed, it does react with Fab fragment in your systems, as it does in the myeloma proteins? Do you know whether these proteins have been studied sufficiently for subclass characteristics that might suggest that the invariant rather than the variable part of the Fab fragment is involved?

DR. HANNESTAD: I was fortunate to be present at a seminar at the National Institutes of Health in January of 1969 at which the subject was antibody activity of homogeneous γ-globulins. The interesting point is that it is the macroglobulins that contain most of the reported activities, except for one γG myeloma protein reported by Eisen. This particular protein was very interesting in that it showed a high degree of specificity for DNP, and this high degree of specificity, I think, is only compatible with a true antigen-antibody reaction. This antibody could distinguish between mono- and trinitrophenol, for instance, and nitrophenol without being conjugated with an amino acid. I don't think such specificity can be exhibited by genetic or subclass structures.

DR. BARNETT: Would you tell us the conditions of salt and pH at which you performed your analyses with DNP and with DNA?

DR. HANNESTAD: The reaction with DNA was not visible in phosphate-buffered saline. When the phosphate-buffered saline was diluted 1:2 in distilled water, the reaction became clearly visible. Likewise, the reaction was clearly visible in the barbital buffer (pH 8.6, ionic strength 0.06) used for immunoelectrophoresis. Thus, it is quite apparent that salt concentration and pH markedly influence precipitation in this system.

DR. KUNKEL: I attended the same meeting that Dr. Hannestad mentioned, and I think it is fair to point out that Dr. Eisen does not accept many proteins as being anti-DNP unless the binding constant is below 10^{-3}. I think the binding constant here is very critical. In his study of mouse proteins, he reported many proteins that bind DNP, but he only accepted a few as being significant.

DR. HANNESTAD: Yes, but I think also that there was disagreement about this point at that meeting. Obviously, binding constants would be very important if DNA is the homologous antigen; one would expect that γM rheumatoid factors reacting with DNA would show higher binding affinity for DNA than for γG, but it's difficult to measure this.

DR. ZVAIFLER: We have been very impressed with reactions in gel between denatured single-strand DNA and rheumatoid synovial effusions; precipitin reactions are observed which are present almost proportional to the titer of rheumatoid factor activity and to the depression of the complement activity. The reactant appears to come off G-200 in the first elution peak. It is destroyed by mercaptoethanol treatment, and the antigen is also destroyed by DNase treatment. This reaction works very well in agarose and also at pH in excess of 7. Have you had any similar observation? We did not really consider the possibility that this could be rheumatoid factor, but it's a strikingly comparable situation.

DR. HANNESTAD: I have been looking at polyclonal γM rheumatoid factors isolated by specific precipitation with aggregated γG. I have not found any direct precipitation with denatured DNA. I think that if polyclonal γM rheumatoid factors have specificity for denatured DNA, then it is only a small fraction of rheumatoid factors.

BINDING PROPERTIES OF MONOCLONAL γG-ANTIGLOBULIN FACTORS WITH HUMAN γG*

Jean-Charles Cerottini, M.D.,† and Howard M. Grey, M.D.‡

Department of Experimental Pathology
Scripps Clinic and Research Foundation
La Jolla, Calif.

Cryoglobulins, serum globulins that reversibly precipitate in the cold, are found in patients with multiple myeloma, macroglobulinemia, and a variety of connective tissue disorders.[1] Whereas the exact mechanism underlying cryoprecipitation is still unknown, the finding of a high incidence of anti-γ-globulin activity among cryoglobulins[2,3] suggests that cryoprecipitates represent antigen-antibody complexes of such a nature that precipitation of the complexes occurs only at low temperature.

Recent studies indicated that five out of seven human monoclonal γG-cryoglobulins possessed anti-γ-globulin activity.[3] The reactive region of the cryoglobulin molecule was located on the Fab fragment, whereas the γG-globulin determinant(s) recognized by the cryoglobulins was located on the Fc fragment. Specificity of the reaction was demonstrated by the fact that the cryoglobulins combined only with primate γG-globulins and not with other primate immunoglobulins or mammalian γG-globulins. The purpose of the present study was to characterize further the interaction between these monoclonal γG-cryoglobulins and γG-globulin by studying the binding strength of the interaction. For comparative purposes, the relative avidity of human γM-rheumatoid factor and induced rabbit anti-human Fc antibody was also studied.

Materials and Methods

Proteins. Monoclonal γG-cryoglobulins and fragments were prepared according to methods described previously.[3] The γM rheumatoid factor was prepared from the sera of patients with high rheumatoid factor activity. The euglobulin fraction obtained by diluting the serum 15-fold with distilled water was further purified by gel filtration on Sephadex G-200 equilibrated with 0.1 M acetate buffer (pH 4.0).

Induced anti-human γG-globulin antibody was obtained seven and 28 days after a single injection of rabbits with 1 mg of DEAE-cellulose-isolated human γG-globulin in complete Freund's adjuvant. Rabbit antibody γG-globulin fraction was obtained by ammonium sulfate precipitation and DEAE-cellulose chromatography. The $F(ab')_2$ fragment was prepared by pepsin digestion of γG-globulin and purified by gel filtration on Sephadex G-150.[4]

Purified anti-human Fc antibody was prepared by precipitation of Fc fragment with hyperimmune rabbit anti-human γG-globulin antiserum at equivalence. The washed precipitate was digested with pepsin at pH 4.0, and the resultant clear solution was submitted to gel filtration on Sephadex G-150. The main protein

* This is publication no. 339 from the Department of Experimental Pathology, Scripps Clinic and Research Foundation, La Jolla, Calif. This research was supported by United States Public Health Service grant no. AI–07007, Atomic Energy Commission contract no. AT (04–3)–410, and American Heart Association grant no. 67–795.

† Supported by United States Public Health Service training grant no. GM–683.

‡ This study was done during the tenure of an Established Investigatorship of the American Heart Association.

peak eluted contained only rabbit $F(ab')_2$. As determined by ultracentrifugal analysis, most, if not all, of the Fab′ fragment obtained by reduction and alkylation of $F(ab')_2$, reacted with human γG-globulin.

Antigen-Binding Capacity (ABC) Test. Details of the ammonium sulfate method using ^{131}I-labeled Fab and ^{125}I-labeled Fc have been described elsewhere.[4] For the study of the binding properties of $F(ab')_2$ fragment, it was necessary to increase the ammonium sulfate concentration to 44% of saturation to ensure precipitation of most of the fragment. In these circumstances, only the portion of ^{125}I-labeled Fc soluble in 44% saturated ammonium sulfate was used.

Ultracentrifugal Analysis. Analytical ultracentrifugation was carried out according to a method described previously.[3] Sedimentation coefficient and areas were calculated with the aid of a Gaertner comparator.

RESULTS

Specificity of the Anti-γ-Globulin Activity of γG-Cryoglobulins

Previous studies have shown that the antigenic determinant(s) on the γG-globulin molecule which reacted with one cryoglobulin preparation was located on the Fc fragment.[3] To extend these findings, the binding properties of three cryoglobulin preparations were determined by means of an antigen-binding capacity test employing ^{131}I-labeled Fab and ^{125}I-labeled Fc.[4] As shown in TABLE 1, 13–42% of the added Fc was specifically bound to the cryoglobulins, whereas there was no significant binding of Fab fragment. Similar results were found with two γM rheumatoid factors. By means of a minor modification of the antigen-binding capacity test, further experiments showed that the binding activity of the cryoglobulins for Fc fragment was still present in the pepsin-digested $F(ab')_2$ fragments. Because it was advantageous to eliminate the Fc fragment of the cryoglobulins and to carry out reactions at low temperature, only $F(ab')_2$ fragments (which did not have the property of cryoprecipitation) were used for further studies of the binding properties of cryoglobulins.

Relative Avidity of γG-Cryoglobulins

Two methods were used to estimate the relative avidity of cryoglobulins with anti-γ-globulin activity. First, the effect of antigen concentration upon the antigen-binding capacity values was determined.[5] Dilutions of each preparation were incubated at 4° C for 18 hours with various antigen concentrations, ranging from 0.01 to 10 μg of nitrogen in ^{125}I-labeled (I*) Fc. The percentage of radio-

TABLE 1

BINDING PROPERTIES OF γG-CRYOGLOBULINS AND γM RHEUMATOID FACTORS

Immunoglobulin Class	Preparation	Percent Radioactivity Bound to Globulin*	
		^{131}I-Fab	^{125}I-Fc
γG-Cryoglobulin	Man	2.7	42.7
	Cra	1.0	24.9
	Pur	0.7	13.0
γM Rheumatoid factor	Joh	1.1	35.4
	Thi	0.8	41.4

* A mixture of both radioactive fragments (0.01 μg of nitrogen antigen) was incubated with each preparation for 18 hours at 25° C before addition of 40% saturated ammonium sulfate.

activity specifically bound to globulin was calculated after precipitation with ammonium sulfate. The dilution at which 30% of the radio-labeled antigen was bound to globulin was used as a measure of the relative antigen-binding capacity. The antigen-binding capacity values were obtained by multiplying the reciprocal of the dilution by the amount of antigen nitrogen precipitated (ABC-30). For comparative purposes, γG-globulin and F(ab′)$_2$ fragment prepared from early and late rabbit antisera to human γG-globulin were also tested. As shown in FIGURE 1, the antigen-binding capacity value of Man F(ab′)$_2$-cryoglobulin was very much affected by the antigen concentration used for the test, since a tenfold increase in antigen concentration resulted in a tenfold increase in the antigen-binding capacity value. By comparison, even the earliest rabbit anti-Fc antibody available, collected seven days after human γG-globulin injection, demonstrated a higher avidity than the cryoglobulin, since its antigen-binding capacity value increased fivefold with each tenfold increase in antigen concentration. By contrast, the antigen-binding capacity value of rabbit antibody to Fc collected 28 days after

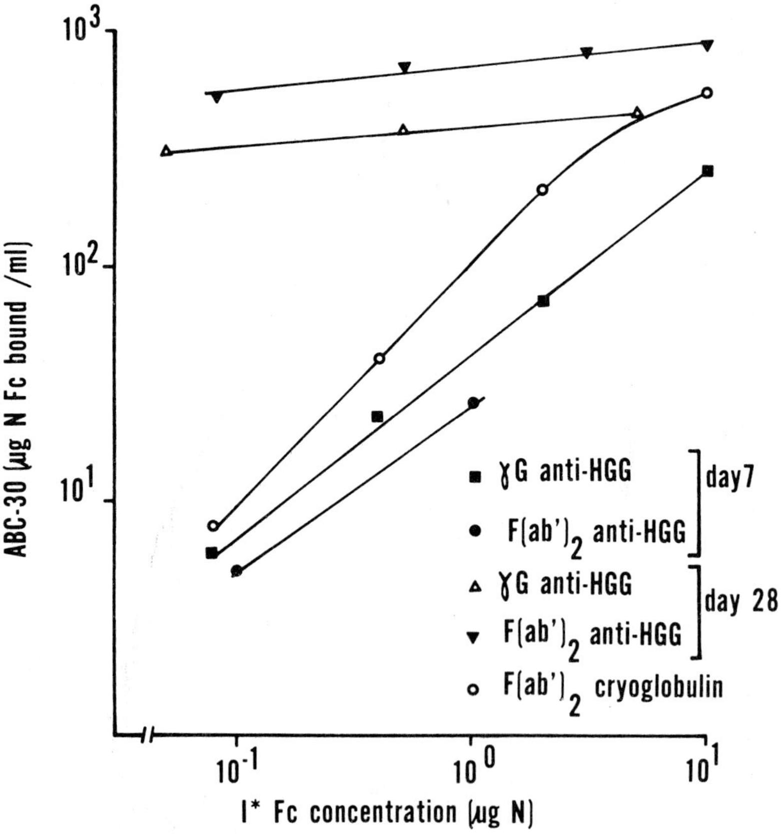

FIGURE 1. Comparison of the effect of antigen (I*Fc) concentration on the binding activity of F(ab′)$_2$ fragment of cryoglobulin Man and rabbit antibody to human Fc fragment obtained early and late during immunization. ABC = antigen-binding capacity; HGG = human γG-globulin.

antigen injection was barely affected by antigen concentration. No significant difference was seen between antibody γG-globulin and its $F(ab')_2$ fragment.

Second, the rate of dissociation of antigen-antibody complexes was also used as an index of the relative avidity of the cryoglobulin in preparations.[5] The whole reaction was carried out at 4° C; 4 ml of I*Fc (0.01) μg of nitrogen/ml) were mixed with 8 ml of $F(ab')_2$ preparation diluted in 10% normal duck serum. The dilution was selected so that about 40% of I*Fc was bound at equilibrium. To determine the amount of nonspecific precipitation of antigen, a control tube containing 5 ml of I*Fc and 10 ml of 10% normal duck serum was used. After incubation overnight, two 1.0-ml aliquots were removed from each tube and incubated with 1.0 ml of 88% saturated ammonium sulfate, as described previously for the antigen-binding capacity test. Then 3 ml of unlabeled Fc (200 μg of nitrogen/ml) was added to each tube in order to provide a large excess of unlabeled antigen over labeled antigen. At intervals of 15, 30, and 60 minutes (or one, five, and 24 hours in the case of "late" rabbit antibody) after the addition of unlabeled antigen, three 1.0-ml aliquots were taken from each tube and treated with the ammonium sulfate solution. After correction for nonspecific precipitation of I*Fc, the percentage of I*Fc precipitated was calculated for the various time intervals after the addition of unlabeled antigen. The time interval necessary for 50% of I*Fc ($T_{1/2}$) to dissociate from the antigen-antibody complex was graphically determined for each preparation. As shown in TABLE 2, I*Fc dissociated very rapidly from complexes formed with cryoglobulins and rheumatoid factors. Again, rabbit anti-Fc antibody collected seven days after antigen injection showed a relatively higher avidity than did cryoglobulins, although its dissociation rate was much faster than that of rabbit antibody collected at a later time after the start of immunization.

TABLE 2

DISSOCIATION RATES OF COMPLEXES BETWEEN I*FC AND CRYOGLOBULINS, RHEUMATOID FACTORS, OR RABBIT ANTI-HUMAN γG-GLOBULIN ANTIBODY

Preparation	$T_{1/2}$*
$F(ab')_2$-Cryoglobulin (Man)	<5
$F(ab')_2$-Cryoglobulin (Pea)	<5
γM Rheumatoid factor (Joh)	<5
γM Rheumatoid factor (Thi)	<5
$F(ab')_2$ Rheumatoid factor (Thi)	5
$F(ab')_2$ Anti-Fc, day 7 (rabbit)	15
$F(ab')_2$ Anti-Fc, day 28 (rabbit)	200
IgG Anti-Fc, hyperimmune (rabbit)	>1,500

* Time, in minutes, required for dissociation of 50% of the I*Fc.

Determination of Association Constant for Fab-Cryoglobulin-γG_1 Myeloma Protein Interaction

Formation of complexes between cryoglobulin and γG-globulin was also quantitatively studied by analytical ultracentrifugation. Constant amounts of Fab fregment of Man cryoglobulin were mixed with varying amounts of a γG_1 myeloma protein. A γG_1 protein was used because previous studies indicated that Man cryoglobulin interacted to a greater degree with proteins of the γG_1 subclass than with the other γG subclasses.[3] Controls included Fab-cryoglobulin alone and γG_1 protein alone, in the same concentrations as the respective reactant

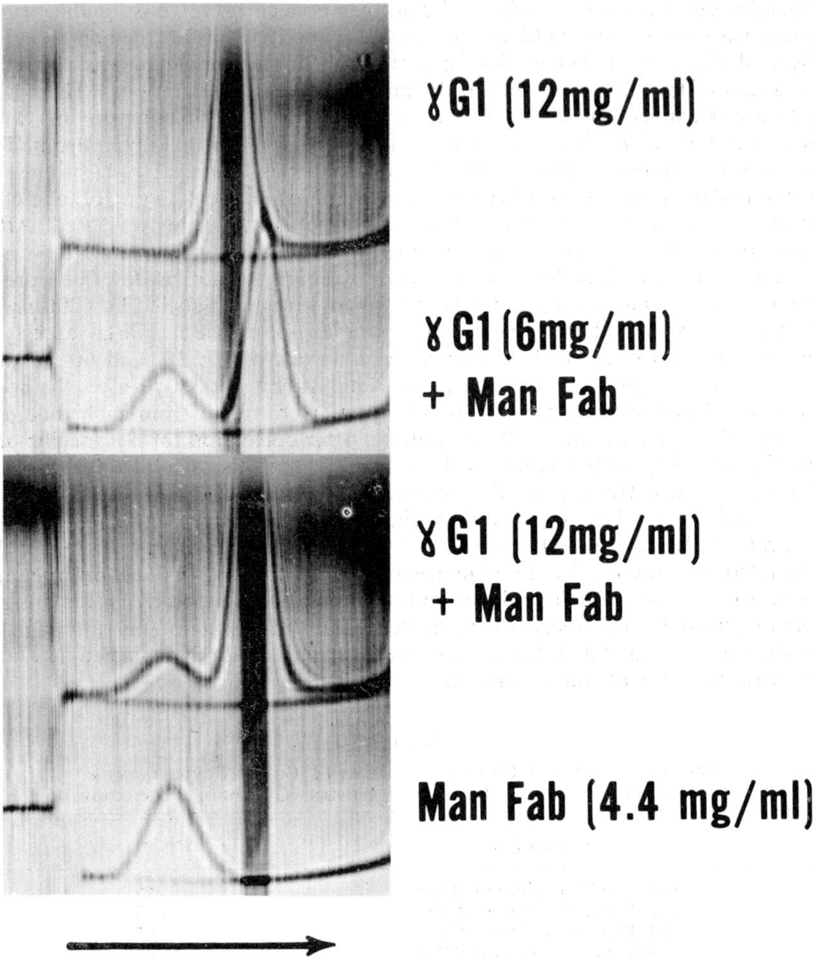

FIGURE 2. Analytical ultracentrifuge analysis of the interaction between Fab fragment of cryoglobulin Man and γG_1 myeloma protein. Pictures were taken 64 minutes after reaching a speed of 52,640 rpm.

TABLE 3

COMPLEX FORMATION BETWEEN FAB FRAGMENT OF MAN CRYOGLOBULIN AND HUMAN γG_1 PROTEIN

Amount of Reactant Mixed ($\times 10^{-5}$ mM)		Fab in Complex (%)	Sedimentation Coefficient of Complex ($S_{20,w}$)	Association Constant (K_A, $\times 10^4$ M)
Cryoglobulin (Fab)	γG_1			
8.8	8.20	42	7.3	0.57
8.8	4.10	26	7.4	0.60
8.8	2.05	16	7.5	0.69
8.8	1.02	1		

TABLE 4

COMPLEX FORMATION BETWEEN FAB′ FRAGMENT OF RABBIT ANTI-FC ANTIBODY AND HUMAN γG_1 PROTEIN

Amount of Reactant Mixed ($\times 10^{-5}$ mM)		Fab in Complex (%)	Sedimentation Coefficient of Complex ($S_{20,w}$)	Association Constant (K_A, $\times 10^4$ M)
Cryoglobulin (Fab′)	γG_1			
8.9	2.80	100	9.7	
8.9.	1.40	100	13.3	
8.9	0.70	57	13.7	>20
8.9	0.35	34	15.0	>15

in the mixture. Complex formation was characterized by a decrease in the concentration of the Fab peak and in an increase in the concentration and the sedimentation coefficient of the faster peak (FIGURE 2). As indicated in TABLE 3, when γG_1 protein and Fab fragment were mixed in a molar ratio of about 1:1, about 50% of Fab fragment complexed with the γG_1 protein. The sedimentation coefficient of the Fab-γG_1 complex was 7.3*s*, only 0.7 Svedberg units greater than that of the peak observed when γG_1 protein was centrifuged alone. Less Fab-cryoglobulin was complexed when lower molar γG_1-Fab ratios were used. Since the percentage of Fab-cryoglobulin bound to γG_1 protein could be determined, and the total concentrations of reactants were known, it was possible to calculate association constants (K_A), assuming a valence of 2 for γG_1. At levels of 16, 26, and 42% binding, the K_A was quite constant, with values of 0.57–0.69 $\times 10^4$ liter/mole (TABLE 3).

For comparative purposes, complex formation between the Fab′ fragment of purified rabbit anti-Fc antibody was studied. When molar antigen-antibody ratios of about 1:6 were used, there was a complete disappearance of the 3.5*s* peak, indicating that all Fab′ antibody was combined to γG_1 protein (TABLE 4). About one third of Fab′ antibody was in complex when a molar antigen-antibody ratio of 1:26 was used, indicating that the valence of γG_1 protein was at least 10 in this system. The sedimentation coefficients of the complexes formed with rabbit Fab antibody were much higher than those observed with Man cryoglobulin, reflecting the difference in the number of γG_1 sites with which each preparation interacted. Due to the high valence of the antigen, it was not possible to calculate absolute association constants for rabbit Fab-γG_1 interaction, but the ultracentrifugation data indicated that the K_A was considerably higher than 15 $\times 10^4$ liter/mole, i.e., at least 20-fold higher than that of the cryoglobulin.

DISCUSSION

The present study was undertaken to characterize further the interaction of monoclonal γG-cryoglobulins with human γG-globulin. By means of a direct binding test, it was demonstrated that cryoglobulins combined with the Fc fragment, but not the Fab fragment, of γG-globulin. Cryoglobulin reactivity with Fc fragment was present in the pepsin-digested $F(ab')_2$ fragment, as well as in the papain-digested Fab fragment. In this respect, the γG-cryoglobulins behaved similarly to the γM-cryoglobulins obtained from patients with mixed cryoglobulinemia.[6,7]

Binding characteristics of these monoclonal γG-cryoglobulins were compared with those of human 19S and 7S rheumatoid factors and of rabbit antibody to Fc fragment obtained early and late during immunization. Three tests were used to measure the strength of interaction between γG-globulin or its Fc fragment and these various anti-γ-globulin preparations. These were: the effect of antigen concentration on the extent of binding; the dissociation rate of protein-I*Fc complexes; and the ultracentrifuge analysis of the degree of complex formation. All three of these test systems gave similar results, namely, that the binding between the cryoglobulins or the rheumatoid factors and γG-globulin or its Fc fragment was very weak compared with that exhibited by induced rabbit antibodies. In particular, determination of the association constant for the interaction of Fab-cryoglobulin with γG-globulin indicated a value of about 0.6×10^4 liter/mole. For the calculation, it was assumed that each heavy chain of γG-globulin contained one determinant, i.e., γG-globulin had a valence of 2. Similar studies have demonstrated that the binding of a Waldenström macroglobulin antibody with γG-globulin was also weak,[6] although the association constant values were slightly higher than those found in our study.

The low avidity of interaction of the human rheumatoid factors is quite interesting and points out the similarity at the immunochemical level between autoimmunity and termination of neonatally induced tolerance. When induced tolerance to serum proteins was broken by injection of cross-reacting antigens, some of the antibodies that were produced cross-reacted with the previously tolerated antigens, but, as with the rheumatoid factors, the interaction was quite weak.[8,9] Whether the mechanism of rheumatoid factor formation or other autoantibodies is similar to that described for termination of induced tolerance is, of course, unknown.

The weakness of the interaction between the monoclonal γG-cryoglobulins and Fc fragment is similar to that observed between certain mouse and human myeloma proteins and the dinitrophenyl (DNP) ligand, where most of the proteins that interact with DNP do so with an association constant of 10^4 liter/mole or less.[10] Since this low association constant is similar to that observed between albumin and certain dyes, the question has been raised whether or not the reaction between myeloma proteins and certain ligands is of the same type as is observed between induced antibody and antigen. On the one hand, it seems that these low-avidity reactions are of a cross-reacting nature, and that there exists some unknown antigen which would exhibit a high-avidity interaction with the myeloma proteins. On the other hand, the variable regions of immunoglobulin molecules may consist of multiple regions that can exhibit some stereospecificity for binding ligands. In the case of the γG-cryoglobulins studied, one of these regions, which are quite distinct from the site involved in "true" antigen-antibody reactions, may weakly interact with the Fc fragment. Obviously, localization of the reactive sites to specific regions within the Fab fragment must be ascertained for both myeloma proteins and induced antibodies before this question can be adequately answered.

References

1. Meltzer, M. & E. C. Franklin. 1967. Cryoglobulins, rheumatoid factors and connective tissue disorders. Arthritis Rheum. **10:** 489.
2. Meltzer, M., E. C. Franklin, K. Elias, R. T. McCluskey & N. Cooper. 1966. Cryoglobulinemia. A clinical and laboratory study. II. Cryoglobulins with rheumatoid factor activity. Amer. J. Med. **40:** 837.
3. Grey, H. M., P. F. Kohler, W. D. Terry & E. C. Franklin. 1968. Human monoclonal γG-cryoglobulins with anti-γ-globulin activity. J. Clin. Invest. **47:** 1875.
4. Cerottini, J.-C. 1968. An antigen-binding capacity test for human immunoglobulin G (lgG) fragments. J. Immunol. **101:** 433.
5. Minden, P. & R. S. Farr. 1967. The ammonium sulfate method to measure antigen-binding capacity. *In* Handbook of Experimental Immunology. **:** 463. F. A. Davis Co. Philadelphia, Pa.

6. STONE, M. J. & H. METZGER. 1968. Binding properties of a Waldenström macroglobulin antibody. J. Biol. Chem. **243:** 5977.
7. CHAVIN, S. I. & E. C. FRANKLIN. 1969. Studies on antigen-binding activity of macroglobulin antibody subunits and their enzymatic fragments. J. Biol. Chem. **244:** 1345.
8. GREY, H. Unpublished observations.
9. LINSCOTT, W. D. & W. O. WEIGLE. 1965. Anti-bovine serum albumin specificity and binding affinity after termination of tolerance to bovine serum albumin. J. Immunol. **95:** 546.
10. EISEN, H. N. Personal communication.

GENERAL DISCUSSION

DR. KUNKEL: If you had a type of rheumatoid factor with a high binding affinity for γ-globulin, you might not find it at all in the circulation. Low-affinity complexes might be expected in the circulation, and high-affinity complexes would be swept away.

DR. CEROTTINI: I agree. If, indeed, there is a protein with a very high affinity for γG determinants, the immune complexes will be eliminated immediately.

DR. J. D. CAPRA (*Rockefeller University, New York, N. Y.*): This is a fine demonstration of γG proteins that are monoclonal with rheumatoid factor activity. Some years ago it was demonstrated that in hyperglobulinemic purpura the complexes seen in the circulation are 7S γG rheumatoid factors that interact with γ-globulin. In Dr. Kunkel's laboratory, we have been investigating these with aggregated γ-globulin to isolate them. By the criteria of individual antigenic specificity, restriction of subgroup, and genetic analysis, and some preliminary sequence studies, most of these factors have proved to be monoclonal. This is, perhaps, another example of a γG protein that is monoclonal and has rheumatoid factor activity.

DR. GOLDBERG: We recently studied a cryoglobulin with a very high rheumatoid factor activity, and we labeled it with ^{131}I to determine its half-life, catabolism, and serum synovial transport in patients with rheumatoid arthritis and other forms of arthropathy. It appeared that the γM which we isolated consisted of at least two populations, one of high affinity and one of relatively low avidity. When this γM rheumatoid factor was injected, there was a very rapid initial falloff, followed by a very slow decline, suggesting that initially there had been a sequestration of the very avid antibody, and that what had remained was the low-avidity-type rheumatoid factor. It was interesting that it was this low-avidity rheumatoid factor which appeared to exist in a state of equilibrium between the serum and synovial joint spaces.

Thus, it appeared that there was a varying avidity in this γM, which was monoclonal—at least it had one type of light chain. Whether this differing avidity existed *in vivo* or whether we induced it in our isolation procedures is questionable.

DR. CEROTTINI: In my preparation, when the dissociation rate was studied, for example, it was very easy to test for the presence of various populations with regard to their binding avidity. The cryoglobulins studied were homogeneous in this respect, i.e., we did not find a detectible subpopulation with a high avidity.

UNIDENTIFIED SPEAKER: We have measured direct average binding constants between isolated rheumatoid factors and normal γG-globulins. In each case, they are about 3×10^5. Would your use of the Fab fragment for your experiment explain the difference? My values are considerably higher than yours.

DR. CEROTTINI: If instead of the Fab fragment you use $F(ab')_2$, you get about the same result.

RHEUMATOID FACTORS AND THE STRUCTURE AND FUNCTION OF γM ANTIBODIES*

S. I. Chavin, M.D., and E. C. Franklin, M.D.
Department of Medicine, Rheumatic Diseases Study Group, New York University School of Medicine New York, N. Y.

The existence of γM antibodies in normal serum and of their counterparts in Waldenström's macroglobulinemia has been known for over 30 years.[1] Only in the past ten years, however, have intensive studies been initiated to elucidate the structure and function of these proteins. As is often the case, these basic studies were stimulated to a large extent by clinical observations such as the discovery that certain antibodies like rheumatoid factors and cold agglutinis resided in macroglobulin fractions, and received further impetus when many other antibodies were shown to be associated with this fraction.[1] It is now generally accepted that rheumatoid factors usually are γM antibodies reacting with antigenic determinants located on the Fc portion of the γ chains of the immunoglobulins, although they may on occasion be found in the γG and γA fractions or the naturally occurring 8S γM molecules.

The present paper deals with recent studies of macroglobulins and, in particular, certain general conclusions derived from studies of the γM rheumatoid factor. Because a full appreciation of the function of these molecules requires a knowledge of their structure, we must begin with a brief review of some relevant structural studies.

Structure of γM-Globulins

Virtually all of the structural work on γM molecules has been carried out on Waldenström macroglobulins, primarily because of the homogeneity of these proteins, their ease of isolation in large amounts, and the ever-increasing evidence that these proteins are identical to their normal counterparts in structure and that they often possess antibody activity. As in the case with the γG-globulins, γM-immunoglobulins can be divided into several subclasses with respect to the structure of their heavy (μ) chains. Several laboratories have each found two immunologically distinguishable subclasses,[2-5] and at least two of these pairs are not identical.[2] Since all of the groups appear to exist in all normal sera, they are probably not allotypic variants. In our laboratory, approximately one-third of 40 proteins tested gave a precipitin reaction with a selected antiserum, whereas the remainder failed to react. It has not yet been possible to obtain an antiserum specific for the other subclasses. It is of some interest that the subunits and isolated μ chains from the reactive proteins failed to give a precipitin line, although they did inhibit the precipitation of the intact protein. These immunological differences are associated with differences in the two-dimensional fingerprints of these proteins[6] and reflect differences in the primary structures of the Fd fragment of the μ chain. On the basis of fingerprint analysis, it seems likely that additional subgroups exist.

The γM molecule exists predominantly as a polymer, with a molecular weight of 900,000 made up of five monomeric subunits, each with a molecular weight

* Supported by United States Public Health Service grants nos. AM-1431 and AM-5064, New York Health Research Council grant no. 1-274, and funds from the Arthritis Foundation of New York.

of about 180,000.[7] There are frequently small amounts of higher-molecular weight polymers with sedimentation coefficients of 26S and 32S. The monomeric subunits are linked to one another by disulfide bonds. While the exact number and location of the intersubunit bonds are not yet established with certainty,[8] it seems likely that there is only a single intersubunit S-S bond,[9,10] located somewhere near the carboxy-terminal end of the μ chains, which links the penultimate half-cysteine residues of the μ chain.[11] That the monomers are not linked by significant nonconvalent bonds is indicated by their tendency to dissociate, even in nondissociating solvents, when the intersubunit S-S bonds are cleaved.

We have begun studies on the location and amino acid sequences of the disulfide bonds of a Waldenström γM protein. Thus far, the only peptide that has been isolated and characterized has the composition (Cysa, Glu, Gly) and appears to be the κ light-chain component of the L-H disulfide bonds, by analogy with work on K-γG and K Bence Jones proteins.[12] In addition, preliminary studies have shown that proteins belonging to the different γM subclasses appear to have cysteine-containing peptides, as indicated by the diagonal technique of Gray and Hartley,[13] which are similar or identical to one another. The only exception is the peptide from the light-chain portion of the light-heavy disulfide bond, which, as expected, differs in proteins with κ and λ light chains. This suggests that the previously mentioned differences in peptide fingerprints do not involve the amino acid sequences surrounding the disulfide linkages, in contrast to the finding in different γG subclasses, for which differences in the location of and sequence around the disulfide linkages have been reported.[14]

It is probable that the five subunits are linked to each other in some sort of stable circular arrangement,[8] because they do not continue to polymerize indefinitely. Although such an arrangement has been demonstrated in the electron microscope for several Waldenström macroglobulins,[15] a comparable pattern was not observed in a preparation of γM antibody to flagelin.[16]

There is abundant evidence that each of the γM subunits is composed of two light and two heavy chains.[17] The light chains are very similar to the light chains of γG molecules, but the μ chains are somewhat heavier than the γ chains, with a molecular weight of about 70,000 and have a different primary structure.[11,18] One recent study[19] has indicated that each subunit may, in fact, be composed of three light chains and two heavy chains, but this finding has yet to be confirmed.

Rheumatoid Factors

While the antigenic determinants toward which classical rheumatoid factor is directed reside primarily in the Fc fragment of human and rabbit γG,[20] the precise structure of these determinants is unknown. A heterogeneous mixture of peptides from an enzymatic digest of human γG has been shown to inhibit a hemagglutination reaction by rheumatoid factor,[21] but the inhibitory peptides have not been isolated. In the Gm system, the F′c fragment, which includes about one-half of the Fc fragment, lacked Gm activity, and it is possible that the tertiary structure of the molecule may be required for full expression of the antigenic activity.[22] Although the existence of the 22S complex in serum initially suggested autoreactivity,[23] this could not be directly demonstrated until the γM fraction was separated from the antigen and allowed to react with autologous γ-globulin coated on a particle.[24]

Specificity

The classical type of rheumatoid factor frequently shows little distinction among either different genetic γ-globulin types or the known γ chain subclasses (with the possible exception of the γ_3 molecules, which appear to have a lesser reactivity than the others[25]). Other types of anti-γ-globulin factors, however, often have much more limited specificity, and can very precisely discriminate among the different genetic groups.[26]

Several different rheumatoid factors appear to react with antigenic determinants that are not detectable in normal native human γ-globulin.[27,28] It is not clear whether these determinants are present in the intact molecules and simply are inaccessible to antibodies, or whether they are determinants that are newly formed in relation to conformational changes in the molecule following enzymatic digestion. It is also not known how, in the course of the normal life of γG molecules, these "hidden" determinants are exposed to the antibody-forming system. Finally, it should be noted that rheumatoid factors occasionally react with determinants on light chains.[29]

It has already been mentioned that rheumatoid factors react with both human and rabbit γ-globulin. We have recently shown that all the monomeric subunits of a rheumatoid factor preparation can react with either human γ-globulin or rabbit γ-globulin, and that there are no subunits which fail to react with either antigen.[30] This type of behavior is characteristic of a cross-reacting system of antigenic determinants, and it suggests that the determinants in the human and rabbit proteins are similar to one another. Nevertheless, the possibility still exists that a few rheumatoid factors react with antigenic determinants that are specific for either human or animal γ-globulin.[31,32]

Interpretations of all studies on the specificity of antibodies are made very difficult by the fact that antibody populations are more or less heterogeneous with respect to many physical, chemical, and immunological properties. This problem has been minimized by the finding, in the past few years, of paraproteins with antibody activity against various types of antigens. Of particular interest in the present context is the work of Stone and Metzger[33] with a Waldenström macroglobulin antibody possessing rheumatoid factor activity. The ability of γG from a number of primates to inhibit the precipitation reaction between the rheumatoid factor and human γG was studied. The γG from hominoids (baboon and chimpanzee) or cercopithecoids (rhesus) was about equal to human γG, but γG from more distantly related primates was either unreactive or much less reactive. The authors concluded that their results were consistent with the interpretation that rheumatoid factor paraprotein is homogeneous with respect to its binding activity and directed against a single antigenic determinant in human γ-globulin.

Binding Capacity of γM Antibodies

While structural studies on γM antibodies have shown that they are very similar to the γG molecules, analyses of antigen-binding activity have shown a striking difference. All γG molecules possess two binding sites per molecule, and most of these molecules participate in precipitation or hemagglutination reactions. On the other hand, γM monomeric subunits bind antigen, but usually fail to give either precipitation or hemagglutination reactions,[34] suggesting that these subunits possess only a single active binding site. These results are consistent with the observation that most γM antibodies which have been studied possess five or six binding sites rather than the ten expected by analysis with γG molecules.[23,30,35,36] Several exceptions to this statement have recently been found,[37-39] indicating that at least some γM antibodies in fact possess the expected ten binding sites. These exceptions will be discussed.

Because of the disparity between the number of binding sites expected and

TABLE 1

MOLAR COMBINING RATIOS OF RHEUMATOID FACTOR SUBUNITS AND FC FRAGMENT OR γG-GLOBULIN

Antigen	Amount of Reactant Mixed (mg/ml)		Amount in Complex (mM × 10^{-5})		Antigen-Antibody Ratio in Complex
	Antigen	Rheumatoid Factor Subunit	Antigen	Rheumatoid Factor Subunit	
Fc Fragment	9.9	5.3	2.8	2.9	1.0
	15.2	5.8	1.8	3.2	0.6
γG-Globulin	22.0	4.0	2.1	2.2	1.0
	9.4	4.9	2.1	2.7	0.8
	12.7	5.2	3.1	2.9	0.9

the number experimentally determined, we undertook a series of experiments to quantitate the binding capacity of the monomeric subunits and enzymatic fragments of rheumatic factor. The experimental details of these studies have already been published,[30] and the results will be summarized briefly. The protein we studied was a 19S rheumatoid factor with κ and λ light-chain determinants, isolated from a patient with mixed cryoglobulinemia. Each monomeric subunit had a single effective antigen-binding site for either 7S γG or a naturally occurring Fc fragment of γG (TABLE 1). There was no evidence of γM antibody subunits that did not bind antigen. Inasmuch as there are five subunits per 19S molecule, the five binding sites in the pentamer are accounted for by the number in the subunits. We prepared Fab_μ fragments by trypsin digestion of the γM subunits. All of the fragments bound antigen. Although the exact number of binding sites on each Fab_μ fragment could not be determined, it is likely to be only one. Since there are two Fab_μ fragments per subunit and ten per molecule, the actual number of binding sites must be two and ten, respectively, albeit only half of these are detected in the intact subunit and pentamer.

Results comparable to ours were obtained by Stone and Metzger[36] with a homogeneous κ-type Waldenström macroglobulin antibody with binding activity for γG. The subunits and the Fab_μ fragments from this protein each had a single binding site. In addition, the authors calculated a K_A of 6×10^4 M^{-1} for the interaction of Fab_μ and γG.

Several results inconsistent with these findings must now be noted, for these suggest that the structure of all γM antibodies may not be alike. Merler and co-workers,[37] studying a γM antibody to a bacterial tetrasaccharide determinant, found a total of ten binding sites. Ashman and Metzger[39] found a γM paraprotein with antibody activity toward nitrophenyl determinants which had ten binding sites. The Scatchard plot was linear, and a K_A of $3.8 \pm 0.1 \times 10^4$ M^{-1} was calculated. Onoue and co-workers[40] originally studied a rabbit γM antibody to p-azobenzenarsonate hapten and found only five binding sites, with an average binding constant of 1×10^5 M^{-1}. A more recent study by these workers,[38] with an antibody to naphthalene sulfonate determinant, showed a discontinuous Scatchard plot with a total of ten binding sites. There appeared to be two populations of antibody-combining sites. Five of these were of high affinity and had an average binding constant of 10^7 M^{-1}, while the remaining five (demonstrated by using a higher concentration of free hapten) were of lower affinity, with a binding constant of 10^5 M^{-1}.

These studies may be summarized as follows: All of the γM antibodies that have been studied appear to have ten potential antigen-binding sites. In several of these (all directed toward haptens), all of the sites can be demonstrated in the pentamers[37,39] and the monomers,[39] and the sites appear to have approximately the same affinities.[39] In one antibody (also directed toward a hapten), there appear to be five sites with high affinity and five with an affinity approximately 100 times less.[38] Finally, in two antibodies,[30,36] only one-half of the sites were demonstrable in the pentamer and monomer, but the remaining sites were detected when the monomer was enzymatically fragmented. It may be significant that the last two studies were done with antigens having molecular weights of 50,000 and 160,000.

The reason for the apparent unavailability of half of the binding sites in some of the intact molecules and their subunits is most puzzling. While it is possible, of course, that there are significant structural differences among different γM antibodies, there is no compelling evidence for such differences, and it seems wiser to seek an explanation which applies to all of these antibodies. There are two possible explanations: The first of these is that the two binding sites on each subunit are related to one another in such a way that only one site can be occupied at a time. Such a mechanism would include the case of steric hindrance between large ligands, such as γG, although it cannot account for the results of Onoue and co-workers[38,40] with a small hapten. The concept of steric hindrance also encompasses the suggestion of Stone and Metzger[36] that the intrinsic association constant of one binding site on a subunit may be reduced when ligand is bound by the second site on the same subunit. Although there is evidence for such negative cooperative effects in enzyme molecules, no such effects have been seen in antigen-antibody systems, and, perhaps more important, they do not occur in all γM antibody-hapten systems.[39]

The second explanation is that half of the binding sites are not as accessible to antigen as are the remainder of the sites. This inaccessibility might be by virtue of a location within the molecule rather than at or near the surface or because the half-molecule within which they reside does not have the optimal conformation when linked to another half-molecule. Such a locational and/or conformational difference (the two qualities are not mutually exclusive) could result in a lower binding affinity, as in the case of Onoue and co-workers.[38] Alternately, it might hinder the sufficiently close approach to a large antigen, and thereby interfere with or altogether prevent ligand binding, as in the case of the rheumatoid factor systems.[30,36]

FIGURE 1 shows a schematic representation of a γM subunit. The general form of the model is similar to one proposed for γG by Edelman and Gally several years ago,[41] but it incorporates several significant new features. The major modification is the Y configuration, adopted by analogy with electron microscopical studies of γG molecules.[16] The interchain disulfide bonds are shown as black bars between the chains, and the intersubunit disulfide bonds are represented by the black bars protruding from the carboxy-terminal half of the μ chains, although their exact number and location are not indicated in this model. The binding sites, represented by the two hatched areas on the lateral surfaces of the Fab fragments, are constituted by portions of both the light and heavy chains.[42] Note that one of the sites is located on the outside of the molecule, while the other faces toward the space between the two arms of the Y. Thus, even though the two halves of the molecule are symmetrical, the dimer itself may be asymmetrical. If we make the further assumption that the two Fab fragments are held relatively close to one another, either by noncovalent bonds or, less likely, by covalent linkages, then the inner binding site may have different physi-

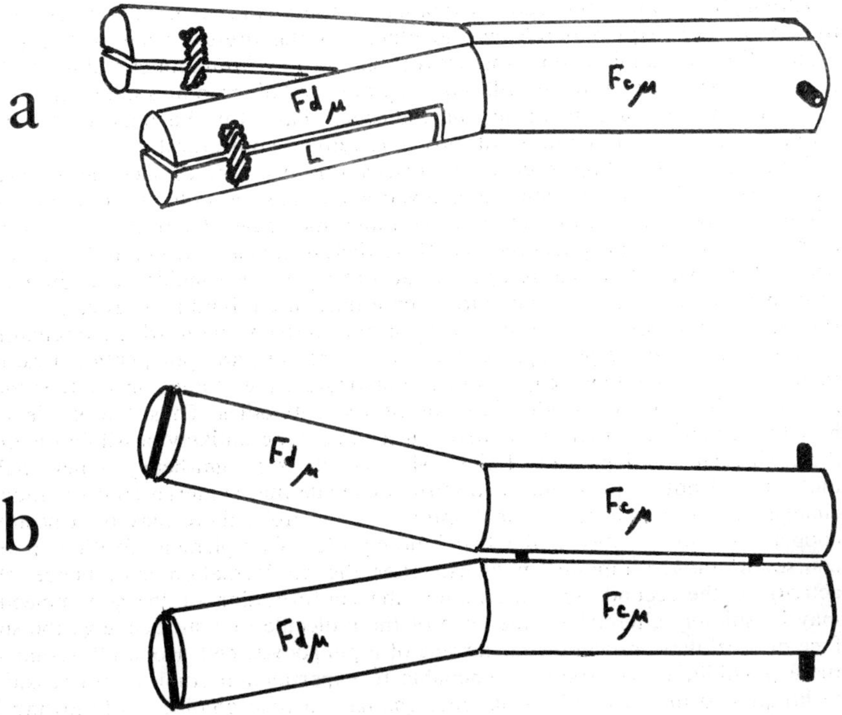

FIGURE 1. Schematic model of γM antibody subunit, viewed from the side (a) and from above (b).

cal and/or kinetic properties than its partner. This type of scheme represents perhaps the simplest structural arrangement that can explain the results. It is quite possible, on the other hand, that a much more subtle or complex basis underlies the differences between the two types of binding sites.

If the second explanation is correct, it may be possible to demonstrate definite functional and/or thermodynamic differences between the two binding sites on a subunit. Such studies should utilize as homogeneous an antibody preparation as is possible, preferably one such as Ashman and Metzger[39] studied. It also would be advantageous to study an anti-hapten system because of the relative ease of measuring binding function and of synthesizing a series of related haptens that differ in selected steric and/or chemical properties. If a binding site is less accessible because it is further removed from the outer surface of the molecule, it may reside in an even more hydrophobic environment than does the normal antigen-combining site.[43] This increased hydrophobicity might favor the binding of more highly nonpolar haptens over less nonpolar or polar ones. Alternately, bulkier haptens might be less avidly bound than smaller ones, for steric reasons, if the binding site were in some type of a crevice. Homologous series of haptens might be used to elicit such differences between the two halves of a monomeric subunit, the differences showing up in the thermodynamic parameters, or as a discontinuity in binding curves. Any such differences would presumably disappear when the isolated half-molecules were examined .

Although we favor this second explanation, there is no experimental evidence to support one explanation over the other. At the present time, virtually no information is available about the conformation of γM-immunoglobulins.[44] This type of information probably will require x-ray crystallographic studies, and until such time as they are available, the molecular basis for the puzzling binding properties of the γM subunits will probably remain conjectural.

It might be interesting to close this discussion on a note of speculation. Why has a large and complex molecule evolved which has ten potential binding sites while only five appear to function in the intact molecule? There may, of course, be no "reason" for this phenomenon. Nevertheless, it is an ancient and venerable belief of biologists that nature operates according to "reasonable" (i.e., human) principles, so it seems reasonable to assume that all ten binding sites can and do function in the organism. Since most of the antigens with which circulating antibodies react are large (e.g., cells, bacteria, proteins, and polypeptides) rather than very small haptens (e.g., azobenzenarsonate), the studies on haptens may not be pertinent to the *in vivo* function of γM antibodies. Thus, the problem is how the second site might be rendered accessible. One unlikely possibility is that the biologically active form of the γM molecule is a light-heavy dimer (half-molecule). Another possibility is that the molecule may undergo conformational changes in the course of its functioning. For example, there may be a positive cooperative effect between the two binding sites. Complement fixation in the course of antigen binding may also alter the conformation and, hence, the activity of the second site. Alternately, the conformation of the γM molecule may be suitably altered by adherence of the molecule to a surface, e.g., the surface of a cellular antigen or the surface of a phagocytic cell. Hopefully, some of these possibilities will soon be amenable to experimental studies with sensitive techniques to measure conformational changes in macromolecules following ligand binding.

Summary

Structural studies on γM-immunoglobulins and their subunits have been briefly reviewed. The subunits are linked to one another by disulfide bonds. There probably is a single bond between each pair of subunits, and this is probably located near the carboxy-terminal end of the μ chain.

Monomeric subunits of a rheumatoid factor preparation were shown to react equally well with either human γG or rabbit γG, and all of the subunits possessed this activity. These results suggest that the antigenic determinants in the human and rabbit proteins are similar to one another.

Experiments were carried out to quantitate the binding capacity of the monomeric subunits and enzymatic fragments of a rheumatoid factor. It was found that each subunit had a single antigen-binding site. Therefore, there must be two binding sites per subunit, and ten sites per 19S pentamer, although only half of these are accessible to the antigen used in these studies. Work from other laboratories indicates that certain γM antibodies may possess ten active binding sites for haptens.

In order to explain the results with different γM antibodies, a model of the γM subunit was proposed in which one of the antigen-binding sites is fully accessible to the outer surface of the molecule, while the second site is less accessible to this surface. The differences between the two sites are more or less evident, depending on the nature of the antigenic determinant and of the antigen molecule.

It was presumed that in the 19S molecule *in vivo*, all ten binding sites are able to bind antigen. Several mechanisms by which the "inactive" site may be rendered active were suggested. It was proposed that conformation of the molecule is altered during the course of its function in such a way as to render both sites accessible to antigen.

References

1. KUNKEL, H. G. 1960. *In* The Plasma Proteins. F. W. Putnam, Ed. **1:** 279. Academic Press, Inc. New York, N. Y.
2. FRANKLIN, E. C. & B. FRANGIONE. 1967. J. Immunol. **99:** 810.
3. MACKENZIE, M. R. & H. F. DEUTSCH. 1965. J. Immunol. **95:** 87.
4. HARBOE, M., J. DEVERILL & H. C. GODAL. 1965. Scand J. Haemat. **2:** 137.
5. WOLLHEIM, F. A. & R. C. WILLIAMS, JR. 1966. Acta Med. Scand. **179** (Suppl. 445): 115.
6. FRANKLIN, E. C. & B. FRANGIONE. 1968. Biochemistry **7:** 4203.
7. MILLER, F. & H. METZGER. 1965. J. Biol. Chem. **240:** 3325.
8. MILLER, F. & H. METZGER. 1965. J. Biol. Chem. **240:** 4740.
9. CHAVIN, S. I. 1968. Unpublished experiments.
10. MORRIS, J. E. & F. P. INMAN. 1968. Biochemistry **7:** 2851.
11. ABEL, C. A. & H. M. GREY. 1967. Science **156:** 1609.
12. EDELMAN, G. M., *et al.* 1969. Proc. Nat. Acad. Sci. In press.
13. GRAY, W. R. & B. S. HARTLEY. 1963. Biochem. J. **89:** 59P.
14. FRANGIONE, B., C. MILSTEIN & J. R. L. PINK. 1969. Nature **221:** 145.
15. CHESEBRO, B., B. BLOTH & S. E. SEVAG. 1968. J. Exp. Med. **127:** 399.
16. VALENTINE, R. C. & N. M. GREEN. 1967. J. Molec. Biol. **27:** 615.
17. MILLER, F. & H. METZGER. 1966. J. Biol. Chem. **241:** 1732.
18. WIKLER, M., H. KOHLER, T. SHINODA & F. W. PUTNAM. 1969. Science **163:** 75.
19. SUZUKI, T. & H. F. DEUTSCH. 1967. J. Biol. Chem. **242:** 2725.
20. FRANKLIN, E. C. 1961. Proc. Tenth Int. Congr. Rheum. (Rome) **2:** 804.
21. HENNEY, C. S., R. JEFFERIS & D. R. STANWORTH. 1968. Biochim. Biophys. Acta **154:** 295.
22. IRIMAJIRI, S., E. C. FRANKLIN & B. FRANGIONE. 1968. Immunochemistry **5:** 383.
23. FRANKLIN, E. C., H. J. MÜLLER-EBERHARD, H. HOLMAN & H. G. KUNKEL. 1957. J. Exp. Med. **105:** 425.
24. ALLEN, J. C. & H. G. KUNKEL. 1966. Arthritis Rheum. **9:** 758.
25. NORMANSELL, D. E. & D. R. STANWORTH. 1968. Immunology **15:** 549.
26. FUDENBERG, H. H. 1962. Progr. Allergy **7:** 1.
27. OSTERLAND, C. K., M. HARBOE & H. G. KUNKEL. 1963. Vox Sang. **8:** 132.
28. WILLIAMS, JR., R. C. & T. G. LAWRENCE, JR. 1966. J. Clin. Invest. **45:** 714.
29. WILLIAMS, JR., R. C. 1964. Proc. Nat. Acad. Sci. **52:** 60.
30. CHAVIN, S. I. & E. C. FRANKLIN. 1969. J. Biol. Chem. **244:** 1345.
31. WILLIAMS, JR., R. C. & H. G. KUNKEL. 1963. Arthritis Rheum. **6:** 665.
32. BUTLER, JR., V. P. & J. H. VAUGHAN. 1965. Immunology **8:** 144.
33. STONE, M. J. & H. METZGER. 1969. J. Immunol. **102:** 222.
34. HILL, W. C. & J. CEBRA. 1965. Biochemistry **4:** 2575.
35. LINDQVIST, K. & D. C. BAUER. 1966. Immunochemistry **3:** 373.
36. STONE, M. J. & H. METZGER. 1968. J. Biol. Chem. **243:** 5977.
37. MERLER, E., L. KARLIN & S. MATSUMOTO. 1968. J. Biol. Chem. **243:** 386.
38. ONOUE, K., A. L. GROSSBERG, Y. YAGI & D. PRESSMAN. 1968. Science **162:** 574.
39. ASHMAN, R. F. & H. METZGER. 1969. Fed. Proc. **28:** 695.
40. ONOUE, K., Y. YAGI, A. L. GROSSBERG & D. PRESSMAN. 1966. Immunochemistry **2:** 401.
41. EDELMAN, G. M. & J. A. GALLY. 1964. Proc. Nat. Acad. Sci. **51:** 846.
42. SINGER, S. J. & R. F. DOOLITTLE. 1966. Science **153:** 13.
43. YOO, T.-J. & C. W. PARKER. 1968. Immunochemistry **5:** 143.
44. DORRINGTON, K. J. & C. TANFORD. 1968. J. Biol. Chem. **243:** 4745.

Discussion

DR. SCHUR: I have two questions. First, when you isolate your Fab fragments, could you get ten fragments per mole of whole 19S rheumatoid factor? Second, if you applied the method of Singer, i.e., plotting one over the valence versus the total antigen, would you find that the true valence at infinite antigen excess is 1?

DR. CHAVIN: In answer to the first question, we did not quantitate the yield of Fab fragments. We found approximately what we expected, but that is all that I can say. In answer to the second question, we did not quantitate the binding capacity that way. This is something which Stone and Metzger did for their rheumatoid factor protein.

DR. HANNESTAD: You found that the γM subunit complexed with rabbit γG, but the Fab fragment did not complex. Perhaps the most reasonable explanation for this situation be that two active sites were required to show complex formation, thus making complex formation feasible with the monomeric subunit; the avidity is too low with the Fab fragment, which therefore does not show any complex formation.

DR. CHAVIN: I don't know the answer to this question now; we were very puzzled that the Fab fragment from a protein that reacts fully with rabbit γ-globulin failed to show complex formation. I cannot explain it. We have certainly found that the avidity in general is very low, as have others, and it is possible that somehow the second binding site must be present or two binding sites must be present in a single molecular species in order to get complex formation; however, I don't really understand why this would be necessary.

PART III. POSSIBLE BIOLOGICAL FUNCTIONS OF RHEUMATOID FACTORS

INTERACTIONS AMONG RHEUMATOID FACTORS, γG ANTIBODIES, LYMPHOCYTES, AND PHAGOCYTES

Ronald P. Messner, M.D.,* Erskine M. Caperton, Jr., M.D., Richard A. King, M.D., and Ralph C. Williams, Jr., M.D.*

Arthritis Unit, University of Minnesota Hospitals Minneapolis, Minn.

It has now been clearly established that anti-γ-globulins are indeed antibodies with specificity for autologous γ-globulin. Besides the originally described 19S human rheumatoid factors,[1,2] over the past few years various types of anti-γ-globulins of different immunoglobulin classes,[3-5] showing an interesting heterogeneity of specificites,[6-9] have been reported. The real task now at hand seems to be definition of the physiological role of human anti-γ-globulins. In approaching this problem, we have turned to studies on the interaction of isolated human or rabbit anti-γ-globulins with two basic cellular phenomena, phagocytosis and lymphocyte transformation. It was hoped that these studies would elucidate mechanisms that might be modified, or in some way directed, through interactions between circulating or tissue-bound anti-γ-globulins and cells which participate directly in tissue lesions of disease.

METHODS

Lymphocyte-transformation studies were performed according to the method of Sell and Gell[10] with normal human lymphocytes. Details of the phagocytosis test system have been previously described.[11,12] Bacteria, isolated γG and, in some instances, rheumatoid factor preparations were tumbled with washed normal human leukocytes. Phagocytosis was measured by a decline in the number of surviving bacteria during two hours of incubation. Highly purified preparations of normal polymorphonucleocytes, obtained by the method of Boyum,[13] or leukocyte mixtures harvested from dextran sedimentation of blood were used as the phagocytic cells. Opsonically active γG was obtained by DEAE-cellulose column chromatography[14] of sera from patients with subacute bacterial endocarditis or repeated septicemia secondary to the intravenous use of narcotics. The bacteria used in the phagocytosis test were isolated from the blood of the same patients as the γG opsonins.

Rheumatoid factors were separated from the serum of patients with classic rheumatoid arthritis by Sephadex G-200 gel filtration in 0.1 M acetate buffer at pH 4.1. These preparations were absorbed with the test bacteria prior to their addition to the phagocytic system. Highly purified rheumatoid factors were obtained by Sephadex G-200 gel filtration of cryoprecipitates isolated from the serum of patients with mixed cryoglobulinemia.[15] Reduction of γG-globulin with 0.1 M mercaptoethanol was performed according to previously described techniques.[16] The amidination technique of Ljaljevic and co-workers was employed.[17] Anti-γ-globulin activity was measured by the latex fixation[18] and Ripley coat agglutination tests.[19]

* Present address: Department of Medicine, Bernalillo County Medical Center, University of New Mexico, Albuquerque, N. M.

Results

Lymphocyte Transformation

Work in our laboratories during the last year has demonstrated that human 19S anti-γ-globulins are capable of inducing transformation of human lymphocytes.[20] Pooled 19S fractions from Sephadex G-200 gel filtration of serum from patients with rheumatoid arthritis were adjusted to approximately equal reactivity in the latex fixation test (1:640–1:1280) and added to cultures of human lymphocytes. Significant stimulation of a threefold increase over baseline incorporation of tritiated thymidine into DNA was noted in three of ten cultures stimulated with aliquots of one rheumatoid factor preparation. Aliquots of a rheumatoid factor preparation from a second patient stimulated only one of the ten test donor lymphocytes. Control 19S preparations from individual or pooled normal sera had no stimulating effect. Rabbit antisera to human γG with agglutination titers equal to the human rheumatoid factor preparations showed greater stimulating effect with the donor lymphocytes. Definition of the active fractions in rabbit anti-human γG antiserum was achieved by DEAE-chromatography with an initial buffer at pH 8.0 (0.01 M), followed by gradient elution. The major lymphocyte-stimulating fractions were noted in peak I, which contained only rabbit γG-globulin (FIGURE 1).

As a foil or contrast to the effect of isolated human 19S anti-γ-globulins, a series of lymphocyte-transformation experiments was performed with γM frac-

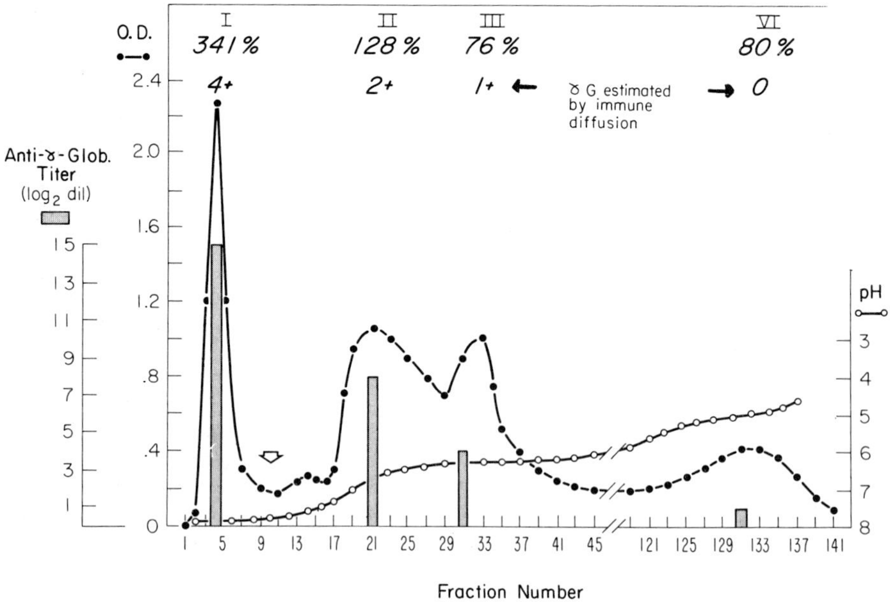

FIGURE 1. DEAE column separation of whole, unabsorbed rabbit antiserum to human γG, showing relative titers of various fractions against cells coated with human γ-globulin. The column separation utilized an initial buffer of pH 8.2, and 0.02 M phosphate buffer for the first peak (I); then a continuously increasing salt-decreasing pH gradient was begun (arrow). Fractions I, II, III, and VI were tested by lymphocyte transformation; only fraction I, constituting the main fall-through γG peak, showed significant lymphocyte-transforming capacity (341%).

TABLE 1

ATTEMPTS TO STIMULATE NORMAL HUMAN LYMPHOCYTES WITH ISOLATED γM AND WHOLE SERUM CONTAINING HIGH TITERS OF COLD AGGLUTININS

Preparation Added to Lymphocyte Culture	Result of DNA-Tritiated Thymidine Incorporation (%)*	Cold Agglutinin Titer	
		With Erythrocytes	With Lymphocytes
Pokeweed mitogen	533		
Nis whole serum at 4° C	154	5,120	2,560
Nis whole serum	143		
Nis γM, 4° C	107	2,560	2,560
Nis γM + fresh normal serum at 4° C	130		
Fresh normal serum alone at 4° C	108		
Joh whole serum at 4° C	250	20,480	2,560
Joh whole serum	147		
Joh γM, 4° C	178	10,240	2,560
Joh γM + fresh normal serum at 4° C	112		

* Percentage represents stimulation relative to that recorded as 100% against cells alone. Threefold stimulation (300%) was considered positive.

† Reciprocal titer.

tions and whole sera from two patients with high-titer cold agglutinins (anti-I). Lymphocytes were preincubated at 4° C for 30 minutes with isolated γM or whole serum containing cold-agglutinin activity before starting the culture. Although slight stimulation occurred, a significant rise in tritiated thymidine incorporation of threefold or better was not achieved with either cold agglutinin (TABLE 1). The results were unchanged when fresh normal serum was added to the cultures as a source of complement. Significant stimulation was obtained with pokeweed mitogen positive controls. Reactions of the cold agglutinins with the lymphocytes were confirmed by agglutination of the cells at 4° C (TABLE 1). Increasing the duration of preincubation at 4° C resulted in inconsistent culture results and considerable cell death as monitored by Trypan blue dye exclusion.

Phagocytosis

Patients with subacute bacterial endocarditis have been shown to develop high titers of opsonic γG antibodies. These opsonins can promote phagocytosis of the infecting organism *in vitro* in the absence of complement.[11] In addition, serum of about one-half of patients with subacute bacterial endocarditis contains anti-γ-globulin factors similar to rheumatoid factors.[12,21] Anti-γ-globulin factors disappear after effective therapy and are thus presumed to be a response to the infection. This natural model has provided a means of studying both the mechanism of γG-mediated phagocytosis of bacteria and the interactions of anti-γ-globulin factors (rheumatoid factors) with γG opsonins and phagocytic cells. Various 19S preparations containing rheumatoid factor activity, isolated from serum of patients with rheumatoid arthritis and subacute bacterial endocarditis, have been shown to inhibit the opsonic action of the γG antibodies. The 19S preparations from normal human sera without rheumatoid factor activity had no antiopsonic effect. Experiments in which bacteria were washed after preincubation with γG before adding rheumatoid factor or rheumatoid factor before adding γG indicated that the inhibiting effect depends on combination of rheumatoid factor with γG attached to the bacteria. Positive latex fixation reactions with material eluted from bacteria washed after incubation with γG and rheumatoid factor and fluorescent studies with anti-human γM and γG antisera confirmed the presence of γG and rheumatoid factor on the bacteria.

These results suggested that human rheumatoid factor inhibits opsonization by interference with or alteration of sites on the Fc fragment of human γG which are required for binding of the bacteria-γG complex to the surface of the phagocytic cell. Supporting evidence for the dependence of γG-mediated phagocytosis on structures present on Fc fragment has been acquired by pepsin digestion of γG opsonins from patients with subacute bacterial endocarditis.[16] The $F(ab')_2$ fragments retain ability to agglutinate the test bacteria, but not to fix complement or promote phagocytosis of the organisms.

Similar results showing reduction of opsonic activity were obtained by Shands and co-workers[22] and by Rowley and his associates[23] after enzymatic digestion of rabbit antibacterial γG antibodies. Thus, it appears that binding of bacteria to phagocytic cells by γG opsonins is similar to binding of erythrocytes to macrophages by γG antibodies directed against erythrocytes,[24–28] in that both require attachment of the Fc fragment to the surface of the phagocytic cell. The following experiments were therefore undertaken, with two objectives: (1) to clarify the cell types active in phagocytosis mediated by antibacterial γG opsonins, and (2) to further define the mechanism through which rheumatoid factors inhibit the opsonic activity of antibacterial γG antibodies.

TABLE 2

EFFECT OF RHEUMATOID FACTORS ON ACTIVITY OF OPSONIC γG WITH HIGHLY PURIFIED POLYMORPHONUCLEAR LEUKOCYTE PREPARATIONS

Source of *Staphylococcus aureus**	Source of Rheumatoid Factor†	Source of Rheumatoid Factor‡	Source of γG Opsonin§	Bacteria Phagocytized and Killed (%)¶
EID	—	—	none	0
	—	—	EID	98
	N 19S	—	EID	96
	HAN	RA†	EID	83
	IDZ	RA	EID	66
	BRA	cryo‡	EID	10
	JAN	cryo	EID	5
FRA	—	—	none	0
	—	—	no. 7	89
	IDZ	RA	no. 7	70
	BRA	cryo	no. 7	43
	JAN	cryo	no. 7	46
FRA	—	—	none	0
	—	—	FRA	93
	N 19S	—	FRA	90
	IDZ	RA	FRA	89
	BRA	cryo	FRA	0
	JAN	cryo	FRA	0

* Patients EID and FRA had subacute bacterial endocarditis.
† N 19S = normal 19S (control); HAN, IDZ, BRA and JAN = patients.
‡ RA = patients with rheumatoid arthritis; cryo = patients with mixed cryoglobulinemia.
§ None = control; no. 7 = drug addict with septicemia.
¶ At 120 minutes.

The capacity of polymorphonucleocytes to phagocytize and kill bacteria coated with γG opsonins was demonstrated by employing highly purified cell preparations containing 97–99% polymorphonucleocytes. Isolated immune γG from two patients with subacute bacterial endocarditis and one with septicemia secondary to the intravenous use of narcotics proved highly effective as opsonins for *Staphylococcus aureus* with these cells (TABLE 2). In each experiment, bacteria were not phagocytized by the polymorphonucleocytes in the absence of γG opsonin. Addition of γG opsonin to the system resulted in phagocytosis and killing of 89–98% of the organisms. When rheumatoid factors obtained from patients with rheumatoid arthritis or isolated from cryoprecipitates obtained from patients with mixed cryoglobulinemia were added with bacteria which had been preincubated with γG opsonin, inhibition of the opsonic effect was noted (TABLE 2). Substituting leukocyte mixtures containing approximately 65% polymorphonucleocytes,

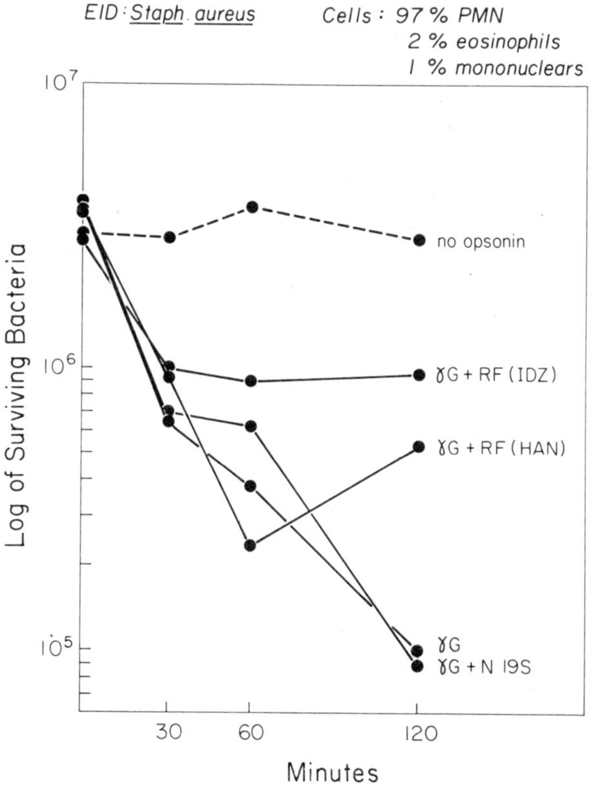

FIGURE 2. Comparison of the inhibiting activity of two rheumatoid factors (RF) on the opsonic activity of γG isolated from a patient (EID) with subacute bacterial endocarditis (causative agent, *Staphylococcus aureus*). Highly purified polymorphonuclear (PMN) leukocytes containing only 1% mononuclear cells were used as the phagocytic cells. The organism was not killed in the absence of opsonin, but was rapidly phagocytized and killed in the presence of isolated γG. Addition of RF (IDZ) inhibited the opsonic effect of γG at 60 and 120 minutes; RF (HAN) inhibited only the terminal portion of the curve. Pooled 19S fractions from normal (N) serum had no effect on phagocytosis.

40% lymphocytes, and 5% monocytes in place of purified polymorphonucleocyte preparations did not alter these results. Control 19S preparations from pooled normal human serum showed no inhibition.

Variation was noted in the ability of individual rheumatoid factor (RF) preparations to inhibit the opsonic effect of different γG preparations (TABLE 2). The same concentration of RF(IDZ) which inhibited the opsonic activity of γG(EID) by 33% had only slight effect on γG(no. 7) and no effect on γG(FRA); RF (HAN), which had a latex titer equal to RF(IDZ), had significantly less inhibitory activity on γG(EID) (FIGURE 2). To investigate this phenomenon, tests were made of the reactivity of three rheumatoid factor preparations with one of the γG opsonin preparations (TABLE 3). All three rheumatoid factors agglutinated latex particles coated with FRA γG. Agglutination of anti-Rh antibody Ripley coated erythrocytes by all three rheumatoid factors was inhibited by FRA γG. Although reactivity with FRA γG could be demonstrated with all three rheumatoid factor preparations, RF(IDZ), which had the lowest titers, had no antiopsonic effect.

Amidination of 68% of the free amino groups of FRA γG or Cohn fraction II with ethylacetimidate did not alter its reactivity with the rheumatoid factor (TABLE 3), but did abolish the opsonic activity of FRA γG (FIGURE 3). All three rheumatoid factor preparations also agglutinated latex particles coated with FRA γG which had been treated with 0.1 M mercaptoethanol. The titer of RF(JAN) was higher with reduced FRA γG than the untreated material, while the titers of RF(BRA) and RF(IDZ) were unchanged. In contrast to reactivity with rheumatoid factors, opsonic activity was diminished by mild reduction (FIGURE 3). Agglutination of the test bacteria by FRA γG was not altered by either treatment.

Naturally occurring human anti-γ-globulin factors directed against pepsin-digested γG were also examined for activity in the phagocytic test system. Sera containing high titers of agglutinating activity for erythrocytes coated with pepsin-

TABLE 3

REACTION OF RHEUMATOID FACTOR PREPARATIONS WITH FRA γG, RIPLEY ANTI-RH ANTIBODY, AND COHN FRACTION II

Test	Rheumatoid Factor*		
	BRA	JAN	IDZ
Latex fixation			
FII	1,280	640	160
Amidinated FII	2,560	640	160
FRA γG	1,280	160	80
Amidinated FRA γG	1,280	160	80
Ripley coat agglutination	2,048	16	8
Inhibition of Ripley agglutination			
FRA γG	32†	64	8
Amidinated FRA γG	32	64	8
Inhibition of >50% of opsonic activity of FRA γG	2	undil.	n.i.

* Reciprocal titer of rheumatoid factor preparation for all results except inhibition of Ripley agglutination tests, which are recorded as the reciprocal titer of the inhibitor; starting dilution of inhibitor = 1 mg/ml. undil. = undilute; n.i. = no inhibition.

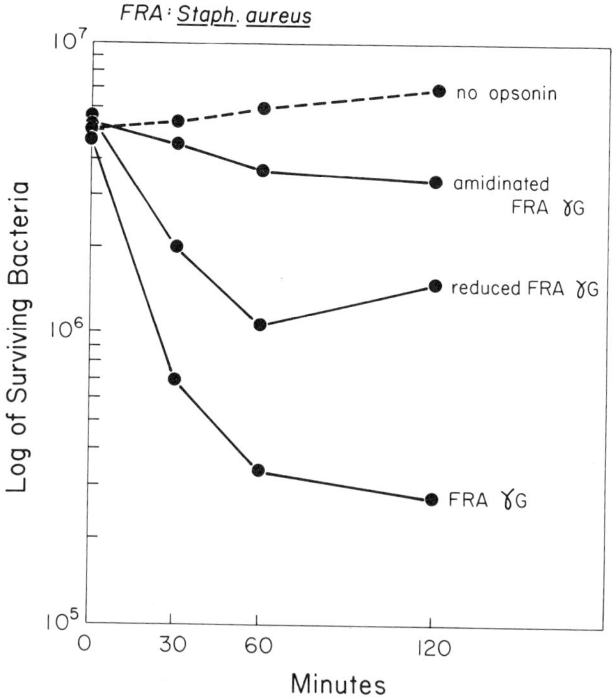

FIGURE 3. Comparison of the opsonic activity of amidinated and reduced immune γG-with the untreated γG-globulin. Opsonic activity of γG for *Staphylococcus* aureus from patient FRA (subacute bacterial endocarditis) was significantly diminished by mild reduction with 0.1 M mercaptoethanol and almost completely abolished by amidination of 65% of the free amino groups of the γG molecules with ethylacetimidate.

digested Ripley anti-Rh antibody were separated by Sephadex G-200 gel filtration. Titers of pepsin agglutinator in the three 7S preparations used ranged from 1:16 to 1:128. No significant difference in phagocytosis was noted when these preparations were added to the system after preincubation of bacteria with whole or pepsin-digested γG opsonin.

In a second set of experiments, rabbit antisera directed against human $F(ab')_2$ and Fc were used in place of human rheumatoid factor as inhibitors of opsonic activity. Rabbit anti-human $F(ab')_2$ and Fc, absorbed with the test bacteria and adjusted to equal titers in agglutination of Ripley coated erythrocytes, gave equal inhibition of the opsonic activity of human γG for *Staphylococcus aureus.*

Discussion

Lymphocyte Stimulation

Studies of the effect of 19S human anti-γ-globulin factors on human lymphocyte cultures have confirmed that these factors are capable of inducing blast transformation. The results with human components are thus analogous to the studies of Sell,[10,29,30] who has shown stimulation of rabbit lymphocytes by sheep and rabbit anti-γ-globulin antisera, and Oppenheim and co-workers,[31] who demonstrated a similar effect of monkey antisera to human γG, γM, γA, and κ and λ light chains on human lymphocytes. Naturally occurring human rheumatoid factors appear to be much weaker stimulators of human lymphocytes than 7S rabbit anti-human γG. In this regard, it was interesting to find that another naturally occurring human 19S antibody directed against an antigen present on the lymphocyte surface, the I antigen, failed to cause significant stimulation. Whether these differences are due to characteristics of the antibodies or the cell surface receptors remains to be clarified, as does the relationship of the lymphocyte-stimulating activity of rheumatoid factor to its ability to terminate tolerance of γG[32] or to inhibit the number of antibody-producing spleen cells after immunization of animals with γG.[33]

Phagocytosis

Human anti-staphylococcal γG antibodies exerted opsonic activity on *Staphylococcus aureus* when tested either with mixtures of leukocytes containing polymorphonucleocytes, lymphocytes, and monocytes roughly in proportion to their presence in whole blood or with highly purified polymorphonucleocytes. With both cell preparations, rheumatoid factors from patients with rheumatoid arthritis and highly purified 19S anti-γ-globulin factors from patients with mixed cryoglobulinemia inhibited the opsonic action of γG antibodies. A rough correlation was found between the latex titer either with fraction II or opsonic γG-coated particles and the antiopsonic effect.

Chemical modification of γG opsonin with ethylacetimidate or 0.1 M mercaptoethanol provided information suggesting the mechanism of inhibition. Amidination of 65% of the free amino groups of human γG opsonins has been shown to abolish the opsonic effect without altering electrophoretic mobility, reactivity with rabbit anti-heavy- and light-chain antisera, or ability to combine with staphylococcal antigens.[34] Mild reduction with mercaptoethanol also abolishes opsonic activity without altering the antibody-combining site.[16] The fact that both of these treatments did not alter the reactivity of rheumatoid factors with a single γG opsonin but did abolish its opsonic activity indicates that the Fc structures responsible for opsonic activity and reactivity with the rheumatoid factors differ. Thus, inhibition of opsonic activity by rheumatoid factor is not due to direct combination of rheumatoid factor with the opsonic site, but more likely a result of interference by the large 19S γM molecule with contact between Fc opsonic sites and cell surface receptors. Evidence that rabbit anti-human $F(ab')_2$ and Fc antisera exert equal inhibitory effects on γG opsonins supports this concept of steric interference.

Since amidination occurs only at α and ε-amino groups,[35,36] these results also imply that free amino groups were necessary for opsonic activity of the γG opsonin, but not for attachment of the anti-γ-globulin factors. Intact sulfhydryl bonds have been shown to be necessary for opsonic activity,[16] but not for reactivity with anti-γ-globulin factors.[37] Results presented here confirm these observations.

Preliminary experiments with anti-γ-globulins directed against sites on γG revealed by pepsin digestion were disappointing. It was postulated that these γG antibodies might restore opsonic activity to pepsin-digested γG opsonins by attaching piggy-back to the digested opsonin on the bacteria and supplying the missing Fc fragment. Failure of the initial experiments does not rule out this possibility. Titers of the pepsin agglutinators may have been below the critical level necessary for expression of their action in the phagocytosis test system.

The potent opsonic effect of heat-labile serum factors on bacteria has been well documented by a number of investigators. Previous work from our laboratory has demonstrated antagonistic, competitive effects of rheumatoid factor and heat-labile serum factors on phagocytosis of bacteria.[12] These antagonistic effects may depend partly on competition of C′1q and rheumatoid factor for sites on the Fc fragment of γG opsonins,[37] but also may involve bypassing the blocking effect of rheumatoid factor on the attachment of Fc opsonic sites to cell receptors. A few molecules of C′1q fixed to antibodies on the bacterial surface may activate the complement sequence.[38] Other complement components may then fix to the bacteria and initiate phagocytosis by attaching to separate complement receptors on the surface of the phagocytic cells.[26,28] Once established, this opsonic system could compensate for the functional loss of the Fc opsonic sites and insure phagocytosis of the organism. In fresh whole serum, the antiopsonic effect of rheumatoid factor on γG opsonins is obscured by the opsonic effect of heat-labile serum factors.[12] The influence of rheumatoid factor on phagocytosis in fresh whole blood has been investigated by Parker and Schmid [39] with heat-aggregated γG as the antigen. In this system, ingestion of γG aggregates is enhanced by preincubation with serum containing rheumatoid factor activity. In contrast to earlier work showing antagonistic effects of rheumatoid factor on complement,[40–42] recent work has indicated that under certain experimental conditions rheumatoid factor can fix complement,[43,44] and that this ability to react with complement may be related to the density of the γG antigen.[45] Thus, it is possible that the influence of rheumatoid factor or phagocytosis may vary, depending on whether phagocytosis under the particular conditions in question is mediated directly by the activity of γG opsonic sites or through heat-labile opsonic factors. In the latter case, it may also depend on the physical state or density of γG-globulin in the system. Under certain conditions rheumatoid factor might facilitate rather than antagonize the heat-labile opsonsins (FIGURE 4).

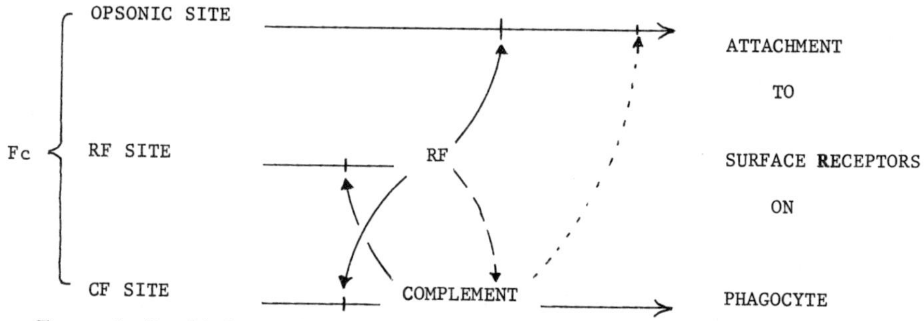

FIGURE 4. Possible interactions between the Fc fragment of γG-globulin rheumatoid factors (RF) and complement in the initial step in phagocytosis. Solid lines indicate pathways for which substantial experimental evidence exists. The dashed line is based on evidence that under certain experimental conditions rheumatoid factors are capable of fixing complement. The dotted line suggesting that C′1q attached to the Fc fragment might block the opsonic site is based on theoretical grounds alone. CF = complement fixation site.

SUMMARY

Evidence has been presented indicating that when phagocytosis of bacteria is mediated by attachment of structures on the Fc portion of γG antibodies (opsonic sites) to receptors on the surface of phagocytic cells, rheumatoid factor may inhibit phagocytosis by combining with Fc sites distinct from the opsonic sites. It has been suggested that the role rheumatoid factor plays in phagocytosis *in vivo* may depend on interaction with components of the complement system.

REFERENCES

1. FRANKLIN, E., H. HOLMAN, H. MÜLLER-EBERHARD & H. G. KUNKEL. 1957. An unusual protein component of high molecular weight in the serum of certain patients with rheumatoid arthritis. J. Exp. Med. **105**: 425.
2. EDELMAN, G. J., H. G. KUNKEL & E. C. FRANKLIN. 1958. Interaction of the rheumatoid factor with antigen-antibody complexes and aggregated gamma globulin. J. Exp. Med. **108**: 105.
3. FRANKLIN, E. C. 1961. Interaction of rheumatoid factor and gamma globulin. Proc. 10th Int. Congr. Rheum. (Rome) **2**: 804.
4. HEIMER, R. & F. M. LEVIN. 1966. On the distribution of rheumatoid factors among the immunoglobulins. Immunochemistry **3**: 1.
5. BIENENSTOCK, J., G. GOLDSTEIN & T. B. TOMASI, JR. 1969. Urinary γA rheumatoid factor. J. Lab. Clin. Med. **73**: 389.
6. FUDENBERG, H. & H. G. KUNKEL. 1961. Specificity of the reaction between rheumatoid factors and γ-globulin. J. Exp. Med. **114**: 257.
7. WILLIAMS, JR., R. C. & H. G. KUNKEL. 1965. Observations on anti-gamma globulin factors in human sera and antibodies against autologous gamma globulins produced in rabbits. Ann. N. Y. Acad. Sci. **124**: 860.
8. OSTERLAND, C. K., M. HARBOE & H. G. KUNKEL. 1963. Anti-gamma globulin factors in human sera revealed by enzymatic splitting of anti-Rh antibodies. Vox Sang. **8**: 133.
9. ALLEN, J. C. & H. G. KUNKEL. 1964. Rheumatoid factors with hidden auto-specificity. Arthritis Rheum. **7**: 725.
10. SELL, S. & P. G. H. GELL. 1965. Studies on rabbit lymphocytes *in vitro*. I. Stimulation of blast formation with an anti-allotype serum. J. Exp. Med. **122**: 423.
11. LAXDAL, T., R. P. MESSNER, R. C. WILLIAMS, JR. & P. G. QUIE. 1968. Opsonic, agglutinating and complement-fixing antibodies in patients with subacute bacterial endocarditis. J. Lab. Clin. Med. **71**: 638.
12. MESSNER, R. P., T. LAXDAL, P. G. QUIE & R. C. WILLIAMS, JR. 1968. Serum opsonin, bacteria, and polymorphonuclear leukocyte interactions in subacute bacterial endocarditis: anti-γ-globulin factors and their interaction with specific opsonins. J. Clin. Invest. **47**: 1109.
13. BOYUM, A. 1968. Isolation of mononuclear cells and granulocytes from human blood. Scand. J. Lab. Clin. Invest. **21**(Suppl. 97): 77.
14. FAHEY, J. L., P. F. MCCOY & M. GOULIAN. 1958. Chromatography of serum proteins in normal and pathologic sera: The distribution of protein-bound carbohydrate and cholesterol, siderophillin, thyroxin-binding protein, B_{12} phosphatases, radio-iodinated albumin and myeloma proteins. J. Clin. Invest. **37**: 272.
15. MELTZER, M. & E. C. FRANKLIN. 1966. Cryoglobulinemia: A study of twenty-nine patients. I. IgG and IgM cryoglobulins and factors affecting cryoprecipitability. Amer. J. Med. **40**: 828.
16. QUIE, P. G., R. P. MESSNER & R. C. WILLIAMS. 1968. Phagocytosis in subacute bacterial endocarditis. Localization of the primary opsonic site to Fc fragment. J. Exp. Med. **128**: 553.
17. LJALJEVIC, M., J. LJALJEVIC & C. W. PARKER. 1968. Modification of the amino groups of rabbit γG-globulin. I. The effect on skin sensitizing activity in guinea pig skin. J. Immunol. **100**: 1041.
18. SINGER, J. M. & C. M. PLOTZ. 1956. The latex fixation test. II. Application to the serologic diagnosis of rheumatoid arthritis. Amer. J. Med. **21**: 888.
19. WALLER. M. & S. D. LAWLER. 1962. A study of the properties of the Rhesus antibody (Ri) diagnostic for the rheumatoid factor and its application to Gm grouping. Vox Sang. **7**: 591.
20. KING, R. A., R. P. MESSNER & R. C. WILLIAMS, JR. 1968. Possible adjuvant effect of rheumatoid factors – an autologous immunostat? Arthritis Rheum. **11**: 828.
21. WILLIAMS, JR., R. C. & H. G. KUNKEL. 1962. Rheumatoid factor, complement and conglutinin aberrations in patients with subacute bacterial endocarditis. J. Clin. Invest. **41**: 66.
22. SHANDS, JR., J. W., H. STALDER & E. SUTER. 1966. Clearance of salmonella typhimurium in mice and immunity to mouse typhoid: A comparison of the activities of hyperimmune rabbit γ-globulin and Porter's fragment I obtained by papain hydrolysis. J. Immunol. **96**: 68.
23. ROWLEY, D., M. THÖNE & H. ISLIKER. 1965. Opsonic requirements for bacterial phagocytosis. Nature **207**: 210.

24. BERKIN, A. & B. BENACERRAF. 1965. Properties of antibodies cytophilic for macrophages. J. Exp. Med. **123:** 119.
25. RABINOVITCH, M. 1967. Studies on the immunoglobulins which stimulate the ingestion of glutaraldehyde-treated red cells attached to macrophages. J. Immunol. **99:** 1115.
26. LAY, W. H. & V. NUSSENZWEIG. 1968. Receptors for complement on leukocytes. J. Exp. Med. **128:** 991.
27. LOBUGLIO, A. G., R. S. COTRAN & J. H. JANDL. 1967. Red cells coated with immunoglobulin G: binding and sphering by mononuclear cells in man. Science **158:** 1582.
28. HUBNER, H., M. H. POLLEY, W. D. LINSCOTT, H. H. FUDENBERG & H. J. MÜLLER-EBERHARD. 1968. Human monocytes: distinct receptor sites for the third component of complement and immunoglobulin G. Science **162:** 2181.
29. SELL, S. 1967. Studies on rabbit lymphocytes *in vitro*. V. The induction of blast transformation with sheep antisera to rabbit IgG subnits. J. Exp. Med. **125:** 289.
30. SELL, S. 1968. Studies on rabbit lymphocytes *in vitro*. VII. The relationship between heterozygosity and homozygosity of lymphocyte donor and percent blast transformation induced by antiallotype sera. J. Exp. Med. **127:** 1139.
31. OPPENHEIM, J. J., G. N. ROGENTINE & W. D. TERRY. 1969. Transformation of human lymphocytes by monkey antisera to human immunoglobulins. Immunology **16:** 123.
32. AZAR, M. M. 1966. The effect of active and inactive rheumatoid factors on tolerance to human γ-globulin in Swiss mice. J. Immunol. **97:** 96.
33. BROWN, J. C. & W. V. EPSTEIN. 1969. Influence of human rheumatoid factor on numbers of antibody producing cells. Arthritis Rheum. **12:** 1.
34. MESSNER, R. P., C. W. PARKER & R. C. WILLIAMS, JR. 1969. Chemical modification of γG antistaphylococcal antibodies: effect on opsonic activity. Clin. Res. **17:** 372.
35. WOFSY, L. & S. J. SINGER. 1963. Effects of amidination reaction on antibody activity and on the physical properties of some proteins. Biochemistry **2:** 104.
36. HUNTER, M. J. & M. L. LUDWIG. 1962. The reaction of imidoesters with proteins and related small molecules. J. Amer. Chem. Soc. **84:** 3491.
37. WIEDERMANN, G., P. A. MIESCHER & E. C. FRANKLIN. 1963. Effect of mercaptoethanol on complement binding ability of human 7S gamma-globulin. Proc. Soc. Exp. Biol. Med. **113:** 609.
38. POLLEY, M. J. & H. J. MÜLLER-EBERHARD. 1967. Chemistry and mechanism of action of complement. Progr. Hematol. **5:** 2.
39. PARKER, R. L. & F. R. SCHMID. 1962. Phagocytosis of particulate complexes of γ-globulin and rheumatoid factor. J. Immunol. **88:** 519.
40. HEIMER, R., F. M. LEVIN & M. F. KAHN. 1963. Inhibition of complement fixation by human serum. J. Immunol. **91:** 866.
41. DAVIS, J. S. & A. J. BOLLET. 1964. Protection of a complement sensitive enzyme system by rheumatoid factor. J. Immunol. **92:** 139.
42. GOUGH, W. W. & J. S. DAVIS. 1966. Effects of rheumatoid factor on complement levels *in vivo*. Arthritis Rheum. **9:** 555.
43. DAVIS, J. S. 1969. Complement fixation by IgM rheumatoid factor. Clin. Res. **17:** 72.
44. ZWAIFLER, N. 1969. Complement fixation reactions of gamma globulin and serum containing rheumatoid factor. Clin. Res. **17:** 74.
45. SCHMID, F. R. & M. J. ROCHA. 1969. Complement fixation by IgM antibody (rheumatoid factor): dependence on antigen concentration. J. Lab. Clin. Med. **72:** 1014.

DISCUSSION OF THE PAPER

UNIDENTIFIED SPEAKER: If you knew nothing about the disease rheumatoid arthritis, would you at the moment be able to predict the susceptibility of the rheumatoid arthritic to handle infection, excluding drugs that doctors administer?

DR. MESSNER: I don't think so. In the subacute bacterial endocarditis patients that we studied, we found that there was no difference in the clinical course, whether they had rheumatoid factor or not.

UNIDENTIFIED SPEAKER: Didn't Dr. Williams' paper in 1962 state that people with recurrent subacute bacterial endocarditis tend to have a low rheumatoid factor response?

DR. MESSNER: The presence of rheumatoid factor correlated roughly with the duration of the disease and the absolute level of γG, but the clinical course, other than duration, showed no particular correlation.

DR. AUSTEN: In interpreting your *in vitro* experiments on the rheumatoid factor and complement interaction with the γG antibody on microorganisms, I think it is important to know the concentration of the reactants involved. Would you specify the dilution of the complement source used in order to provide some idea of the amount available. Also, what was the dilution of the rheumatoid factor, as well as its titer. I realize that specificity is an additional variable, but I suspect that the amount of rheumatoid factor employed obtain the inhibitory effect was rather high.

DR. MESSNER: The γG opsonins we use are usually in a concentration of 0.5–2/mg/ml. This is diluted again by a factor of 5 when it is added to the system. The rheumatoid factors are usually used in a concentration of approximately 1 mg/ml. These are 19S preparations from rheumatoid sera, or, in the case of the cryoproteins, a much more potent material. We have obtained inhibition of the opsonin with as little as 0.5 mg/ml of the 19S preparation, which had a latex titer in the final mixture of approximately 1:20, although most rheumatoid factors will not inhibit at that strength. Most need titers in the range of 1:640 to 1:1,280 to cause this inhibition.

In general, the final dilution in the complement system that we studied will show this inhibitory effect with rheumatoid factor to a dilution of about 1:300, so that the ranges of dilutions, either of the titer of latex activity or the dilution of the serum, are within reason.

DR. AUSTEN: I don't agree, because you need 0.5 mg/ml of rheumatoid factor with a titer of perhaps 1:640. In addition, you are diluting your complement source by 1:300, whereas in most of our work it is undiluted.

DR. MESSNER: That's true, but if you dilute the 1:640 by a factor of 5, you are working with a rather low titer, and titers of 1:10,000 or 1:20,000 in latex activity in human serum are not unusual.

DR. AUSTEN: I don't question the results, but I do want to be careful about the biological interpretation.

THE INTERACTION OF SOLUBLE IMMUNE COMPLEXES WITH RHEUMATOID FACTORS

Robert W. Lightfoot, Jr., M.D., Ronald E. Drusin, M.D.,
and Charles L. Christian, M.D.

Department of Medicine
Columbia University College of Physicians and Surgeons
New York, N. Y.

The preparation of dinitrophenol-protein conjugates possessing a limited number of haptenic groups per protein molecule has provided a model for studying the behavior of low-valence antigens in immunological systems. The tendency of these antigens not to precipitate when reacted with antibody and the properties of the soluble immune complexes thus formed have been reported previously.[1] This paper reports our observations on the reactivity of rheumatoid factors with these complexes.

The conjugates to be considered are four dinitrophenol-rabbit serum albumin (DNP-RSA) preparations with average haptene:protein ratios of 1.6, 2.5, 4.1, and 8.2, respectively. The RSA was labeled with iodine-125(^{125}I) prior to conjugation with DNP. Antiserum was prepared by injecting rabbits via the toe pads with keyhole limpet hemocyanin heavily conjugated with DNP, and the euglobulin fraction was isolated by ammonium sulfate fractionation followed by Sephadex G-200 gel chromatography.

The DNP 1.6-RSA and DNP 2.5-RSA formed negligible amounts of immune precipitate with antibody. Approximately 10% of DNP 4.1-RSA precipitated at equivalence, and 48% of DNP 8.2-RSA. Only DNP 8.2-RSA precipitated with antibody in gel diffusion. The precipitin curve for DNP 8.2-RSA, a relatively high-valence antigen, in the presence of various co-factors is shown in FIGURE 1. There was no substantial difference between antigen precipitability with antibody in the presence of buffer, heated normal human serum, or a complement-rich normal human serum stored at −70° C. In contrast, the presence of heated rheumatoid serum having a latex fixation titer of 1:16,000 resulted in precipitation of over 75% of the antigen present near equivalence and a substantial increase in precipitation in the region of antigen excess.

In contrast were the results obtained with DNP 4.1-RSA, presumably containing antigen molecules of lower valence, as shown in FIGURE 2. Precipitation with antibody in the presence of buffer and heated normal human serum was negligible, while the presence of fresh-frozen human serum resulted in an increased precipitation of antigen. Again, rheumatoid serum increased precipitin formation, although not to the degree seen with DNP 8.2-RSA. It should be noted that, at the peaks shown, there was four times as much antigen precipitated in the presence of rheumatoid serum as was precipitated with fresh normal serum.

Curves for the total amount of protein nitrogen precipitated were similar to those shown for antigen precipitation. TABLE 1 shows the amount of nitrogen precipitated with antibody and various cofactors at the points of peak precipitation shown in FIGURES 1 and 2. For DNP 8.2-RSA, approximately 9 μg grams of nitrogen precipitated whether buffer, heated normal serum, or fresh normal serum was present. Heated rheumatoid serum caused twice as much protein to be precipitated. Using DNP 4.1-RSA as antigen, fresh normal human serum effected precipitation of as much protein as with DNP 8.2-RSA, although there was much less antigen precipitated. Because of this, the effect of rheumatoid serum on the total amount of protein precipitated was relatively less striking. Presumably, complement components affixed to the immune complexes are responsible for the marked increase in protein precipitated in the presence of fresh normal serum, an effect that is negligible when antigens of higher valence are used. Purified rheumatoid factor was prepared by absorption onto aggregated human γ-globulin followed by acid elution and density-gradient separation. This preparation gave results similar to whole rheumatoid serum, confirming the role of rheumatoid factors in the previously noted phenomena.

Another aspect of the interaction between rheumatoid factors and immune complexes was demonstrated with the antigens DNP 1.6-RSA and DNP 2.5-RSA. When antigen DNP 1.6-RSA was reacted with antibody at 37° C for 30 minutes and stored at 4° C overnight, no visible precipitate formed. The soluble complexes in the supernatant were subjected to sucrose-density-gradient centrifugation, with the results shown in FIGURE 3. In the control tube, minimal amounts of antigen were deposited in the immune precipitate. There was also no radioactive pellet deposited at the bottom of the gradient tube following ultracentrifugation. In the presence of rheumatoid serum, again no immune precipitate formed; however, there was a shift of the antigen in the supernatant from the zone of heavier complexes into the pellet. This reactivity is shown more graphically in FIGURE 4, in which the arithmetic difference of counts per minute with

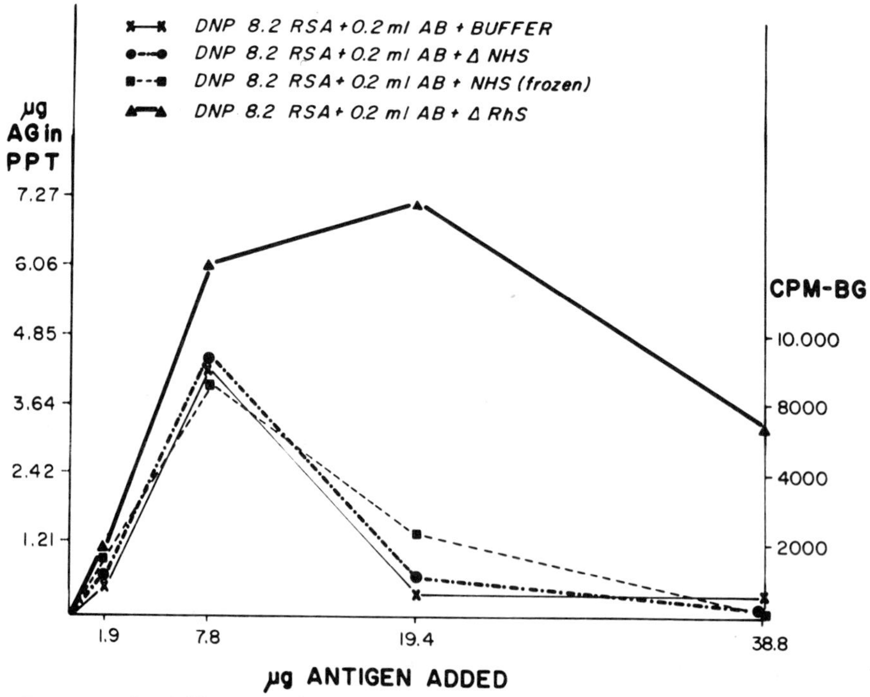

FIGURE 1. Precipitin curve of DNP 8.2–RSA with rabbit anti-DNP-globulin and various cofactors. Abbreviations: NHS = normal human serum; Δ NHS = heated normal human serum; Δ RHS = heated rheumatoid serum; AB = antibody; AG = antigen; PPT = immune precipitate; CPM–BG = counts per minute minus background.

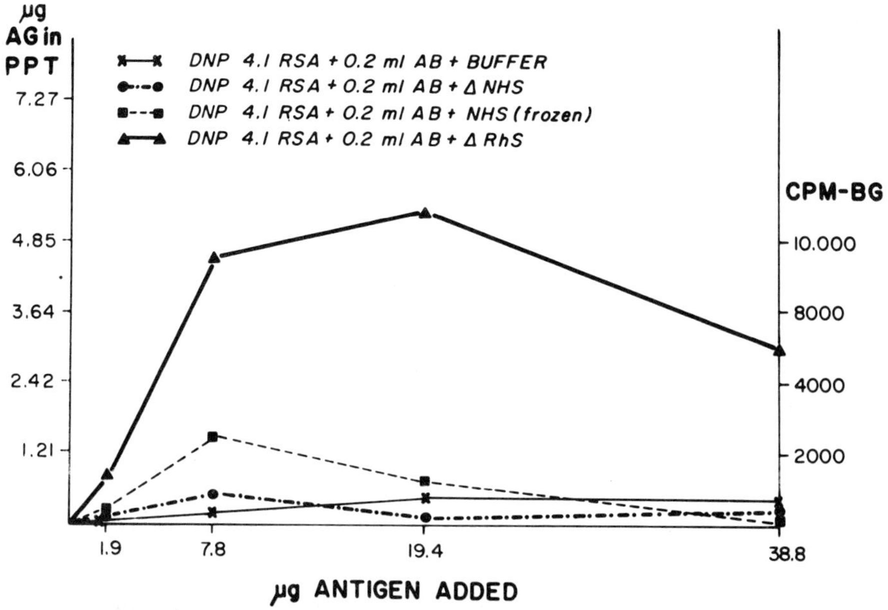

FIGURE 2. Precipitin curve of DNP 4.1–RSA with rabbit anti-DNP-globulin and various cofactors. Abbreviations as in FIGURE 1.

and without rheumatoid serum is obvious. It is clear that any antigen found in the pellet came from the gradient zone corresponding to complexes having antibody:antigen ratios of 5:2 or greater, with a possible contribution from those with a ratio of 2:1. Incubating the reagents for as long as eight days at 4° C did not alter the distribution of complexes from that shown in FIGURE 3. DNP-RSA reacted with rheumatoid serum in the absence of anti-DNP antibody sedimented at tube 20, as did DNP-RSA alone.

Density-gradient analysis with DNP 2.5-RSA as the antigen gave the results shown in FIGURE 5. Distribution in the control was similar to that with DNP 1.6-RSA, with a minimal amount of antigen in the pellet and precipitate regions. However, the reaction with rheumatoid serum resulted not only in a shift of antigen into the pellet but also in the formation of significant amounts of immune precipitate. Again, the rheumatoid factor reactivity is found primarily with the more heavily sedimenting complexes.

TABLE 1

NITROGEN PRECIPITATION WITH ANTIBODY AND VARIOUS COFACTORS*

Cofactor	Antigen DNP 4.1	Antigen DNP 8.2
Buffer	0.13	9.5
Heated normal human serum	1.5	8.9
Fresh normal human serum	8.6	9.8
Heated rheumatoid serum	13.4	18.6

* Values given as micrograms of protein nitrogen precipitated at the peaks shown in FIGURES 1 and 2.

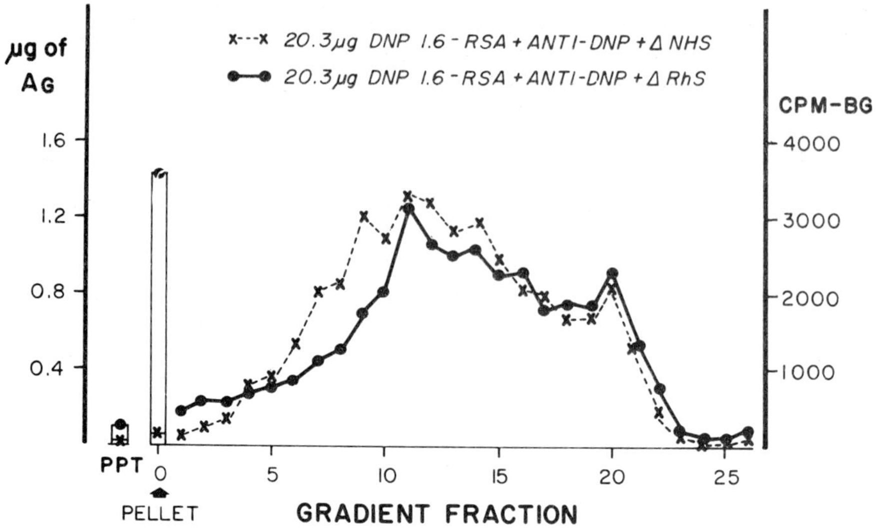

FIGURE 3. Distribution of antigen DNP 1.6–RSA reacted with anti-DNP in the presence of normal or rheumatoid serum. α_2 = Macroglobulin marker sediments between tubes 6 and 11. Prior studies utilizing double-isotope labeling have given estimated antibody:antigen ratios of 5:2, 2:1, 1:1 at the peaks in tubes 9, 11, and 14, respectively. Abbreviations as in FIGURE 1.

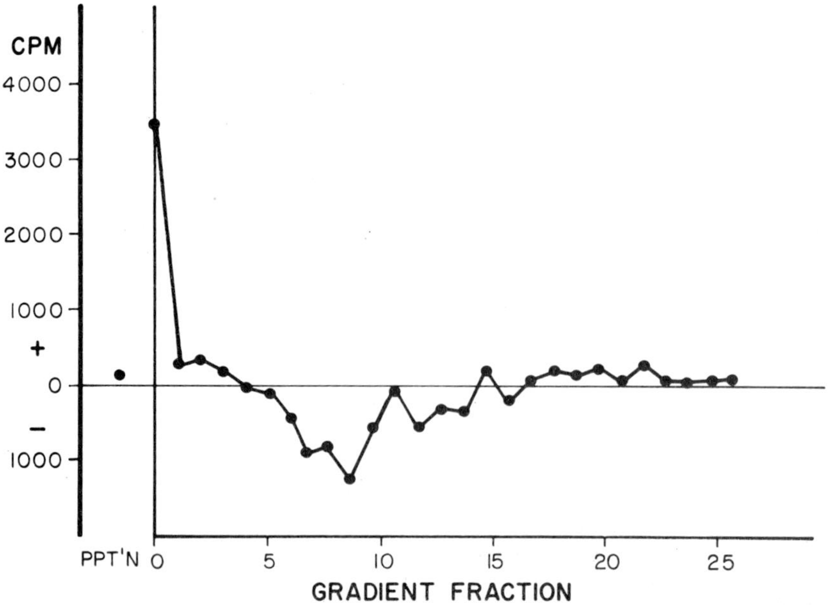

FIGURE 4. Arithmetic difference in counts per minute (CPM) between the gradient curves for DNP 1.6–RSA shown in FIGURE 3.

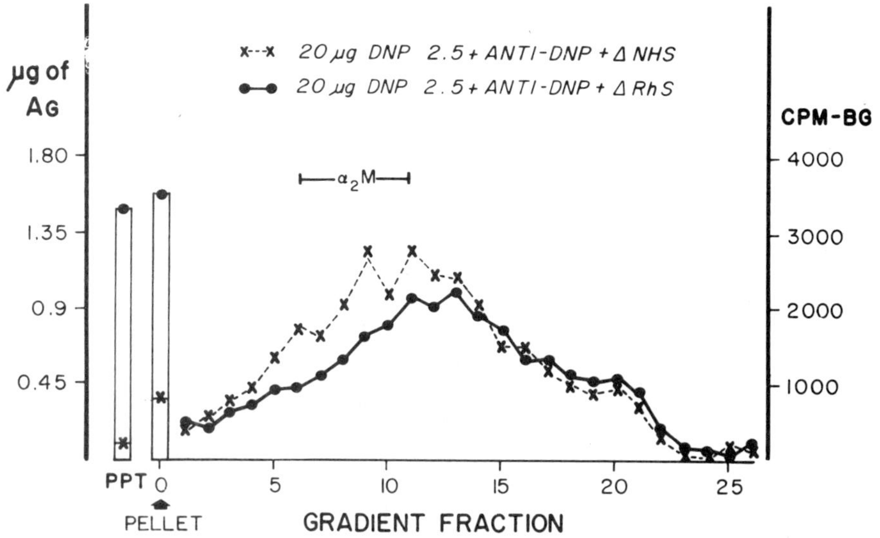

FIGURE 5. Distribution of DNP 2.5–RSA reacted with anti-DNP in the presence of normal or rheumatoid serum. See FIGURE 3. Abbreviations as in FIGURE 1.

These observations are in agreement with a prior report of Edelman and his associates on the reactivity of rheumatoid factors with complexes rendered soluble by large excesses of antigen.[2] The effect of heat-labile serum factors, presumably complement components, on precipitation was marked when antigens of lower valence were employed and negligible with higher-valence antigens. The preferential reactivity of rheumatoid factors with the heavier soluble complexes correlated closely with the complement-fixing ability of these complexes. When gradient fractions were adjusted to contain equivalent amounts of antigen, the bulk of complement fixation was found in complexes sedimenting at or below 19S. Davis and Bollet have previously suggested that rheumatoid factors may exert a protective effect when present in patients with an immune complex disease such as lupus erythematosus.[3] Presumably, reaction with rheumatoid factors would render these complexes less soluble and promote their phagocytosis by tissue macrophages and by the reticuloendothelial system, thus preventing a dissemination of them and lessening the immunopathological sequelae of circulating immune complexes. We have previously reported that the rate of intravascular clearance of soluble complexes prepared as described herein is directly related to their size, those heavier than 19S being cleared more rapidly than lighter ones.[4] In preliminary experiments, rheumatoid serum did not accelerate the clearance of DNP 1.6-RSA in passively immunized mice. Similar work using antigens of higher valence is in progress.

References

1. DRUSIN, R. E., R. W. LIGHTFOOT, JR. & C. L. CHRISTIAN. 1968. Studies of soluble immune complexes. Arthritis Rheum. **11:** 821.
2. EDELMAN, G. M., H. G. KUNKEL & E. C. FRANKLIN. 1958. Interaction of the rheumatoid factor with antigen-antibody complexes and aggregated gamma globulin. J. Exp. Med. **108:** 105.

3. DAVIS, IV, J. S. & A. J. BOLLET. 1966. Complement levels, rheumatoid factor, and renal disease in systemic lupus erythematosus (SLE). Arthritis Rheum. **9:** 499.
4. LIGHTFOOT, JR., R. W., R. E. DRUSIN & C. L. CHRISTIAN. 1969. The *in vivo* fate of artifically-prepared immune complexes. Fed. Proc. **28:** 307.

General Discussion

DR. LITWIN (*New York, N. Y.*): Many of the rheumatoid sera also have high titers of pepsin agglutinators, that is, antiglobulins against pepsin-treated γ-globulin. I think they tend to have a little higher titers than normal sera, even though these are found very frequently in normals. Harboe has suggested that in some cases they will react with immune precipitates. I suspect the suitable control for this would be a normal serum with a high titer of pepsin agglutinator to be assured that your rheumatoid agglutinator was the reactant.

DR. LIGHTFOOT: We have not attempted this.

DR. BARNETT: In your laboratories you've been interested in complex-induced nephritis in actively immunized animals. The size of the complex is very critical in such cases. Have you investigated the interrelationships of antiglobulin in that system?

Also, as you know, in those infectious diseases in lower animals which we used to call persistent-tolerant infections, and which we now refer to as persistent infection because they apparently have lifelong viremia, the infectious material is associated with IgG, and this infectious material is precipitated *in vitro* by anti-IgG. Have you any information from your own laboratory or from the laboratories of others on the role of rheumatoid-like anti-IgG's in such *in vitro* or *in vivo* experiments related to persistent viremia.?

DR. LIGHTFOOT: I'm unaware of any data that we have on the role of rheumatoid factors in diseases exhibiting persistent viremia. With regard to your first question concerning rheumatoid factors in our rabbits, to the best of my knowledge, we have not attempted any therapy of the disease with rheumatoid factors.

DR. AUSTEN: McFarland, in the *Journal of Clinical and Experimental Immunology,* recently indicated that he could potentiate a nephritoxic nephritis model by the infusion of rheumatoid arthritis serum. To twist Dr. Barnett's question a little bit, why don't you see if these mice that you are trying to facilitate have any lesions?

DR. LIGHTFOOT: In the kidney? It might take more antigen than we give for the ordinary clearance determination in order to detect lesions in the kidney. I did some preliminary work to see if more counts were deposited at the end of clearance, for example, in the kidney in those mice receiving soluble complexes as opposed to those receiving the higher-valence antigens; there results were not especially noteworthy. The problem is that soluble complexes are cleared so slowly; with the iodine label, it is hard to compare an antigen that is cleared very slowly with one that is cleared very rapidly because of blood levels. I hope to eliminate this problem by using a tag, perhaps radioactive serum albumin or chromium-tagged red cells.

DR. AUSTEN: I don't think you should make any judgment on this type of study until you've tried it. Dr. Epstein's case report on mixed cryoglobulinemia and nephritis demonstrated a lot of gamma-M in the glomerulus. The immunofluorescent pictures that McFarland shows are very striking, and he didn't use much serum. I think you should try this.

DR. SCHUR: According to the study reported by Koffler and his colleagues, when γ-globin was eluted off the kidneys of patients dying of lupus nephritis, no rheumatoid factors or pepsin agglutinators were found.

RELATION OF RHEUMATOID FACTOR TO INTRACELLULAR INCLUSIONS*

John H. Vaughan, M.D., Ralph F. Jacox, M.D.,
George Abraham, M.D., and Richard Clark, M.D.

Department of Medicine
University of Rochester School of Medicine and Dentistry
Rochester, N. Y.

Previous presentations have indicated that rheumatoid factor-like activities may arise in diseases other than rheumatoid arthritis. We have also heard that these factors may conceivably have a protective value. In this paper we shall review investigations that have sought evidence of whether rheumatoid factors may contribute to the pathogenesis of rheumatoid arthritis.

Ten years ago, Harris and Vaughan transfused normal volunteers with plasmas and leukocytes from patients with well-established seropositive rheumatoid arthritis.[1] These studies were justified at the time by knowledge that prior investigators had injected joint fluids from patients with rheumatoid arthritis into normal individuals and found no transfer of disease, thus appearing to rule out a readily transferred infectious agent as the cause of the disease. Harris and Vaughan assumed that any possible ill effect from the transfusions would last no longer than the time it would take the recipient to metabolize the transfused elements. In their studies, one patient was retransfused several times, so that he had circulating levels of anti-γG activities for as long as six weeks. No grossly evident ill effect was seen after any of the transfusions, even when an added effort to facilitate development of arthritis was made by the mild trauma of injecting one knee with sterile saline. Mild inflammation over one olecranon bursa was seen in a recipient who enthusiastically submitted his elbows to frictional trauma on table tops, chair arms, and other paraphernalia. On biopsy, the inflammation was judged to be nonspecific and reflective more of the enthusiasm than of the rheumatoid factor. The conclusion was drawn that the anti-γ-globulins of rheumatoid arthritis can have only very weak pathogenetic significance if any.

In 1963, Baum and co-workers[2] reported the injection of rheumatoid factors into rats. Euglobulins made from the sera of patients with rheumatoid arthritis and containing large amounts of anti-γG-globulins induced a vasculitic reaction in the mesenteric vessels of the rats. In control studies, euglobulin preparations made from normal individuals induced no vasculitic lesions, even when 19S protein from a patient with a Waldenström macroglobulinemia was added to them.

Shortly thereafter, Delbarre and his associates[4] in France and Hollander and his colleagues[4] in Philadelphia described intracytoplasmic inclusions in the leukocytes of the joint fluids of patients with rheumatoid arthritis. These inclusions were shown to contain γ-globulins, and latex-agglutinating activity was exhibited in lysates from the leukocytes. On the assumption that γ-globulin complexes were present in the inclusions and that these might provoke an inflammatory reaction in the joints, the Philadelphia group[4,5] injected γG-globulins into uninvolved joints of patients with seropositive disease, provoking an arthritis that was not seen in patients with osteoarthritis, who were used as controls. It is puzzling that other laboratories have had difficulty in reproducing these results, but as yet there seems to be no adequate reason for questioning their authenticity.

* Supported in part by United States Public Health Service training grants nos. T1–AI–28 and T1–AM–5188 and research grants nos. AM–02443 and FR–44.

The possible role of pyrogens seems to have been ruled out. The peculiar need to utilize joints completely free of effusion in the injection experiments may explain the failures of others to confirm the results of the Philadelphia group.

The "RA cell" or "ragocyte" of the synovial fluid grossly resembles the glitter cell so commonly encountered in pyelonephritis. Indeed, various investigators have pointed out that leukocytes containing intracytoplasmic γ-globulin inclusions can be found in a wide variety of diseases other than rheumatoid arthritis, in the peripheral blood as well as in the synovial fluids. Much confusion has existed, therefore, as to the real meaning of "ragocytes." If they are to have particular meaning in rheumatoid arthritis, they must have characteristics peculiar to rheumatoid arthritis. Further, they should be shown to have appropriate correlations with other serum factors that might be biologically related.

We began a survey of our arthritis population at the University of Rochester with these problems in mind. In our first evaluation (TABLE 1), we were interested in determining in our patients how well the presence of intracytoplasmic inclusions in joint-fluid leukocytes related to diagnosis, the seropositive state, and the level of joint-fluid complement activity. The joint-fluid complement was ex-

TABLE 1

RELATION OF INTRACYTOPLASMIC INCLUSIONS IN JOINT-FLUID LEUKOCYTES TO COMPLEMENT TITERS AND TO SERUM ANTIBODIES TO IGG-GLOBULINS OR LEUKOCYTE NUCLEI IN THE INITIAL SERIES

Serum No.*	Joint-Fluid Inclusions†				C'H_{50} Fluid/Serum (%)	Serum Antibodies	
	IgG	IgA	IgM	C'3		LFT‡	ANA§
1.	4	0	4	1	15	≥5,120	—
2.	1	0	1		4	≥5,120	+
3.	4	0	4	0	6	≥5,120	—
4.	4	1	2		4	≥5,120	—
5.	3				6	≥5,120	—
6.	4	3	2		27	≥5,120	—
7.	2	1	3		18	≥5,120	—
8.	0	0	0		33	≥5,120	—
9.	3		1		8	2,560	—
10.	4		3		12	1,280	—
11.	2	0	2		6	40	+
12.	2	0	0	2	28	20	+
13.	2	0	0	0	30	—	—
14.	1		0	0	35	—	—
15.	2	0	1	0	40	—	—
16.	4	0	0	1	42	—	—
17.	0	0	0	0	53	—	—
18.	0	0	0	0	45	—	—
19.	3		0		35	—	+
20.	0	1	0	1	55	—	—
21.	1	0	0	0	32	—	—
22.	2	0	0	0	15	—	—
23.	3	0	1	1	40	—	—
24.	0	0	0	0	59	80	—
25.	0	0	0		30	—	—

* Sera nos. 1–18 were from adult rheumatoid arthritis patients, nos. 19 and 20 were from juvenile arthritis patients, and nos. 21–25 were from degenerative arthritis patients.

† Proportion of cells exhibiting intracytoplasmic inclusions with fluorescein-labeled antisera; scale: 4 = >75% of cells staining; 3 = 50–75% of cells staining; 2 = 25–50% of cells staining; and 1 = <25% of cells staining.

‡ Latex titer (reciprocal) for anti-IgG activity.

§ Antinuclear antibody by immunofluorescence with leukocyte nuclei.

TABLE 2

MEAN STAINING REACTIONS AND COMPLEMENT TITERS IN THE INITIAL SERIES

	Joint-Fluid Inclusion*			$C'H_{50}$ Fluid/Serum (%, average)
	IgG	IgA	IgM	
Seropositive rheumatoid arthritis	2.8	0.6	2.0	14
Other Arthritis	1.4	0.1	0.1	39

* Average scores; see footnotes to TABLE 1.

TABLE 3

PRESENCE OF ANTI-γG ACTIVITY IN INTRACYTOPLASMIC INCLUSIONS IN THE SECOND SERIES*

Serum no.†	Patient	Joint-Leukocyte Inclusions				Serum Antibodies	
		γG	γA	γM	a-HγG	LFT	ANA
1.	F.B.	4	4	4	3	>5,120	+
2.	M.H.	4	2	1	–	>5,120	+
3.	T.M.	4	4	4	1	>5,120	–
4.	A.Po.	–	–	–	–	>5,120	+
5.	M.V.	4	2	3	1	>5,120	–
6.	J.C.	1	–	–	–	>5,120	–
7.	D.J.	4	4	4	4	5,120	–
8.	E.B.	4	2	3	3	5,120	–
9.	G.B.	4	2	4	1	2,560	–
10.	D.B.	4	4	4	3	2,560	–
11.	F.P.	Tr	–	1	–	2,560	–
12.	E.A.	Tr	–	1	–	640	–
13.	R.D.	–	–	–	–	–	–
14.	A.Pi.	–	–	–	–	–	–
15.	B.C.	–	–	–	–	–	–
16.	H.B.	–	–	–	–	–	–
17.	J.F.	–	–	–	–	–	–
18.	M.M.	–	–	–	–	–	–
19.	T.B.	–	–	–	–	–	–
20.	E.G.	–	–	–	–	–	–
21.	G.R.	–	–	–	–	–	–
22.	L.O.	1	Tr	–	–	–	–
23.	L.C.	–	–	–	–	–	–
24.	C.F.	–	–	2	–	–	–
25.	J.Do.	–	–	Tr	–	–	–
26.	M.B.	–	–	–	–	–	–
27.	C.K.	–	–	2	–	–	–

* See footnotes to TABLE 1.

† Sera nos. 1–16 were from patients with adult rheumatoid arthritis, nos. 17–19 were from patients with juvenile rheumatoid arthritis, nos. 20–22 were from patients with septicemia, and nos. 23–27 were from miscellaneous patients.

pressed as a ratio of titer in the fluid to titer in the serum, since it is probable that the joint-fluid complement arrives there by diffusion from the serum, and that its level in the fluid is a resultant between that which diffuses into the joint and that which is consumed locally. It is evident (TABLE 1) that the joint-fluid complement titers of patients who were seropositive were relatively lower than those who were seronegative. It is also evident that a greater proportion of the joint-fluid cells from the seropositive patients contained inclusions (TABLES 1 and 2) than did those from patients with seronegative arthritides. γM-Globulins were especially characteristic of the inclusions of the seropositive group, as would be expected if the anti-γG antibodies of the rheumatoid factors were contained in the inclusions. γA-Globulins were also present more frequently in the inclusions in the seropositive group.

A second series of patients was then examined primarily to determine directly whether anti-γG activities were present in the inclusions (TABLE 3), but also simply to expand the first series. It can clearly be seen that anti-γG activity, as evidenced by staining of the inclusions with fluorescein-labeled aggregated γG-globulins, was present only when γM was also seen in the inclusions. In this series, the four seronegative patients with rheumatoid arthritis provided cells that were completely negative for inclusions. Also, in the other control arthritides, inclusions were exhibited remarkably infrequently. In studies not yet reported, Dr. Jovan Kacaki in our laboratories has noted that the inclusions in patients with seropositive rheumatoid arthritis usually contain all four subtypes of the γG-globulin class (γG_1, γG_2, γG_3, and γG_4).

We have been left by these observations with the following conclusions: The presence of anti-γG activity in the sera of patients with rheumatoid arthritis is highly related to the presence of large numbers of joint-fluid cells containing γ-globulin inclusions, the presence of γM-globulins and anti-γG activity in the inclusions, and low joint-fluid complement titers. Although inclusions are seen in seronegative arthritides, they are fewer in number and involve fewer cells than in the seropositive group. When the data of both series are summarized together and analyzed for significance (TABLE 4), our major conclusions are substantiated statistically. Not displayed in TABLE 4, but evident from an inspection of TABLES 1, 3, and 4, is the fact that there was also a high degree of correlation between presence of inclusions, particularly γM inclusions, and lowered joint-fluid complement titers.

During our studies, we have been struck by another observation. If a patient with rheumatoid arthritis is seropositive, he is apt to be so in high titer or not at all (FIGURE 1). The numbers of patients with anti-γG titers in the 20–160 range was small relative to those who were entirely negative or of high titer. This same pattern has been seen by Epstein with the FII tanned cell method of assaying anti-γG-globulin activity[6] and by other workers using sensitized-sheep cells.[7,8] This grouping in the high-titer range contrasts distinctly with the distribution of titers of anti-γG-globulin activity seen in general populations, in which a plot such as that in FIGURE 1 shows a maximum frequency ($>$ 95%) at 0 titer, a sharp fall to less than 5%, and then progressively less for each titer range thereafter. Rheumatoid arthritis seems, therefore, to involve selectively those patients

TABLE 4

CORRELATIONS BETWEEN JOINT-FLUID INCLUSIONS AND COMPLEMENT TITERS IN THE COMBINED SERIES

		Rheumatoid Arthritis			
		Seropositive	Seronegative	Arthritides	p
Inclusions	Present	22	4	11	<0.01
	Absent	2	6	11	
IgM inclusions	Present	19	1	5	<0.001
	Absent	3	9	17	
$C'H_{50}$ ratio	$<30\%$	19	1	4	<0.001
(fluid/serum)	$<30\%$	3	7	18	

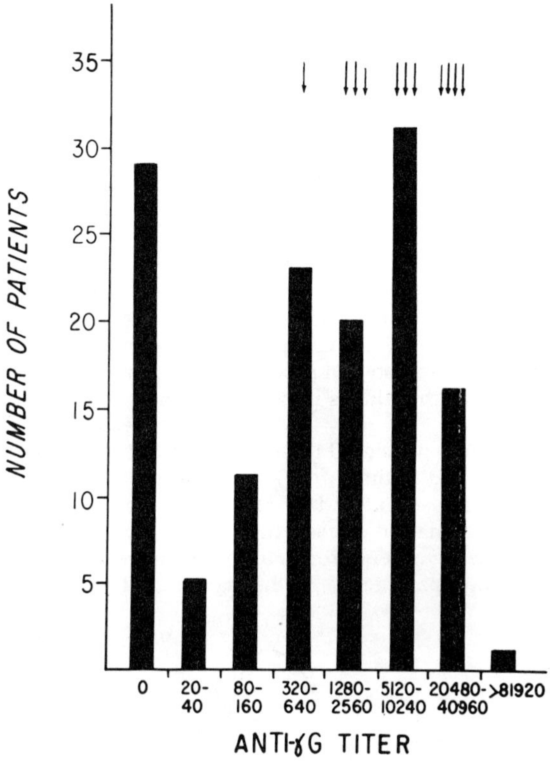

FIGURE 1. Cumulative incidences of anti-γG activity (latex tests) in rheumatoid arthritis. Patients with rheumatoid arthritis and necrotizing vasculitis are indicated by the arrows above. (From Vaughan *et al.*[10] Reproduced by permission of the Transactions of the Association of American Physicians.)

in the general population who have particularly high titers. One might wonder whether this distribution for the rheumatoids is not an artifact produced by a greater predisposition of patients with higher titers to consult physicians in hospitals. Ball and Lawrence, however, found the same phenomenon in a general-population study.[9]

A further point is indicated by the arrows in FIGURE 1. Those patients with rheumatoid arthritis who have the highest titers of anti-γG activities in their serum are those who are likely to have the most severe manifestation of disease, the complication of necrotizing vasculitis. Seronegative patients do not develop this complication. When the serum complement titers of seropositive patients with and without this complication were compared, those with the vasculitis had the lower serum complement titers (TABLE 5). The complement titers of the patients with vasculitis are not out of the range of normal individuals and proved to be significantly lower than those of patients with rheumatoid arthritis without vasculitis. In fact, it was even noted that there was a significant difference by t-test of the mean values of the complement titers of the seronegative patients as compared with the seropositive patients, with or without vasculitis. Taken together with the report by Pernis and co-workers[10] of the finding by immunofluorescence of γ-globulins, rheumatoid factor, and complement in the walls of

TABLE 5

SERUM COMPLEMENT TITERS IN RHEUMATOID ARTHRITIS

	No.	C′H$_{50}$
Seronegatives	29	120 ± 23*
Seropositives		
Without vasculitis	96	112 ± 22†
With vasculitis	11	93.6 (range, 77–118)†

* $p < 0.05$ by t-test.
† $p < 0.05$ by χ^2 analysis.

arteries of a patient with rheumatoid arthritis and vasculitis, it is hard to ignore the likelihood that the γ-globulin complexes in rheumatoid arthritis are indeed capable of complement fixation and precipitation in the peripheral vasculature as well as in the joints, and that this is important in the pathogenesis of seropositive rheumatoid arthritis.

The principal dilemma presented by this concept is: Why don't all seropositive states exhibit rheumatoid arthritis? What about the leukocyte inclusions that can be seen in other disease states? If γ-globulin complexes have any meaning in the pathogenesis of rheumatoid disease, they must have quantitative or qualitative differences from those of other seropositive states in which rheumatoid arthritis is not present. Possibly, persistence of the rheumatoid factor anti-γG activity is

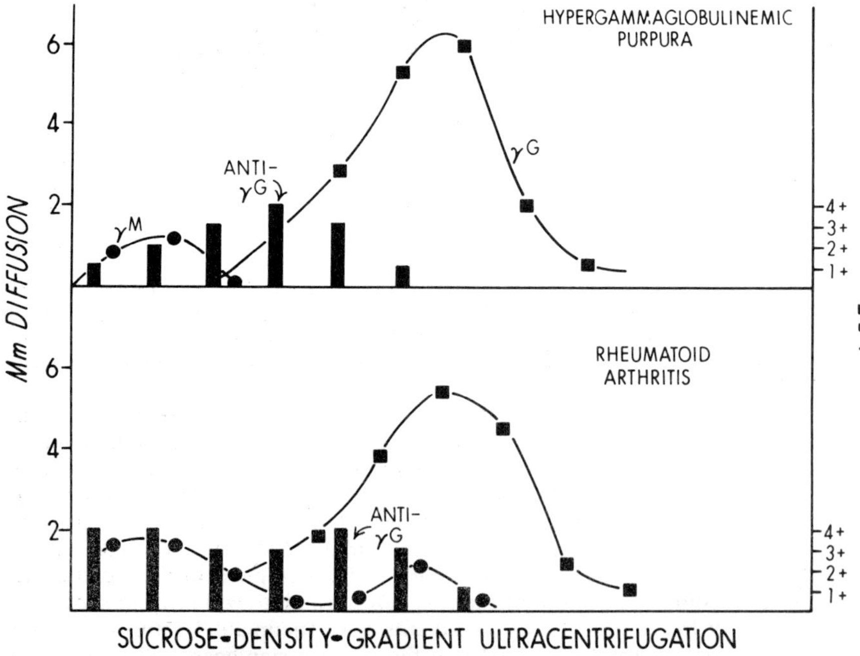

FIGURE 2. Examples of distribution of γG- (●) and γM- (■) globulins and anti-γG activities by a slide latex fixation test (LFT). Sucrose-density-gradient ultracentrifugation of sera from patients with hypergammaglobulinemic purpura and rheumatoid arthritis. Quantities of immunoglobulins are indicated by millimeters of diffusion in radial analysis. The bottom of the tube is at the left.

TABLE 6

SUSCEPTIBILITY OF ANTI-γG-GLOBULIN ACTIVITIES IN VARIOUS DENSITY-GRADIENT REGIONS TO REDUCTION BY 2-MERCAPTOETHANOL*

Serum	>19S Pool	7S-19S Pool	≤7S Pool
Rheumatoid Arthritis			
Ha.	−7	−3	+1
Dy.	−7	−3	−1
An.	−4	−3	0
Be.	−6	−4	0
Ve.	−6	−2	−3
Le.	−6	−5	−2
He.	−2	n.t.	0
Ne.	−4	−2	0
Ro.	−3	n.t.	0
McD.	−6	−4	+1
Hypergammaglobulinemia			
Mi.	−1	0	0
Bo.	−1	−1	0
Ro.	−1	−1	0
Di.	−2	n.t.	+1
Be.	−3	−1	0
Ti.	−3	0	+2
Mar.	0	+1	0
Gu.†	−5	−3	−2
Ross.†	−3	0	+1
Ar.‡	−2	0	0
Matz.‡	−1	−1	−1
Boy.§	−2	0	0

* All values indicate reduction in titer: $\log_2$; n.t. = no titer in unreduced sample.
† Hypergammaglobulinemic purpura accompanying sicca syndrome.
‡ Hypergammaglobulinemic purpura accompanying sicca syndrome with arthralgias.
§ Hypergammaglobulinemic purpura accompanying systemic lupus erythematosus.

important, so that patients with long continued presence of complexes in high titer are more "at risk" than are patients with complexes for only shorter periods. Possibly, differences in classes of immunoglobulin carrying anti-γG activities, specificities for particular configurations on the γG molecule, avidities, or solubilities may be important.

In an exercise to learn something more about such possibilities, we recently began a comparison of the sera of patients with hypergammaglobulinemic purpura with those of patients with rheumatoid arthritis. In FIGURE 2, archetypes of the patterns in sucrose-density-gradient ultracentrifugation are shown for sera from the two disease entities. The predominant anti-γG activity in hypergammaglobulinemic purpura sediments intermediately between 19S and 7S while peaks of anti-γG activity are seen above and below this point in the rheumatoid arthritis serum. When pools from the 19S, intermediate, and 7S regions of the centrifugations of the individual hypergammaglobulinemic purpura sera were exposed to 2-mercaptoethenol, all but one showed relative resistance (TABLE 6). The 19S and intermediate regions from the rheumatoid arthritis sera showed much greater losses of titer, as expected from γM anti-γG found in this disease. Other studies have confirmed that the hypergammaglobulinemic purpura sera have little anti-γG activity in the γM class of immunoglobulins. Further comparative studies, including abilities of the complexes formed by anti-γG of various immunoglobulin classes to fix complement, need to be carried out.

TABLE 7

IMMUNOPATHOGENIC CONCEPTS FOR SEROPOSITIVE RHEUMATOID ARTHRITIS

Etiology	Role for "Rheumatoid Factors"
Infection	
An "RA-specific" microbe	Aggravate an independently derived chronic infection
A series of nonspecific, unrelated microbes	Convert acute, transient inflammatory response to chronic inflammation
No infection	
A metabolically abnormal IgG-globuiln	Initiate inflammation on basis of normal antibodies vs. abnormal IgG-globulins
A metabolically abnormal IgM-globulin	Initiate inflammation on basis of abnormal antibodies vs. normal IgG-globulins

It might be helpful to conclude with a presentation of several possible ways of looking at the pathogenesis of seropositive rheumatoid arthritis (TABLE 7). Seropositive rheumatoid arthritis may be due to an as yet undefined microbial agent specific for rheumatoid arthritis. The presence of anti-γG-globulins, in such instance, may aggravate the damage in tissues already damaged by chronic infection by forming complexes which are deposited there. It is also possible that no microbe specific for rheumatoid arthritis exists, but that the disease may be the consequence of a series of nonspecific, unrelated microbial infections; anti-γG globulins evolving as a natural consequence of these may convert otherwise acute, transient inflammatory responses into a chronic inflammatory process.

If the hypothesis is made that infection does not cause seropositive rheumatoid arthritis, one may conceive that the production of anti-γG-globulins is due to exposure of the antibody-forming systems to structurally abnormal γG-globulins which arise perhaps from some defect in γG-globulin synthesis or catabolism. No evidence yet exists, however, for such a role of structural abnormality in γG-globulins in rheumatoid arthritis. The alternative that the anti-γG-globulins are themselves abnormal immunoglobulins must remain a possibility, but this is the least tenable of all the hypotheses. What relation seronegative rheumatoid arthritis has to seropositive rheumatoid arthritis is not clear, but it is evident that these need not be the same fundamental disease.

References

1. HARRIS, J. & J. H. VAUGHAN. 1961. Transfusion studies in rheumatoid arthritis. Arthritis Rheum. **4**: 47.
2. BAUM, J., P. STASTNY & M. ZIFF. 1964. Effects of the rheumatoid factor and antigen-antibody complexes on the vessels of the rat mesentery. J. Immunol. **93**: 985.
3. DELBARRE, F., A. KAHAN, B. AMOR & G. KRASSININE. 1964. Value of the synovial ragocyte in the diagnosis of rheumatic diseases. Presse Med. **72**: 2129.
4. HOLLANDER, J. L., D. J. MCCARTY, JR., G. ASTORGA & E. CASTRO-MURILLO. 1965. Studies on pathogenesis of rheumatoid joint inflammation. I. "R.A. cell" and working hypothesis. Ann. Intern. Med. **62**: 271.
5. RESTIFO, R. A., A. J. LUSSIER, A. J. RAWSON, J. H. ROCKEY & J. L. HOLLANDER. 1965. Studies on pathogenesis of rheumatoid joint inflammation. III. Experimental production of arthritis by intra-articular injection of purified 7S gamma globulin. Ann. Intern. Med. **62**: 285.
6. EPSTEIN, W. V. & E. P. ENGLEMAN. 1959. The relation of rheumatoid factor content of serum to clinical neurovascular manifestations of rheumatoid arthritis. Arthritis Rheum. **2**: 250.

7. VAUGHAN, J. H. 1959. Serum responses in rheumatoid arthritis. Amer. J. Med. **26:** 596.
8. KELLGREN, J. H. 1969. The epidemiology of rheumatoid factor. 4th Nuffield Conf. Rheum., Ditchley Park, London.
9. BALL, J. & J. S. LAWRENCE. 1961. Epidemiology of the sheep cell agglutination test. Ann. Rheum. Dis. **20:** 235.
10. PERNIS, B., C. B. BALLABIO & G. CHIAPPINO. 1963. Presenza del fattore reumatoide nelle lesioni vascolari in casi di artrite reumatoide aggravata (maligna): Studio con anticorpi fluroescenti. Rheumatisimo **15:** 187.
11. VAUGHAN, J. H., E. S. MONGAN & R. F. JACOX. 1968. Trans. Ass. Amer. Physicians **81:** 231.

General Discussion

DR. MACKENZIE (*Cincinnati, Ohio*): Utilizing the Williams Messner observations, we started absorbing out these latex factors in subacute bacterial endocarditis sera with the patient's own microbes. In ten out of ten streptococci viridans cases in which we isolated the organism, the latex factor could be absorbed out only by the patient's own streptococci viridans, i.e., by the affecting organism alone. Other streptococci viridans, staphylococci, *Escherichia coli,* etc., do not remove this latex factor, which seems to be specific for the infecting agent. This may be part of our problem in dealing with these antiglobulins, because they may indeed be very specific anti-antibodies for the infecting microbe, i.e., for this specific antibody.

DR. VAUGHAN: Dr. MacKenzie, I wonder if the specific infecting agent in this system is most effective in absorbing out rheumatoid factor activity, because the serum of an individual recently infected with this specific agent must have more antibody against the particular organism you are using for absorption. This might mean that, in effect, you are absorbing with more antigen-antibody complex than you are with some unrelated organism.

DR. MACKENZIE: I think that is a possibility, except that we've had the opportunity to study a few relatively new patients and isolate a new strain of streptococci viridans from their throats. After one month of infection, each patient should show a lot of antibody against streptococci viridans, yet the new strains are ineffective in absorbing out the antiglobulin. Thus, it seems that we are really dealing with a microbe-specific phenomenon.

DR. WILLIAMS: I think there is a difference between isolating something from the throat and isolating something from the blood; isolating a microbe from the blood means that the patient has had the infection for four or five months and has a high-avidity antibody. What Dr. Vaughan probably meant, Dr. MacKenzie, was that this specificity that you've demonstrated was against the high-avidity antibody present in the native serum.

Dr. Vaughan, have any of these hypergammaglobulinemic purpura patients that you've studied showed any synovial effusion? Were you able to look at the joint fluids? Also, your intermediate-sedimenting anti-γ-globulin factors were not reduced very much by mercaptoethanol. Do you conclude that these are γG rheumatoid factors or A?

DR. VAUGHAN: I can't answer you about the joint fluids. These sera have come from Rochester, Minnesota, and this is a cooperative study with Dr. Robert Kyle. I have not seen any of these patients, but I have read a good number of their case records. Arthritis is not a prominent or even frequent manifestation of disease in these patients; purpura, on the other hand, is. In regard to your second question, of course the intermediate antibody need not be γG. There is good evidence that intermediate antibody may be γA in some of these patients with rheumatoid arthritis. We have seen one instance among the hypergammaglobulinemic purpura patients in which the major anti-γ-globulin activity was γA rather than γG, and certainly mercaptoethanol does differentiate between these two classes.

DR. BARNETT: Your paper and some other work that has been reported point out the importance of looking at the heterogeneity of antiglobulins in regard to their specificity for antigen and their relationship to presenting symptoms. You illustrate differences between the sera of hyperglobulinemic purpura patients and those of rheumatoid arthritis patients. We have been interested in the study of synovial fluids from rheumatoid arthritis patients. Synovial fluid cryoprecipitates fell into two major subdivisions: Either γG alone was detectable in the cryoprecipitates, or both γG and γM was present. Those patients with only γG in their cryoprecipitates had rheumatoid factor activity in the cryoprecipitate that was resistant to mercaptoethanol. Those with both γG and γM had rheumatoid factor activity that was destroyed by mercaptoethanol. In both groups of patients, ragocytes that had γM inclusions were demonstrable. This points out the problem of how we should look at the patient. If we study cryoprecipitates or synovial fluid, we may get one picture and set of relationships; if we study the serum, we get another viewpoint; and if we look at ragocytes, we apparently get a third.

DR. VAUGHAN: And if you chill the joint fluid, you get still another! Whether what you precipitate from a joint fluid at 4° C is really related to what is going on in the way of precipitation and phagocytosis *in vivo* is another question.

DR. EPSTEIN: Most of the foregoing has been directed to bacterial infection. There is a report in the literature of the infectivity of herpes simplex virus when coated with IgG antibody. When an anti-IgG is then added, the herpes simplex is no longer infectious. Is there any more information available concerning the ability of anti-IgG to alter the infectivity of virus?

DR. ASH: The studies you refer to about herpesvirus were done in our laboratories, and we were able to take herpes simplex virus in an *in vitro* system and coat it with an anti-herpes antibody and produce a persistent infectivity. This persistent fraction was resistant to neutralization by antiviral antibody, but was highly sensitive to neutralization with the anti-γ-globulin antibody.

DR. VAUGHAN: Persistent in what way?

DR. ASH: Persistent in that it was resistant to neutralization by antiviral antibody. We obtained what we refer to as a persistent fraction.

DR. VAUGHAN: Still infective in tissue culture or in the whole animal?

DR. ASH: This was *in vitro,* by plaque reduction. In addition to this, we have also found that we could show specificity in terms of allotypic specificities with this technique. Recently, we have found that there is a complement-dependent antibody that interacts with the herpes antigen. If you treat this antibody with mercaptoethanol to remove its complement specificity, and then coat the virus with this antibody and treat it with rheumatoid factor, you can restore its reacivity with complement.

DR. VAUGHAN: That's interesting. I would like to make one further comment about a possible viral agent or other infectious agent in rheumatoid arthritis. It is apparent, at least to me, that such a postulated agent cannot be one of the "garden variety" of viral agents that we know so well. Joint studies with Dr. Barnett to find the routine type of viral agents in joint tissues, etc., in patients with rheumatoid arthritis came to nought. Herpesvirus is so easy to grow that, if it were a causative agent in arthritis, we should have been able to prove it long ago. The same may be said of adenovirus. One could name a whole series of organisms. Perhaps the virologists have some suggestions for us on what line of research to pursue.

DR. ASH: Do you ever study these rheumatoid arthritic patients to determine what their levels of antibody to herpes and other viruses are?

DR. VAUGHAN: Our virologists ask us what virus to look for and how many to look for. We've been frustrated in our further thoughts about it.

DR. ASH: The reason I mention herpes is that you suggested a microbial etiology. One of the possibilities you noted was an agent which was probably innocuous, but which might influence the development or progression of the disease. Herpesvirus has been described as a rather ubiquitous agent in our society, to the extent that it is found in about 95% of the population. Perhaps in nonrheumatoid states it is quite innocuous; possibly in connection with rheumatoid arthritis one might find an elaboration of the disease. The study of herpes antibody or other common virus diseases would be a logical approach to this problem.

THE ROLE OF RHEUMATOID (ANTIGLOBULIN) FACTORS IN HEMOLYTIC ANEMIA*

Leonard S. Goldberg, M.D., and Eugene V. Barnett, M.D.

Department of Medicine
University of California School of Medicine
Los Angeles, Calif.

Autoimmune hemolytic anemias are characterized by anti-erythrocyte antibodies that usually belong to one class of immunoglobulins. Warm-antibody hemolytic anemia is associated with γG-type autoantibodies, whereas antibodies of the γM class are responsible for chronic cold-agglutinin disease. The transient cold-agglutinin hemolytic anemia present in patients with infectious mononucleosis, however, is frequently caused by a mixed γG-γM cold agglutinin. In the mixed cold agglutinin, neither the γG or γM component alone is capable of destroying the red blood cell; the presence of both is required for cold-agglutinin activity. The hemolytic mechanism appears to depend on the sensitization of erythrocytes with γG at 4° C, and the subsequent interaction of the sensitized red cells with a cold-reactive γM-antiglobulin (FIGURE 1).

γG-γM Hemolytic Mechanism

The data presented here consists of the observations made in our laboratory[1] and the confirming studies of Capri and co-workers.[2] The sera studied were from patients with infectious mononucleosis. Eluates were obtained from type O red cells exposed to the patient's serum at 4° C; fetal or adult erythrocytes were used, depending on the specificity of the cold agglutinin in whole serum. Cold-agglutinin activity of the eluate was markedly reduced by absorption with antisera monospecific for either γG or γM. Absorption with antiserum to γA did not significantly alter the titer. The presence of γG and γM was confirmed by the method of quantitative complement fixation. Components of the eluates were isolated by either DEAE-cellulose chromatography or by sucrose-density-gradient ultracentrifugation. Neither the γG or γM component alone had cold-agglutinin activity. When the two components were recombined, cold-agglutinin activity was restored. The addition of γG or γM isolated from normal serum to either component of the mixed cold agglutinin did not restore cold-agglutinin activity.

The γG component behaved as an incomplete cold agglutinin in that it sensitized red cells at 4° C, but not at 37° C. The majority of the γG cold agglutinins had specificity for the i erythrocyte antigen, although specificity for the I antigen was noted in one patient. The γG-sensitized red cells were agglutinated by the γM component at 4° C. Furthermore, the γM-antiglobulin reacted strongly with erythrocytes sensitized with anti-CD serum Ripley when tested at 4° C, but not at 37° C. The majority of the cold-reactive antiglobulins were also detected with latex particles coated with aggregated γG, but only when the test was performed at 4° C.[3] Thus, the interaction of the γG component with the red cells and the subsequent interaction of the γG-sensitized cells with the γM-antiglobulin occurred exclusively at 4° C. The mixed cold agglutinin does not appear to fix complement, since Coombs tests using antiserum to β_{1C} were negative.

* Supported in part by United States Public Health Service grant no. GM–15759.

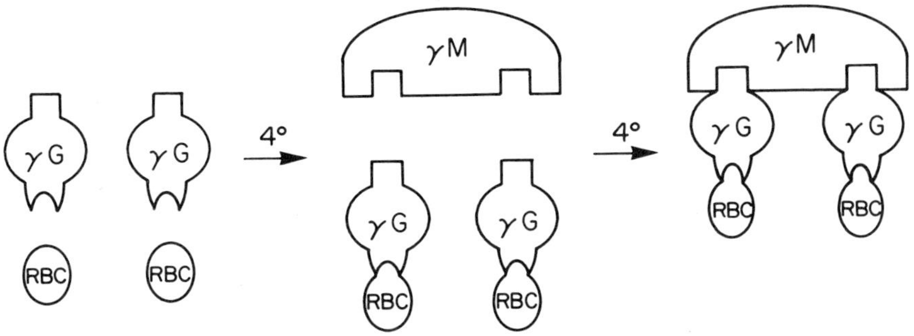

FIGURE 1. Mixed γG-γM cold agglutinin. Interaction of γG with erythrocytes (RBC) and subsequent interaction of γG-sensitized erythrocytes with γM-antiglobulin occurs at 4° C.

Discussion

Recent observations indicate that the transient cold-agglutinin hemolytic anemia present in patients with infectious mononucleosis is frequently caused by a mixed γG-γM cold agglutinin. Mixed cold agglutinins were detected in 66% of the 50 cases studied by Capri and co-workers;[2] in those cases with overt, severe hemolysis, the mixed γG-γM cold agglutinin was usually the causative agent. The sequence of events leading to the formation of mixed cold agglutinins is not understood. It may be that the incomplete γG-antibody is initially produced and becomes antigenic when attached to the erythrocyte surface. The γG complexed to the red cell then induces formation of the peculiar γM-antiglobulin, which is reactive only at reduced temperatures. However, the presence of the incomplete γG-antibodies does not invariably induce production of antiglobulins; in the 50 cases previously noted, 90% of the sera contained an incomplete γG-antibody, whereas only 66% showed the mixed γg-γM cold agglutinin. Thus, the factors responsible for the formation of the γG as well as γM components of these peculiar cold agglutinins remain to be deliniated.

A similar anti-antibody mechanism has also been proposed in a patient with moderately severe warm-antibody hemolytic anemia.[4] On initial evaluation (1961), the patient's erythrocytes were shown to be sensitized with γG, and his serum contained an antiglobulin in high titer (TABLE 1). The antiglobulin activity

TABLE 1

STUDIES IN A PATIENT WITH SUSPECTED MIXED γG-γM WARM AGGLUTININ*

Test	1961	1962	1968
Hematocrit	27%	49%	51%
Reticulocyte count	20%	1.4%	1%
Direct Coombs test			
γ	4+	4+	3+
β_{1C}	N.D.	N.D.	2+
Antiglobulins			
Latex	1:28,000	0	±1:20
Ripley†	4+	0	0

* The 1961 studies were performed before corticosteroid therapy. The 1962 and 1968 studies were performed one month and six years, respectively after therapy was discontinued. N.D. = not done.

† Erythrocytes sensitized with anti-CD serum Ripley.

was restricted to the γM fraction of serum, and this fraction agglutinated the autologous γG-sensitized red cells *in vitro*. Following corticosteroid therapy, the antiglobulin disappeared and the hemolysis subsided, although the direct Coombs test remained strongly positive. When reevaluated in 1968 (six years after the discontinuation of corticosteroids), there was no evidence of hemolysis and no detectable serum antiglobulins, although the strongly positive Coombs test persisted.[5] These findings suggested that the interaction of the antiglobulin with the γG-sensitized cells may have been the mechanism responsible for hemolysis.

Summary

Antiglobulins that coexist with γG-sensitized red cells *in vivo* can assume a pathogenic role in hemolytic anemia. The interaction of a γM antiglobulin with γG-sensitized erythrocytes appears to be responsible for the hemolysis induced by the mixed γG-γM cold agglutinin; a similar anti-antibody mechanism may exist in certain patients with warm-antibody hemolytic anemia.

References

1. GOLDBERG, L. S. & E. V. BARNETT. 1967. Mixed γG-γM cold agglutinin. J. Immunol. **99:** 803.
2. CAPRA, J. D., P. DOWLING, S. COOK & H. G. KUNKEL. 1969. An incomplete cold reactive γG antibody with i specificity in infectious mononucleosis. Vox Sang. **16:** 10.
3. CAPRA, J. D., R. J. WINCHESTER & H. G. KUNKEL. 1969. Cold-reactive rheumatoid factor in infectious mononucleosis and other diseases. Arthritis Rheum. **12:** 67.
4. FIALKOW, P. J., H. H. FUDENBERG & W. V. EPSTEIN. 1964. "Acquired" antibody hemolytic anemia and familial aberrations in gamma globulins. Amer. J. Med. **30:** 188.
5. GOLDBERG, L. S. & H. H. FUDENBERG. 1968. Warm antibody hemolytic anemia: Prolonged remission despite persistent positive Coombs test. Vox Sang. **15:** 443.

General Discussion

DR. AUSTEN: Did you study the fixation of the complement system at 4° C?

DR. GOLDBERG: No, we did not.

DR. AUSTEN: I think that is relevant inasmuch as fixation occurs at certain temperatures, depending on the nature of the γM antibodies. In the last patient that you described with warm-antibody hemolytic anemia, I noticed that you tested sera over a number of years. Do you have β_{1C} levels in that patient on the initial specimen?

DR. GOLDBERG: No, we do not. I initially saw that patient in 1968, and I don't think any 1961 serum is left, although I may be incorrect.

DR. VAUGHAN: In your anti-red cell antibody, the γG component had specificity for the i antigen. This is usually poorly represented on adult red cells. Did your patient have more of the i antigen than is usual for a normal adult population?

Also, did you do any studies on the thermal amplitude of your system, that is, how many of these combinations would take place at various temperatures, considering that the blood in the capillaries of ambient patients usually doesn't go below 28° C, at the lowest?

DR. GOLDBERG: The patients appeared to have more i antigen than you would expect. This was attributed to their high reticulocyte counts. As you know, reticulocytes are relatively rich in the i antigen, whereas the mature red cell tend to have more of the I antigen.

In regard to the thermal amplitude, we tested it at three temperatures: 37° C, room temperature, and at 4° C. At room temperature, there was very little attachment of the γG to the red cell surface. It seemed much like the descriptions of the complete γM cold agglutinin, that is, attachment was greatest at 4° C.

DR. MACKENZIE: When testing your red cells with the γG antibody at 37° C, was there any evidence that the γG was eluted?

DR. GOLDBERG: The γG antibody was eluted from the erythrocytes at 37° C.

DR. MACKENZIE: We have found a cold-acting γG antibody, although not the same as you have been describing. This is a γG antibody which is only detectable, as far as we can ascertain, in the cold. It occurs fairly frequently in autoimmune hemolytic anemia. At 37° C, it undergoes a configurational change and can no longer be detected with the antisera. It is still on the red cell, which can be shown by varying the temperature. I think this may be an explanation of some of the routine Coombs tests reported as "only having complement on the cells." These all have complement on the cells as well.

DR. VAUGHAN: If you were to use labeled red cells coated with IgG, and then add the antiglobulin and administer to a recipient, what would the survival be?

DR. GOLDBERG: I suspect it would agglutinate. Unless a subagglutinating amount were used.

HISTAMINE-RELEASING ACTIVITY OF RHEUMATOID AND NONRHEUMATOID SERUM AND SYNOVIAL FLUID*

I. Broder, M.D., R. Baumal, M.D., Ph.D.,
D. Gordon, M.D., and D. Bell, M.D.

Departments of Medicine, Pathology, and Pharmacology
Faculty of Medicine, University of Toronto
Toronto, Canada

Introduction

Rheumatoid factors are a heterogeneous family of immunoglobulins possessing specificity for different sites on the γ-globulin molecule.[1–5] Some rheumatoid factors are directed against determinants on γ-globulin which are normally hidden and become exposed following aggregation either by physicochemical procedures or by the union of antibody with antigen.[6,7] In view of this specificity, it is possible that the formation of some rheumatoid factors is stimulated by the presence of aggregated γ-globulin or of antigen-antibody complexes. The present studies have been concerned with determining whether such materials are present in the serum and synovial fluid of patients with rheumatoid arthritis. This problem has been pursued through the use of a biological assay for aggregated γ-globulin and soluble antigen-antibody complexes, based on the capacity of these reagents to release histamine from the isolated perfused guinea pig lung. By means of this system, a factor resembling a soluble antigen-antibody complex has been detected in rheumatoid serum and synovial fluid.

Materials and Methods

A more complete description of the materials and methods has been published previously.[8–11]

Bioassay

Heart-lung preparations obtained from normal guinea pigs were perfused at 37° C with Tyrode solution through a cannula inserted into the pulmonary artery. The effluent drained from the left atrium and was collected in sequential fractions. Materials to be tested for histamine-releasing activity were injected into the pulmonary artery cannula. The content of histamine in the perfusion effluent was assayed by measuring contraction of the guinea pig ileum.

Histamine-Releasing Agents

The preparations of soluble complexes used in these studies contained bovine plasma albumin as antigen and antibody produced by rabbits. Soluble complexes were prepared by solubilizing the equivalence precipitate in ninefold antigen excess. Antibody to γ-globulin was obtained by immunizing rabbits with human Cohn fraction II. Aggregated γ-globulin was prepared by heating human Cohn fraction II at 63° C for ten minutes, and was purified on Sephadex G-200. Anaphylatoxin was generated from guinea pig serum by incubation with agar.

* This work was supported by the Canadian Arthritis and Rheumatism Society and by the Medical Research Council of Canada.

Chemical and Serological Techniques

Standard methods were used for gradient and analytical ultracentrifugation, gel filtration on Sephadex G-200, starch-block electrophoresis, ammonium sulfate fractionation, reduction and alkylation, and the detection of rheumatoid factor by latex agglutination.

Clinical Studies

Serum and synovial fluid were obtained from patients who were in the active stage of one of a variety of diseases. These specimens were characterized by a number of procedures, and their behavior in the guinea pig lung was compared with that of soluble complexes, aggregated γ-globulin, anaphylatoxin, and antibody to γ-globulin. Statistical analyses were performed by means of the student's t-test and the χ^2 method; p values of 0.05 or less are considered to be statistically significant.

Results

The Inhibitory Effect of γ-Globulin on the Histamine-Releasing Activity of Soluble Antigen-Antibody Complexes and Aggregated γ-Globulin

Both soluble antigen-antibody complexes and aggregated γ-globulin have been shown to liberate histamine from the isolated perfused guinea pig lung.[9,12] Appreciable amounts of histamine were released from lungs injected with microgram quantities of these reagents purified from other serum components. However, the same degree of sensitivity did not apply when soluble complexes or aggregated γ-globulin were present in serum, since the relatively high concentration of normal γ-globulin in serum produced inhibition of histamine-releasing activity. This was shown by a study in which soluble antigen-antibody complexes were mixed with the different starch-block fractions of normal rabbit serum. The histamine-releasing activity of the soluble complexes was inhibited only by the γ-globulin fraction, and no difference was found with either the slow- or fast-migrating γ-components (Table 1). Similar results have been obtained with aggregated γ-globulin and reagents which were all of human origin.

Separation of Soluble Antigen-Antibody Complexes and Aggregated γ-Globulin from the Inhibitory γ-Globulin in Serum

The foregoing study suggested that in order to achieve maximal sensitivity for the detection of soluble complexes in serum, it was necessary to separate the

Table 1

Influence of Fractions of Normal Rabbit Serum on the Histamine-Releasing Activity of Soluble Immune Complexes*

Electrophoretic Fraction	Residual Histamine-Releasing Activity (%)
Albumin	82 ± 37
α-Globulin	167 ± 45
β-Globulin	112 ± 28
α-Globulin	
Fast	3 ± 2
Slow	4 ± 1
Total	5 ± 2

* The histamine-releasing activity of a dose of soluble complexes containing 0.5 μg of antibody nitrogen was compared when injected alone and when mixed with 12.8 μg of the different starch-block fractions of normal rabbit serum. Each entry represents the mean and standard error of nine observations.

complexes from the inhibitory γ-globulin fraction of serum. This separation was achieved by the use of gel filtration on Sephadex G-200 at pH 8 (FIGURE 1). The soluble complexes used in this study contained bovine plasma albumin as antigen and ^{131}I-labeled antibody. When these soluble complexes were added to normal rabbit serum and then fractionated on Sephadex G-200, it was observed that both antigen[8] and antibody were eluted in the Sephadex excluded fraction, and only this fraction showed histamine-releasing activity. In further studies, it was shown that the histamine-releasing activity of soluble complexes was inhibited by the Sephadex middle fraction of normal rabbit serum. Similar results were obtained with aggregated γ-globulin and reagents which were all of human origin. Therefore, fractionation on Sephadex G-200 resulted in a separation of soluble complexes and aggregated γ-globulin from the component of serum which inhibited their histamine-releasing activity. By the use of this sepa-

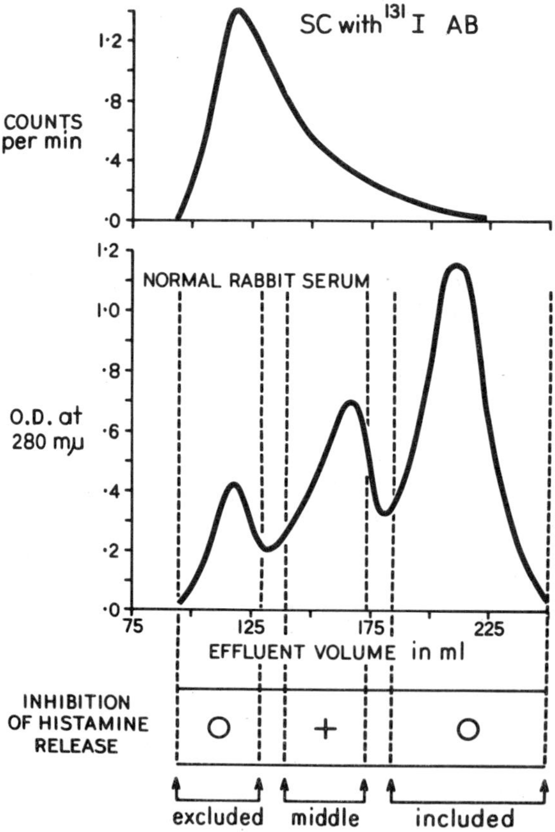

FIGURE 1. Separation of immune complexes from the fraction of serum inhibitory to histamine-releasing activity. Soluble immune complexes were prepared containing ^{131}I-labeled antibody. The labeled complexes were added to normal rabbit serum and then fractionated on Sephadex G-200 at pH 8. In separate studies, the excluded, middle, and included fractions of normal rabbit serum were used in amounts of 1440, 480, and 1440 μg, respectively, to determine whether they inhibited histamine release by a dose of soluble complexes containing 1.6 μg of antibody nitrogen.

ration procedure, there was an approximately tenfold increase in sensitivity, with the result that histamine release was detectable by soluble complexes originally present in serum at a concentration of 3.2–8 μg of antibody nitrogen per milliliter.

Characterization of Other Histamine-Releasing Factors Obtained from Serum

Anaphylatoxin and antibody to γ-globulin have also been found to release histamine from the perfused guinea pig lung.[9] Since it is conceivable that either of these agents might be present in serum or synovial fluid, it was necessary to establish criteria by which they could be distinguished from soluble complexes and aggregated γ-globulin. These criteria have been published previously.[9] Anaphylatoxin differed from soluble complexes and aggregated γ-globulin in many respects; the chief distinguishing characteristics consisted of a failure of anaphylatoxin to be recovered in the excluded fraction following gel filtration on Sephadex G-200 at pH 8 and the lack of inhibition of anaphylatoxin in the presence of γ-globulin. Antibody to γ-globulin could also be differentiated from soluble complexes and aggregated γ-globulin, since it was eluted in the middle fraction obtained from Sephadex G-200 and it was inhibited by γ-globulin in a manner different from that of soluble complexes and aggregated γ-globulin.

Rheumatoid factors belonging to either the human IgM or IgG classes failed to release histamine from the perfused guinea pig lung.[9,10] This behavior was in marked contrast to a number of experimentally induced antibodies to γ-globulin which were found to be potent histamine releasers.[9] Human rheumatoid factors did not activate histamine release even when the lungs were pretreated with normal human γ-globulin. These negative findings may have resulted from an inability of the rheumatoid factor to gain access to the determinants on the γ-globulin present in the lung.

Detection of a Histamine-Releasing Factor in Human Serum and Synovial Fluid

Serum from healthy persons, and serum and synovial fluid from patients with various diseases were fractionated on Sephadex G-200. It was found that the Sephadex-excluded fraction of serum showed histamine-releasing activity in 68 out of 186 patients with rheumatoid arthritis, in four out of 20 patients with disseminated lupus erythematosus, and in one patient with anaphylactoid purpura (TABLE 2). In addition, the Sephadex-excluded fraction of synovial fluid showed histamine-releasing activity in 29 out of 40 patients with rheumatoid arthritis (TABLE 3). The histamine-releasing activity in the synovial fluid was almost invariably found to be greater than in the serum from the same patient.[10] Moreover, this activity was often not detected in serum but was shown to be present in the synovial fluid of the same patient.[11] The Sephadex middle and included fractions from all of the sera and synovial fluids tested were devoid of activity. The Sephadex-excluded fractions of specimens obtained from all of the patients with other diseases and from healthy persons failed to demonstrate histamine-releasing activity (TABLES 2 and 3). Since the histamine-releasing factor was found most frequently in patients with rheumatoid arthritis, we have named it the rheumatoid biologically active factor (RBAF).

Properties of the Rheumatoid Biologically Active Factor

Studies were carried out to characterize the RBAF present in rheumatoid sera and synovial fluids. A large number of sera and synovial fluids have been ex-

TABLE 2

HISTAMINE-RELEASING ACTIVITY IN HUMAN SERA*

	No. of Sera	
	Tested	Active
Rheumatoid arthritis	186	68
Systemic lupus erythematosus	20	4
Anaphylactoid purpura	1	1
Healthy	30	0
Ankylosing spondylitis	14	0
Charcot's joint	1	0
Degenerative joint disease	13	0
Gout	8	0
Monarticular arthritis, idiopathic	3	0
Psoriatic arthritis	6	0
Reiter's syndrome	5	0
Glomerulonephritis, acute	10	0
Hepatitis, lupoid	2	0
Polymyositis	4	0
Polyarteritis	3	0
Scleroderma	13	0
Serum sickness, horse	10	0
Sjögren's syndrome	2	0
Infectious mononucleosis	2	0
Postcardiotomy syndrome	10	0
Rheumatic fever, acute	5	0
Urticaria, chronic	4	0
Miscellaneous: anaphylactic death (penicillin), 1; Behcet's syndrome, 1; crib death, 1; erythema multiforme with arthritis, 1; erythema nodosum, 1; macroglobulinemia, 1; multiple myeloma, 1; post-myocardial infarction syndrome, 1; steatorrhoea with arthritis, 1; temporal arteritis, 1; Wegener's syndrome, 1	11	0

* A 1-ml sample of each serum was fractionated on Sephadex G-200 at pH 8. One-quarter of the excluded fraction was tested for histamine-releasing activity.

TABLE 3

HISTAMINE-RELEASING ACTIVITY IN HUMAN SYNOVIAL FLUID*

	No. of Synovial Fluids	
	Tested	Active
Rheumatoid arthritis	40	29
Ankylosing spondylitis	1	0
Degenerative joint disease	7	0
Erythema multiforme	1	0
Gout	3	0
Monarticular arthritis, idiopathic	2	0
Psoriatic arthritis	4	0

* A 1-ml sample of each synovial fluid was fractionated on Sephadex G-200 at pH 8. One-tenth of the excluded fraction was tested for histamine-releasing activity.

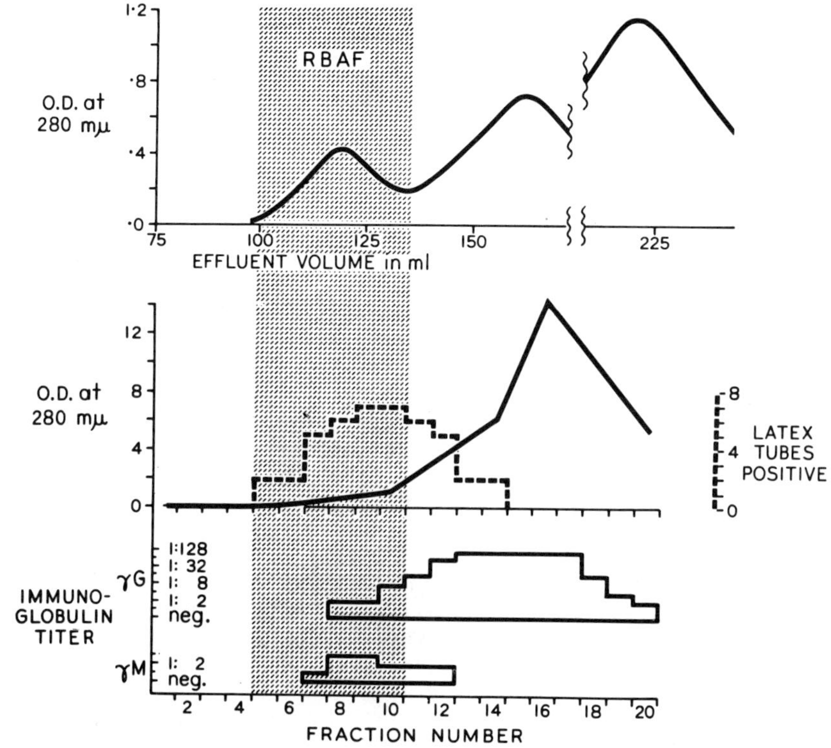

FIGURE 2. Distribution of the rheumatoid biologically active factor (RBAF) in the fractions obtained from Sephadex G-200 (top) and by sucrose-density-gradient ultracentrifugation (bottom). Gel filtration on Sephadex G-200 was performed with 0.1 M trishydroxymethylaminomethane hydrochloride (pH 8) containing 1M sodium chloride as the eluent. Gradient ultracentrifugation was performed with sucrose concentrations varying from 15 to 37%; centrifugation was carried out at 24,000 rpm for 24 hours. Distribution of protein in the effluent from Sephadex G-200 and in the sucrose-gradient fractions was determined at an optical density (O.D.) of 280.

amined, and no differences have been detected in the RBAF, which would indicate an individual specificity. The most significant characteristics of the RBAF were related to its size and to its composition as determined in absorption studies. The RBAF was always found to be associated with the high-molecular weight components of serum on the basis of chromatography on Sephadex G-200 (FIGURE 2). Similar results have been obtained by sucrose-density-gradient ultracentrifugation (FIGURE 2). With the latter method, the RBAF was found in the deeper part of the gradient in a slightly lower distribution than rheumatoid factor and IgM. However, failure to detect the RBAF at a higher level could have resulted from its spread into the lower end of the IgG distribution, which would result in inhibition of histamine-releasing activity.

Absorption studies were performed to determine whether the RBAF contained immunoglobulin. Separate aliquots of rheumatoid sera and synovial fluids containing the RBAF were absorbed at equivalence with goat anti-human IgG, anti-IgA, and anti-IgM. The supernatants were tested for residual histamine-

TABLE 4

ABSORPTION OF HISTAMINE-RELEASING ACTIVITY FROM SERUM AND SYNOVIAL FLUID BY ANTISERUM SPECIFIC FOR HUMAN IMMUNOGLOBULIN CLASSES*

Precipitation at Equivalence with Goat Antiserum	Residual Histamine-Releasing Activity (%)		
	Serum A.J.	Serum A.C.	Synovial Fluid J.C.
Anti-human IgA	94	64	100
Anti-human IgG	0	0	0
Anti-human IgM	100	91	100

* The Sephadex-excluded fractions from RBAF-positive sera and synovial fluids were precipitated at equivalence in separate studies using goat anti-human IgA, anti-IgG, and anti-IgM. The absorbed supernatants were then refractionated on Sephadex G-200, and the residual histamine-releasing activity was determined by comparison with an unabsorbed control. The unabsorbed control was treated in the same manner, except for the addition of a volume of normal goat serum equal to that of the immune goat serum used in the absorbed sample.

releasing activity. The RBAF was completely absorbed by anti-IgG but not by the other antisera (TABLE 4). Similar results were obtained with sera and synovial fluids from a number of different patients.[10] It was concluded that the RBAF was an aggregate, since it contained IgG but behaved as a larger molecule than IgG when examined by Sephadex G-200 and density-gradient ultracentrifugation. Therefore, the RBAF appeared to be either an aggregate of IgG or an aggregate containing IgG plus an unidentified component.

The properties of the RBAF were compared with those of soluble immune complexes and aggregated γ-globulin (TABLE 5). All three reagents were found to be identical in a number of respects, including failure to pass through a dialysis membrane, elution in the excluded fraction from Sephadex G-200 at pH 8, insolubility in 50% saturated ammonium sulfate, and failure to contract the guinea pig ileum. In addition, the histamine-releasing activity of all three was inhibited in the presence of excess γ-globulin or in the absence of calcium. All

TABLE 5

CHARACTERISTICS OF SOLUBLE IMMUNE COMPLEXES, HEAT-AGGREGATED γ-GLOBULIN AND THE RHEUMATOID BIOLOGICALLY ACTIVE FACTOR*

	Soluble Complexes	Aggregated γ-Globulin	RBAF
Dialyzability	0	0	0
50% saturated $(NH_4)_2SO_4$	insoluble	insoluble	insoluble
Sephadex G-200 at pH 8	excluded	excluded	excluded
Ileum contraction	0	0	0
Influence on histamine release			
Excess γ-globulin	inhibiiton	inhibition	inhibition
Calcium lack	inhibition	inhibition	inhibition
0.5 mM succinate	enhancement	enhancement	enhancement
Treatment of lung			
With 0.4 mM idioacetate	inhibition	inhibition	inhibition
With heating to 45° C	inhibition	inhibition	inhibition
Sephadex G-200 at pH 3	excluded + middle fraction	excluded fraction	excluded + middle fraction
Reduction-alkylation	stable	part labile	stable
Freezing	stable	labile	stable
Dialysis at pH 3	stable	stable	part labile

* Soluble immune complexes were prepared from hyperimmune rabbit antibody to bovine plasma albumin. Heat-aggregated γ-globulin was prepared from human Cohn fraction II.

were enhanced in the presence of 0.5 mM succinate, and irreversible inhibition was seen when the lungs were pretreated with 0.4 mM iodoacetate or with heating to 45° C.

The RBAF was similar to immune complexes but differed from aggregated γ-globulin in three respects: The aggregated γ-globulin showed no tendency to dissociate when fractionated on Sephadex G-200 at pH 3, was partially inactivated by reduction and alkylation, and was unstable to freezing. The RBAF and immune complexes were both stable to freezing and to reduction and alkylation, and both showed a tendency to become partially dissociated when passed through Sephadex G-200 at pH 3. However, the RBAF was unique in that it underwent a marked reduction in activity when merely dialyzed at pH 3 and was then restored to pH 7.4; the other agents were stable to the same treatment.

In summary, the RBAF differed from aggregated γ-globulin in several aspects but was similar to soluble complexes in all but one respect. The findings were most consistent with the interpretation that RBAF is a soluble immune complex containing an unidentified acid-labile or dialyzable antigen.

Correlation of the Rheumatoid Biologically Active Factor with Clinical and Laboratory Features of Rheumatoid Arthritis

A total of 127 patients with definite or classical rheumatoid arthritis were assessed in order to determine the relationship between the presence or absence of the RBAF and various clinical and laboratory features of this disease. A detailed description of the study has been published.[11] Some of the more outstanding features of the RBAF-positive and RBAF-negative groups are shown in TABLE 6. It was found that the sera were RBAF-positive in 38 patients and RBAF-negative in 89 patients. The RBAF-positive group exhibited a more severe form of rheumatoid disease, as manifested by a lower grip strength, more advanced x-ray changes, and a higher prevalence of extraarticular features. On the other hand, there was no correlation between presence of the RBAF and the level of existing inflammatory activity, as judged by the articular index method of Lansbury[26] and by the erythrocyte sedimentation rate. Both groups were also similar with respect to the mean titer of rheumatoid factor, as measured by the

TABLE 6

CLINICAL FEATURES OF RHEUMATOID PATIENTS WITH OR WITHOUT THE RHEUMATOID BIOLOGICALLY ACTIVE FACTOR IN THEIR SERA*

	RBAF Positive	RBAF Negative	p value
No. of cases	38	89	
Grip strength (mm Hg)	85	109	0.04
X-Ray stage II + III + IV	95%	75%	0.02
Extraarticular features	89%	67%	0.02
Articular index	68	63	0.62
Erythrocyte sedimentation rate	61	65	0.43
Latex titer (log reciprocal)	3.41	3.38	0.88

* X-Rays of the hands and feet were staged according to the method proposed by the Department of Rheumatology, University of Manchester, Manchester, England, in the Atlas of Standard Radiographs of Arthritis (1963). Extraarticular features included one or more of the following: rheumatoid nodules, splenomegaly, lymph node enlargement, episcleritis, digital vasculitis, skin ulceration, pericarditis, pulmonary fibrosis, and noncompressive neuropathy. The articular index was estimated according to the method of Lansbury.[26]

agglutination of latex particles coated with γ-globulin. These patients are being reassessed in an ongoing study.

Discussion

The present studies have shown that the isolated perfused guinea pig lung could be used successfully in a biological assay to demonstrate the presence of soluble immune complexes and aggregated γ-globulin in serum. The system was extremely sensitive in detecting low concentrations of these reagents in serum, especially when the mixture was first subjected to chromatography on Sephadex G-200. In addition, by using a number of simple tests of specificity, it was possible to distinguish immune complexes and aggregated γ-globulin from other biologically active factors which might be present in human serum. Finally, the bioassay offered the advantage of enabling soluble complexes to be detected even though the identity of the antigen was not known.

The feasibility of using the bioassay to detect soluble complexes formed *in vivo* was shown by a study in which rabbits were injected with fluorescein-labeled bovine plasma albumin.[13] During the stage of immune antigen elimination, a portion of the labeled antigen was present in the ammonium sulfate precipitate fraction of the serum, indicating the presence of soluble complexes. At the same time, a histamine-releasing factor could be detected in the Sephadex-excluded fraction of the serum. The histamine-releasing factor was shown to have the properties of soluble immune complexes. Therefore, the bioassay was successful in detecting soluble complexes formed *in vivo* under circumstances where the complexes were also demonstrable by means of an independent method.

It is known that only human antibody of the IgG-globulin class has the capacity to liberate histamine from guinea pig tissue.[14,15] Therefore, this immunoglobulin must be a part of any soluble complex of human origin if the complex is to be demonstrated by the bioassay. This fact may be responsible for our inability to detect soluble complexes during the course of human serum sickness and acute post-streptococcal glomerulonephritis, two diseases in which complexes are believed to play an important role. Immune complexes containing a class of immunoglobulin other than IgG might be present during these diseases, but would not be detected by the bioassay.

Rheumatoid sera and synovial fluid have been shown to contain a number of different immunoglobulin complexes, and it was therefore of interest to determine whether the RBAF was similar to one of these. A 22S complex containing IgM rheumatoid factor and IgG as antigen has been demonstrated by analytical ultracentrifugation of rheumatoid serum.[1] The RBAF appeared to differ from this complex since some sera which contained the RBAF did not contain these high-molecular weight complexes, and vice versa.[10]

A similar complex composed of IgM rheumatoid factor and IgG as antigen has been demonstrated by immunological methods in rheumatoid serum by Allen and Kunkel,[16] and in rheumatoid synovial fluid by Hannestad.[17,18] The presence of IgM rheumatoid factor in the RBAF was excluded by the finding that the RBAF was stable to reduction and alkylation and could not be absorbed by goat anti-human IgM. Therefore, the RBAF appeared to differ from this type of aggregate.

A second type of complex, containing IgG rheumatoid factor and IgG as antigen, has been demonstrated in rheumatoid serum and synovial fluid by analytical ultracentrifugation.[2,19,20] It appeared unlikely that this complex represented the RBAF since it sedimented on ultracentrifugation at a point intermediate between IgG and IgM. Also, the RBAF was labile to dialysis at pH 3, while the intermediate-sedimenting complex would presumably be stable to the same treatment. A further distinguishing characteristic was the presence in the intermediate complex of rheumatoid factor activity that was stable to reduction and alkylation.[19] However, samples containing the RBAF were shown to lose all rheumatoid factor activity upon reduction and alkylation without loss of histamine-releasing activity.[10] Finally, one rheumatoid serum that contained large amounts of intermediate complex did not contain the RBAF.[10] Therefore, it appeared unlikely that the RBAF was a complex of IgG rheumatoid factor and IgG.

It has been noted previously that some rheumatoid factors possess specificity for soluble immune complexes. Since the RBAF demonstrated the biological, biochemical, and immunological properties of an immune complex, the possibility was considered that it was the antigen of either an IgM or IgG rheumatoid factor. This represents a third type of complex in which rheumatoid factor might be a component. Our failure to absorb the RBAF with anti-IgM might at first suggest that IgM rheumatoid factor is not present in the RBAF. However, this finding could be explained on the basis that a subfraction of IgM rheumatoid factor possessed antibody specificity for the RBAF, and the RBAF was detectable only under conditions of antigen or RBAF excess. In the presence of RBAF excess, the amount of histamine-releasing activity which could be precipitated by anti-IgM would be less than 100%. The design used in the absorption studies to measure loss of histamine-releasing activity was relatively crude and could likely have detected only a large fractional loss. This explanation indicates that a clear answer cannot be given to the question of whether the RBAF is the antigen of an IgM rheumatoid factor. It also remains unresolved whether the RBAF may be the antigen of an IgG rheumatoid factor.

Finally, a fourth type of complex has been described by Marcus and co-workers in rheumatoid synovial fluid.[21,22] This factor contained IgG and DNA and possessed anticomplementary activity. However, it was, to a major extent, cryoprecipitable while the RBAF was not cryoprecipitable. We cannot exclude the possibility that the RBAF represented the portion of this factor which did not precipitate in the cold.

The RBAF is a histamine releaser in the guinea pig lung, and the question whether it is also a histamine releaser in humans is obvious. This question is of considerable importance, since Knicker and Cochrane have shown that the release of vasoactive amines is the initial step in the mechanism of tissue injury by soluble immune complexes.[23] The process activated by the RBAF in the guinea pig lung exhibits the characteristics of anaphylactic histamine release.[24] However, it might be presumed that the RBAF could not activate the same mechanism in humans since only IgE antibodies appear to have this capacity.[25] We have no direct indication that the RBAF contains IgE, and we have found that the RBAF is stable to heating at 56° C for four hours, indirectly suggesting that IgE is not an important component. On the other hand, the RBAF might activate histamine release in humans by a different pathway, such as by complement activation and the generation of anaphylatoxin. Studies are in progress to determine whether the RBAF has the potential to fix complement.

Persons who possessed the RBAF in their serum exhibited a more severe form of rheumatoid disease.[11] This correlation suggested that the RBAF was instrumental in the genesis of the rheumatoid process. However, it was equally possible that the RBAF was a product of severe disease.

Summary

The foregoing studies have defined a factor resembling a soluble antigen-antibody complex present in one-third of rheumatoid sera and in three-quarters of rheumatoid synovial fluids. This factor differed from most other agents identified in rheumatoid serum and synovial fluid. Patients exhibiting the RBAF in their serum suffered from a more severe form of rheumatoid disease than patients in whom the factor was not demonstrable. However, it is not yet clear whether this factor contributes to the genesis of rheumatoid disease or is a byproduct of the disease process.

Acknowledgments

We are grateful to Miss Sheila Bond and to Miss Christine Lawlor for their invaluable technical assistance.

References

1. Franklin, E .C., H. R. Holman, H. J. Müller-Eberhard & H. G. Kunkel. 1957. An unusual protein component of high molecular weight in the serum of certain patients with rheumatoid arthritis. J. Exp. Med. **105:** 425.
2. Kunkel, H. G., H. J. Müller-Eberhard, H. H. Fudenberg & T. B. Tomasi, Jr. 1961. Gamma globulin complexes in rheumatoid arthritis and certain other conditions. J. Clin. Invest. **40:** 117.
3. Osterland, C. K., M. Harboe & H. G. Kunkel. 1962. Rheumatoid factors (7S and 19S types) reacting with different portions of the gamma globulin molecule. Arthritis Rheum. **5:** 312.
4. Butler, Jr., V. P. & J. H. Vaughan. 1965. The reaction of rheumatoid factor with animal gamma globulins. Immunology **8:** 144.
5. Heimer, R. & F. M. Levin. 1966. On the distribution of rheumatoid factors among the immunoglobulins. Immunochemistry **3:** 1.
6. Edelman, G. M., H. G. Kunkel & E. C. Franklin. 1958. Interaction of the rheumatoid factor with antigen-antibody complexes and aggregated gamma globulin. J. Exp. Med. **108:** 105.
7. Henney, C. S. & D. R. Stanworth. 1965. The reactivity of rheumatoid factor with human gamma G globulin. Immunology **9:** 139.
8. Baumal, R. & I. Broder. 1968. Studies into the occurrence of soluble antigen-antibody complexes in disease. I. A biological assay for soluble complexes. Clin. Exp. Immunol. **3:** 525.
9. Broder, I., R. Baumal & E. Keystone. 1968. Studies into the occurrence of soluble antigen-antibody complexes in disease. II. Criteria for distinguishing soluble complexes from other macromolecular histamine releasers. Clin. Exp. Immunol. **3:** 537.
10. Baumal, R. & I. Broder. 1968. Studies into the occurrence of soluble antigen-antibody complexes in disease. III. Rheumatoid arthritis and other human diseases. Clin. Exp. Immunol. **3:** 555.
11. Gordon, D. A., D. A. Bell, R. Baumal & I. Broder. 1969. Studies into the occurrence of soluble antigen-antibody complexes in disease. IV. Correlation between the rheumatoid biologically active factor (RBAF) and the clinical features of rheumatoid arthritis. Clin. Exp. Immunol. **5:** 57.
12. Broder, I. & H. O. Schild. 1965. Action of soluble antigen-antibody complexes in perfused guinea-pig lung. Immunology **8:** 300.
13. Baumal, R., I. Broder, D. A. Bell, D. A. Gordon & E .C. Keystone. 1968. An approach to the study of soluble antigen-antibody complexes in clinical disease. Univ. Mich. Med. J. **34:** 30.
14. Buckley, R. H. & R. S. Metzgar. 1966. Reactivity of human IgG antibodies in primate and guinea pig passive anaphylaxis. Int. Arch. Allerg. **29:** 485.
15. Terry, W. D. 1965. Skin-sensitizing activity related to γ-polypeptide chain characteristics of human IgG. J. Immunol. **95:** 1041.
16. Allen, J. C. & H. G. Kunkel. 1966. Hidden rheumatoid factors with specificity for native gamma globulins. Arthritis Rheum. **9:** 758.
17. Hannestad, K. 1967. Presence of aggregated γ-globulin in certain rheumatoid synovial effusions. Clin. Exp. Immunol. **2:** 511.

18. HANNESTAD, K. 1968. Rheumatoid factors reacting with autologous native γG aggregates. Clin. Exp. Immunol. **3:** 671.
19. CHODIRKER, W. B. & T. B. TOMASI, JR. 1963. Low-molecular-weight rheumatoid factor. J. Clin. Invest. **42:** 876.
20. WINCHESTER, R. & H. G. KUNKEL. 1968. High molecular weight complexes involving γ-globulin in joint fluids from rheumatoid arthritis patients. Arthritis Rheum. **11:** 849.
21. MARCUS, R. L. & A. S. TOWNES. 1968. Identification of single-stranded (heat-denatured) DNA as an antigenic determinant in the complement-fixing activity of rheumatoid synovial fluid. Arthritis Rheum. **11:** 497.
22. THOMAS, A. S., C. R. STEWART, JR. & R. L. MARCUS. 1966. Anticomplementary activity of rheumatoid synovial fluid. Arthritis Rheum. **9:** 878.
23. KNICKER, W. T. & C. G. COCHRANE. 1968. The localization of circulating immune complexes in experimental serum sickness. The role of vasoactive amines and hydrodynamic forces. J. Exp. Med. **127:** 119.
24. BAUMAL, R. & I. BRODER. 1969. In preparation.
25. ISHIZAKA, K., T. ISHIZAKA & M. M. HORNBROOK. 1966. Physicochemical properties of reaginic antibody. V. Correlation of reaginic activity with γ-E globulin antibody. J. Immunol. **97:** 840.
26. LANSBURY, J. 1966. Methods for evaluating rheumatoid arthritis. *In* Arthritis and Allied Conditions. J. L. Hollander, Ed. : 269. Lea & Febiger. Philadelphia, Pa.

DISCUSSION OF THE PAPER

DR. EPSTEIN: Dr. Broder's closing statement is, of course, an exact duplicate of a description of rheumatoid factor when the least sensitive systems were available. The specificity of the test for the disease is exactly as we knew it when we used the sensitized-sheep cell test.

DR. WILLIAMS: Recently, we studied some rheumatoid lungs by immunofluorescence and were impressed with the large amounts of γG in some of these specimens. Could you elute this material from guinea pig lung?

DR. BRODER: We have not tried this. I think it presents very great difficulties. Also, the assumption has to be made that the material stays in the lung after it activates histamine release. In other work, using known preparations of soluble labeled immune complexes, we have shown that virtually all of the reagent appears in the eluate from the lung within several minutes of the injection and activation of the histamine release. I think if one attempted to elute these lungs, one would elute many other endogenous guinea pig proteins.

DR. VAUGHAN: I don't think one ought to rule out the possibility that your RBAF is simply an intermediate complex of the γG anti-γG variety. If I recall correctly, your major evidence against the idea that these complexes are responsible for the histamine-release phenomenon is your ultracentrifugation data, in which complexes can be seen in varying quantities that don't correspond to your histamine-releasing capability. We ought to remember that intermediate complexes can also be caused by IgA anti-γG or IgG anti-γG. We must also remember that there are subclasses of γG. molecules which have different biological capabilities.

It is certainly true that when you examine rheumatoid arthritis sera of high titer by sensitive techniques, essentially all of them have intermediate complexes. We also commonly see IgG being brought down into the 19S region by complexing with anti-γ-globulins. I'm quite sure that the IgG variety of anti-γG-globulin can bring them down into the 19S area as easily as can the 19S molecule itself. Thus, I don't think your failure to see histamine release from your Sephadex column fractions in the intermediate area is convincing. There is enough free IgG in that area to be internally inhibiting to the system.

DR. BRODER: I agree in general with the point that you are making, and we have noted this ourselves. We don't feel that we have excluded entirely the possibility that these are complexes of IgG rheumatoid factor and IgG. However, all of the attempts we've made to demonstrate that they might be this type of complex have been negative.

DR. VAUGHAN: You are inclined to define rheumatoid factor as simply the 19S component. I think that most of us would also like to think of IgG anti-γ-globulin as rheumatoid factor.

DR. LITWIN: Can you set up an *in vitro* system using soluble complexes produced between γG rheumatoid factors and γG-globulin which would resemble closely the activity that you're measuring in your system?

DR. BRODER: I think this could be done. We haven't done it.

DR. EPSTEIN: You have some preparations in which the G-200-excluded fraction of rheumatoid serum doesn't release histamine. Can you activate such a nonreactive G-200-excluded fraction by the addition of aggregated γ-globulin? Do you have any techniques by which you can make such an inactive excluded fraction active? Have you tested these preparations on uterine strips from estrogen-treated rats for kinin activity?

DR. BRODER: We have not tested our histamine-releasing fractions for kinin activity, and we have not generated activity in fractions that ordinarily are inactive. We haven't made any effort to do this.

DR. ZVAIFLER: I noted that the sera of only four of 20 systemic lupus patients were positive for this activity. Is there any correlation in this group with the presence or absence of rheumatoid factor activity?

DR. BRODER: These were just sera of diseased people. To date, we have not made a careful study of any of the other disease groups, other than the rheumatoid arthritis group. We are in the process of initiating a careful study of lupus. I can't answer your question at the present time, but I can say that we have seen rheumatoid sera that have been latex test-negative and yet have shown this histamine-releasing activity.

DR. AUSTEN: These are very nice data, and I think that there is support for the idea that this biological activity does represent human IgG. But I think it is worth noting that in all likelihood in this system the mast cells are being directly sensitized. With guinea pig immunoglobulin, this is done only by the immunoglobulin of the γ_1 class, which is heat stable. If you then turn to the heterologous system, it is done by either rabbit γ_2 or human IgG.

If you sensitize first with antibody and then challenge with antigen, you can accomplish this effect with guinea pig γ_1 or with the heterologous rabbit γ_2 or human γ_2. If you then challenge with antigen, the various mediators are released. This can be showed nicely either with the perfused organ system that Dr. Broder mentioned or with lung slices.

In a previous report you had not yet been able to make this factor or the complexes work with lung slices. At that time, it still required the whole organ system. Now that you have removed the competing γ-globulin, is it now possible to make the assay work with the more reproducible lung slices?

DR. BRODER: I'm not sure I'd leave unchallenged your last sentence that the lung slices are more reproducible. At any rate, using crystalline antigen and complexes that are prepared from the equivalence precipitate resolubilized, in excess crystalline antigen, we have been repeatedly unsuccessful in stimulating histamine release from chopped guinea pig lung. There is a peculiar requirement in activating histamine release by immune complexes in guinea pig tissue that the complex be administered by the vascular route. We are very puzzled by this, but it's very definite. Even if one perfuses the guinea pig lung exhaustively before one chops it to exclude the possibility that there is very much residual endogeneous γ_1-globulin, the outcome is still the same. It would appear that the ileum shows the same peculiarity. With a given antigen-antibody system, we can passively sensitize chopped lung or guinea pig ileum for later responsiveness to antigen given separately, but with the same antigen-antibody system in the form of a purified, soluble-immune complex, there is no activation when the complexes have to come in from the outside. If you administer them by an inside route, such as the vascular route, then they are extremely active. As far as we can determine, it seems to be identical to the mechanism of the so-called anaphylactic histamine release. I don't think we are dealing with the activation of an anaphylotoxin in the guinea pig tissue.

DR. VAUGHAN: Your comment on the reactivity of the Sephadex fractions from seronegative rheumatoid arthritics is very important. Rarely, the sera of patients may behave as seronegative in whole serum, but become seropositive when you isolate the fractions. This is another example of the problem of internal inhibition by the free γG-globulins in the system. Have you done latex tests on the active fractions from seronegative patients? And in that instance, are they latex-positive or are they latex-negative? Also, how many times have you seen this?

DR. BRODER: We've seen this more than once, but I don't think we've seen it more than four or six times. I can't recall the exact figure. We have not taken the fractions from a seronegative serum to check the fractions, but we have taken the excluded fractions with the histamine-releasing activity and reduced and alkylated them; there was absolutely no detectable latex-agglutinating activity after reduction and alkylation. The histamine-releasing activity was absolutely unchanged.

DR. MAUER (*Albany, N. Y.*): Have you had the opportunity to check out your RBAF in the presence of an antihistamine or a histamine depleter with the possibility that the RBAF may be working on *de novo* synthesis of histamine?

DR. BRODER: We were becoming interested in whether there is *de novo* synthesis of histamine in this histamine-releasing system. We have some preliminary information that might suggest that there is some *de novo* synthesis, but I can't give a definite answer to that.

IN VIVO INTERACTIONS OF ANTIGLOBULIN FACTORS

R. T. Schultz, M.D., K. Kano, M.D., and F. Milgrom, M.D.
Department of Microbiology, School of Medicine
State University of New York at Buffalo
Buffalo, N. Y.

The possibility that the antigenic structure of an antibody molecule may undergo alteration as a result of combination of the antibody with its antigen was considered during the course of previous studies of a factor in normal human and rabbit sera which was called anti-antibody.[1,2] Subsequent studies revealed that immunization of rabbits with autologous γ-globulin or autologous alum-precipitated serum resulted in the formation of antibodies that were strongly reactive with the immunoglobulins of some other species but were not reactive with the immunoglobulins of the antibody producer or of other rabbits.[3] It seemed likely, in view of these and other findings, that the occurrence of antiglobulin factors in various human diseases might be explained on the basis of chronic antigenic stimulation leading to the formation of immune complexes and subsequent denaturation of antibody molecules in such a way that they became antigenic. The demonstration of a high incidence of antiglobulin factors in patients with subacute bacterial endocarditis provided good support for this possibility.[4] Also, it has been shown in a number of animal experiments that chronic antigenic stimulation may lead to the formation of these factors.[5-7] In our most recent experiments, the study of the occurrence of antiglobulin factors in the sera of patients who have received a renal allograft has provided data that confirm and extend some of the foregoing observations.

Waller and co-workers[8] were the first to report the occurrence of antiglobulin factors following renal allotransplantation, and their findings have been confirmed by others.[9,10] Between 70 and 90% of patients who have received a renal allograft have shown antiglobulin factors reactive with human immunoglobulins. The incidence of antiglobulin factors reactive with rabbit immunoglobulins has been somewhat lower. The antiglobulin activity usually appeared within three to eight weeks after transplantation.

Studies by means of the technique of mixed agglutination with cell cultures have shown that many patients who receive a renal allograft form antibodies which react with cell surface isoantigens of human tissues.[11] These antibodies are not demonstrable in the patient's serum while the graft is in place and functioning, but are often easily demonstrated after the graft has been rejected and/or removed (TABLE 1). In our experiments, cell culture monolayers of HEp2 cells were used to demonstrate the antibodies to cell surfaces. Sera taken while the grafts were in place showed no antibodies; after the grafts were rejected and/or removed, however, antibodies were demonstrable in high titers in many sera. That these antibodies react with the cell surface antigens of the grafts *in vivo* has been confirmed by the demonstration of antibodies in eluates prepared from the grafted kidneys following their removal (TABLE 2). In this experiment, all of the grafted kidneys had been removed following chronic rejection, and eluates from all of them showed antibodies to cell surface isoantigens. None of the eluates from normal kidneys gave positive results. It would seem very likely, on the basis of these experiments and of experiments in animals with renal allografts,[12] that the antibodies are not demonstrable in the serum while a graft is in place and functioning because under these circumstances the antibodies are continually being absorbed by the graft.

TABLE 1

MIXED AGGLUTION TEST WITH HEp2 CELL CULTURES AND SERA OF SEVEN RECIPIENTS OF RENAL HOMOGRAFTS*

Patient No.	Graft	Reciprocal Titer of Reaction with Serum Samples Tested			
		Before Transplantation	During Normal Function	During Rejection	After Removal of the Graft
1	1st	<30	<30	<30	810
	2nd	810	<30	<30	—
2	1st	<30	<30	810	2,430
	2nd	2,430	—	810	—
3	1st	<30	<30	270	2,430
4	1st	—	—	<30	270
5	1st	<30	<30	<30	<30
	2nd	<30	<30	<30	7,290
6	1st	<30	<30	<30	<30
	2nd	<30	<30	—	—
7	1st	<30	<30	<30	<30
	2nd	<30	<30	<30	<30

* From Williams *et al.*[11] Reproduced, with minor modifications, by permission of the Journal of the American Medical Association.

TABLE 2

MIXED AGGLUTINATION TESTS WITH HEp2 CELL CULTURES AND ELUATES OBTAINED FROM FIVE REJECTED RENAL GRAFTS*

Dilution of Eluate†	Eluates of Grafts Removed from Patients‡					Eluates of Five Normal Human Kidneys
	No. 1	No. 3	No. 4	No. 5	No. 7	
1:1	3+	1+	3+	3+	3+	—
1:3	3+	3+	3+	3+	3+	—
1:9	3+	3+	3+	1+	3+	—
1:27	3+	1+	3+	—	2+	—
1:81	2+	—	—	—	—	—
1:243	±	—	—	—	—	—
Diluent	—	—	—	—	—	—

* From Williams *et al.*[11] Reproduced by permission of the Journal of the American Medical Association.

† Protein concentration of eluates was adjusted to 1 mg/ml.

‡ Patient number as in TABLE 1.

TABLE 3

DISPERSION OF AGGLUTINATION OF EH*: EFFECT OF PRE-TRANSPLANTATION SERA ON AGGLUTINATES FORMED BY POST-TRANSPLANTATION SERA†

EH* Agglutinated by Transplantation Sera	Reciprocal Titer of Dispersion							
	Pre-Transplantation Sera					Normal Human Sera		4% Human Fraction II
	N.C.	W.W.	W.E.	W.B.	D.N.	K.J.	K.E.	
N.C.	2	8	4	8	<2	2	4	128
W.W.	8	<2	8	<2	8	16	<2	64
W.E.	16	8	<2	4	2	16	<2	256
W.B.	8	<2	<2	<2	4	8	<2	64
D.N.	<2	4	8	8	<2	8	2	128

* Human O-type Rh-positive erythrocytes sensitized by anti-Rh serum Ripley.

† From Kano and Milgrom.[10] Reproduced by permission from Transplantation.

The occurrence of antiglobulin factors in post-transplantation sera provided an excellent opportunity to test for auto- or isoreactivity of such factors, since in most instances the corresponding pre-transplantation sera were also available for testing. For these studies,[10] the technique of dispersion of agglutination was employed. The patient's pre-transplantation serum was compared with other human sera in regard to its ability to disperse the agglutination of sensitized-human erythrocytes when this agglutination was caused by the patient's own post-transplantation antiglobulin factors. The results are shown in TABLE 3. Results of tests in which the pre- and post-transplantation sera were from the same patient fall along the diagonal line formed by the numbers that are italicized in TABLE 3. Quite apparently, none of the antiglobulin factors in these post-transplantation sera combined with the patient's own pre-transplantation serum, whereas they did react with some other human sera and with fraction II of pooled human serum.

Thus, it would appear that in human renal allotransplantation the histocompatibility antigens of the graft serve as a chronic antigenic stimulus, leading first to the formation of antibodies to these antigens and later to the formation of antiglobulin factors that are more reactive with immunoglobulins in some other human sera than in the patient's own serum. This is similar to what occurs in other conditions in which antiglobulin factors are formed, and suggests that formation of these factors is a common response of man and animals to chronic antigenic stimulation.

Experiments have also been performed which showed that the antiglobulin factors formed following renal transplantation may become fixed to the graft *in vivo*.[13] The procedure of mixed agglutination with tissue sections, which was used for these experiments, may be briefly described as follows: A section of the tissue being tested is mounted on a cover slip and washed in saline. A suspension of human Rh-positive erythrocytes sensitized with incomplete Rh antibody is placed in the concavity of a microculture slide. The cover slip is then placed over the concavity in such a way that the tissue section is immersed in the erythrocyte suspension. The edges of the cover slip are sealed with Vaseline®, and the slide is inverted so that the sensitized erythrocytes settle onto the tissue

TABLE 4

SUMMARY OF STUDIES ON ANTIBODIES BOUND TO ELEVEN RENAL GRAFTS*

Patient Graft	Clinical Status of Graft	Binding of EH† by Tissue Section	Antibodies in Eluates‡ Against Human Cell Cultures	Antibodies in Eluates‡ Against EH†
B.L.	Chronic rejection	+++	+	+
Y.E.	Chronic rejection	+++	+	+
B.C.	Chronic rejection	+++	+	+
M.D.	Acute rejection	+++	+	+
W.B.	Chronic rejection	+++	—	—
S.D.	Good function	+++	+	+
H.P.	Good function	+	+	+
S.G.	Acute rejection	+	+	+
S.S.	Acute rejection	+	+	—
W.W.	Chronic rejection	+	—	—
R.E.	Chronic rejection	+	+	+

* From Kano and Milgrom.[10] Reproduced by permission from Transplantation.
† Human O-type Rh-positive erythrocytes sensitized by anti-Rh serum Ripley.
‡ Protein concentration of eluates was adjusted to 1.0 mg/ml.

section. After a suitable period of incubation, the slide is turned over, and the erythrocytes are allowed to settle to the bottom of the concavity. The slide is then examined under a microscope. Significant numbers of sensitized erythrocytes remaining adherent to the tissue section indicate a positive result, which can be graded according to the degree to which the tissue section is covered by the erythrocytes. Control experiments were performed with a variety of normal and pathological renal tissues, including some from patients with seropositive rheumatoid arthritis.

Eleven of 26 kidney grafts gave positive results when tested by this procedure, and all control tissues gave negative results. The results with the 11 positive specimens are summarized in TABLE 4. Five of seven grafts that were removed following chronic rejection gave strongly positive results, and the remaining two grafts gave weakly positive results. Two grafts that were removed during acute rejection gave weakly positive results, and, of two grafts obtained after the patients had died from other causes but which were still functioning normally just prior to death, one was strongly positive and the other weakly positive. The finding of the antiglobulin factor in the tissues of two well-functioning grafts would suggest that fixation of the factor in tissues may have no pathogenic role, but of course this finding in only two cases does not permit any conclusion. The results of testing of the eluates of these grafts for antibodies to cell surface antigens and for antibodies to human erythrocytes coated with incomplete Rh antibody are also summarized in TABLE 4.

What role these antiglobulin factors may play in the various conditions in which they occur is not at all clear. In our previous experiments, some rabbits that were immunized intravenously with autologous γ-globulin not only formed antiglobulin factors but also developed rather extensive cardiac lesions.[14] The early lesions appeared similar in some respects to those of rheumatic fever. They were focal, subendocardial, and valvular, and were characterized by edema and infiltration with inflammatory cells. The more chronic lesions had many of the characteristics of rheumatoid granulomata. Whether these lesions could be attributed to the altered γ-globulin in the preparations that were injected or to altered γ-globulin in complex with the antiglobulin factors is not certain.

On the other hand, some evidence has appeared that antiglobulin factors may compete with the complement system for reaction with γ-globulin aggregates.

TABLE 5

EFFECT OF SELECTED RHEUMATOID ARTHRITIS AND NORMAL HUMAN SERA ON THE ANTICOMPLEMENTARY TITER OF HEAT-AGGREGATED HUMAN FACTION II*

Serum†	Degree of Complement Fixation by Heat-Aggregated Human F II‡						
	1:1	1:2	1:4	1:8	1:16	1:32	1:64
Buffer	4+	4+	4+	4+	2+	2+	—
RA (E.W.), 1:5	—	—	—	—	—	—	—
RA (M.P.), 1:5	4+	—	—	—	—	—	—
NH (K.W.), 1:5	4+	4+	4+	4+	2+	2+	—
NH (J.S.), 1:5	4+	4+	4+	4+	4+	2+	2+

* From Milgrom and Schultz.[16] Reproduced by permission of the International Archives of Allergy.

† RA = rheumatoid arthritis serum; NH = normal human serum.

‡ Initial concentration of fraction II was 0.25%. Scale: 4+ = no hemolysis of sensitized-sheep erythrocytes that were added to reaction mixture to measure residual complement activity; 2+ = partial hemolysis of subsequently added sheep erythrocytes; — = complete hemolysis of subsequently added sheep erythrocytes.

Studies performed by Heimer and co-workers[15] and in this laboratory[16] have shown that rheumatoid factors, if allowed to prereact with aggregated γ-globulin, inhibit the subsequent fixation of guinea pig complement by the aggregates. An example of one of our experiments is shown in TABLE 5. As shown, seral twofold dilutions of heat-aggregated fraction II had an anticomplementary titer extending out to six tubes. However, when these dilutions of aggregated fraction II were preincubated with a rheumatoid serum at a dilution of 1:5, a marked reduction in titer was noted. The degree of reduction of the titer correlated well with the amount of rheumatoid factor in the serum being tested. Normal serum either did not affect the anticomplementary titer or else increased it slightly. Inhibition of anticomplementariness was not as striking if human or rabbit complement was substituted for guinea pig complement.

The results of studies such as this are difficult to interpret, because the extent to which the phenomena observed *in vitro* are duplicated *in vivo* is uncertain. However, fixation of complement in tissue spaces is often associated with acute inflammation. It is possible that if γ-globulin aggregates are formed or deposited in tissue spaces and antiglobulin factors are also present, competition of the antiglobulin factors with the complement system for reaction with the aggregates might reduce and modify the severity of the resulting inflammatory reaction. In human renal allotransplantation, the antiglobulin factors that have been demonstrated within the grafted tissues may be blocking the cytotoxic effect of the IgG transplantation antibodies.

References

1. MILGROM, F., S. DUBISKI & G. WOZNICZKO. 1956. Human sera with anti-antibody. Vox Sang. **1**: 172.
2. MILGROM, F. 1962. Rabbit sera with "anti-antibody." Vox Sang. **7**: 545.
3. MILGROM, F. & E. WITEBSKY. 1960. Studies on the rheumatoid and related serum factors. I. Autoimmunization of rabbits with gamma globulin. J.A.M.A. **174**: 56.
4. WITEBSKY, E. & F. MILGROM. 1960. Immunological research in rheumatic disease. Presented at the Annual Meeting of the Amer. Rheum. Assoc., Hollywood-by-the-Sea, Florida, June, 1960.
5. MILGROM, F. & S. DUBISKI. 1957. Antigenicity of antibodies of the same species. Nature **179**: 1351.
6. MILGROM, F. & E. WITEBSKY. 1960. Rabbit antibodies against γ-globulins resembling the rheumatoid factor. Fed. Proc. **19**: 197.
7. ABRUZZO, J. L. & C. L. CHRISTIAN. 1961. The induction of a rheumatoid factor-like substance in rabbits. J. Exp. Med. **114**: 791.
8. WALLER, M., R. IRBY, F. MULLINAX & E. C. TOONE, JR. 1965. Connective-tissue disease and rheumatoid factors in patients with renal transplants. New Eng. J. Med. **273**: 12.
9. BRAVO, J. F., J. H. HERMAN & C. J. SMYTH. 1967. Musculoskeletal disorders after renal homotransplantation. A clinical and laboratory analysis of 60 cases. Ann. Intern. Med. **66**: 87.
10. KANO, K. & F. MILGROM. 1968. Anti-γ-globulin factors in human allograft recipients. Transplantation **6**: 111.
11. WILLIAMS, G. M., D. M. HUME, K. KANO & F. MILGROM. 1968. Transplantation antibodies in human recipients of renal homografts. J.A.M.A. **204**: 119.
12. MILGROM, F., B. I. LITVAK, K. KANO & E. WITEBSKY. 1966. Humoral antibodies in renal homograft. J.A.M.A. **198**: 226.
13. KANO, K. & F. MILGROM. 1969. Relation of anti-γ-globulin antibodies to transplantation antibodies in human renal allograft recipients. Transplantation **7**: 281.
14. DIXON, F. J., R. T. SCHULTZ & F. MILGROM. 1965. Cardiac lesions in rabbits injected with autologous gamma globulin Lab. Invest. **14**: 2056.
15. HEIMER, R., F. M. LEVIN, A. PRIMACK, J. M. CORCOS & C. NOSENZO. 1962. Inhibition of complement fixation by human serum. J. Immunol. **89**: 382.
16. MILGROM, F. & R. T. SCHULTZ. 1965. Serodiagnosis of rheumatoid arthritis based on inhibition of anticomplementariness of denatured fraction II. Int. Arch. Allerg. **27**: 338.

General Discussion

DR. VAUGHAN: Have you tried your mixed-cell agglutination system to see whether the antibodies eluted off the kidneys of patients who are transplanted will react with any of the patient's own tissues? Some years ago, Nelson reported that during the course of a renal homograft rejection in dogs, the red cells of the animal that was carrying the graft became positive in the immunoadherent system. He suggested that the antibody reacting with the implanted tissue was able to cross-react with the transplanted animal's own tissues and brought forth this immune-adherence studies as an example of that. Your very sensitive mixed agglutination system affords an excellent opportunity to test that sort of reaction. Have you studied the nonrenal tissues in any of your patients for such reactivity with the antibodies eluted from the transplanted kidneys?

DR. SCHULTZ: We performed this type of experiment in animals and never observed any reaction with cultures of the recipient's cells. In humans, cell cultures of the recipient's origin were not available.

DR. VAUGHAN: It might be especially interesting to look at the synovial tissues with this test system inasmuch as such tissues have shown arthritic manifestations.

Part IV. Possible Biological Functions of Rheumatoid Factor in Synovial Space

RHEUMATOID FACTOR AND THE FIXATION OF COMPLEMENT*

Nathan J. Zvaifler, M.D.

Department of Medicine
Division of Rheumatic Diseases
Georgetown University Medical Center
Washington, D.C.

Introduction

During the past decade, a number of studies have analyzed the influence of rheumatoid factor on complement-fixation reactions. In almost all of these reports, isolated rheumatoid factor, rheumatoid euglobulin preparations, or heat-inactivated serum containing rheumatoid factor has been shown to compete with complement for binding sites on the γ-globulin molecule.[1–5] Initially, it was suggested that these were the same sites. This view became untenable, however, when Weidermann and his colleagues[6] demonstrated that if 7S antibody, or aggregated γ-globulin, was reduced with 2-mercaptoethanol, it lost the ability to fix complement while retaining the capacity to react with rheumatoid factor. From these *in vitro* observations of the competition between γ-globulin and rheumatoid factor developed the idea that rheumatoid factor might have a protective role *in vivo*,[7] namely, that by reacting with aggregated γ-globulin, or antigen-antibody complexes, it could prevent the activation of the complement sequence that would normally ensue, and thus avoid the deleterious effects mediated by the various complement components.

The concept that rheumatoid factor is protective implies that the reaction between rheumatoid factor and γ-globulin does not fix complement. If it did, it could be harmful. Direct testing of this hypothesis has not been possible, since aggregated γ-globulin is too anticomplementary by itself.[8] Such an analysis can be performed, however, if γ-globulin is reduced and alkylated prior to aggregation; the reduced, aggregated γ-globulin retains the ability to react with rheumatoid factor, but it can no longer fix complement. Therefore, any complement fixation observed should result from the interaction of rheumatoid factor with the reduced, aggregated γ-globulin. The present study presents evidence that under appropriate conditions human complement is fixed by the reaction between γ-globulin and serum containing rheumatoid factor, and examines the possible biological significance of these findings.

Materials and Methods

Human γ-globulin (Cohn Fraction II) at a concentration of 10 mg/ml in phosphate-buffered saline was dialyzed for three hours at room temperature against 100 ml of 0.1 M 2-mercaptoethanol. The reduced γ-globulin solution was dialyzed for four hours against a large volume of 0.01 M iodoacetamide, and then overnight in the cold against several changes of phosphate-buffered saline. Aggregation of γ-globulin, either reduced or nonreduced, was accomplished by heating at 63° C for 15 to 20 minutes. The concentration of γ-globulin was

* Supported by United States Public Health Service research grants nos. AM–5140, AM–5042, and AM–12059 from the National Institute of Arthritis and Metabolic Diseases.

always adjusted to 10 mg/ml prior to agggregation, and in experiments utilizing lesser amounts of γ-globulin, dilutions were made of the stock solution. After aggregation, proteins were measured by the Lowry method, against a γ-globulin standard with a known protein concentration determined by micro-Kjeldahl analysis.

Precipitin Reactions

Precipitin reactions were performed according to methods previously described.[9] Increasing concentrations of γ-globulin solution were introduced into ice-cold phosphate-buffered saline (0.15 M, pH 7.2), and then 0.5 ml of a serum with a high titer of rheumatoid factor was added. The final reaction volume was 5.0 ml. The reaction was allowed to proceed at room temperature for three hours and then at 4° C for seven days. Following this, the tubes were centrifuged, and the supernatants were decanted and analyzed for rheumatoid factor. The precipitates were washed twice with ice-cold buffered saline, packed by centrifugation, and analyzed for their nitrogen content by the micro-Kjeldahl method. Rheumatoid factor was measured by the bentonite-flocculation test.[10] A single serum containing a high titer (1:4,096) of rheumatoid factor was utilized for the precipitin studies.

Precipitates of rheumatoid factor and reduced, aggregated γ-globulin were made as follows: Pooled sera containing high titers of rheumatoid factor were inactivated at 56° C for 30 minutes and centrifuged at 2,000 rpm in a refrigerated centrifuge; then 7.5 ml were added to 27.5 ml of iced buffered saline containing 0.01 M EDTA. Subsequently, 15 ml of reduced, aggregated FII (10 mg/ml) was added dropwise. These proportions were chosen to be at or near equivalence. The mixture was kept at room temperature for one hour and then at 4° C for 72 hours. The precipitates that formed were washed three times with phosphate-buffered saline and then suspended at the desired protein concentration.

Complement Fixation Reactions

Quantitative complement fixation was performed by the method of Barbaro and Becker.[11] Hemolysis was measured spectrophotometrically.

Studies with Heat-Inactivated Serum Containing Rheumatoid Factor. An amount of fresh guinea pig serum containing approximately 100 $C'H_{50}$ units, or human serum with 50 $C'H_{50}$ units, was added to iced test tubes containing 0.25 ml of heat-aggregated, reduced γ-globulin (10 mg/ml) and 0.25 ml of heat-inactited human serum containing rheumatoid factor. Sufficient triethanolamine-buffered saline with optimum concentrations of metals and 0.5% gelatin was added to bring the total volume to 1.0 ml. After incubation at 37° C for 60 minutes, 19 ml of ice-cold triethanolamine-buffered saline were added. The tubes were centrifuged in the cold at 2,000 rpm for 15 minutes. Residual complement was determined in the supernatants. Controls of complement alone, complement and rheumatoid factor serum, and complement and aggregated, reduced γ-globulin were incubated with each experiment.

Studies with Preformed Precipitates of Rheumatoid Factor and Reduced, Aggregated γ-Globulin. In experiments with preformed precipitates, 0.25 ml of the rheumatoid factor complexes was incubated with 1.75 ml of fresh human serum at 37° C for two hours or overnight at 4° C. Controls included 0.25 ml of reduced, aggregated FII of an equal protein concentration or 0.25 ml of saline handled in an identical fashion. In some experiments, 1.75 ml of guinea pig serum were substituted as a complement source. Following incubation, the mixtures were centrifuged in the cold, and the supernatants were analyzed for residual total hemolytic complement and residual activity of the second and third components of complement. The C′2 was measured by the method of Austen and Beer,[12] and C′3 by immune adherence.[13] Conversion of C′3 was ascertained by microimmunoelectrophoresis[14] with an anti-human C′3 antiserum prepared in rabbits by the zymosan-adsorption method of Mardiney and Muller-Eberhard.[15] The percentage of complement fixed (% $C'H_{50}$) was calculated as:

$$\frac{C'H_{50}\text{ units fixed}}{\text{total } C'H_{50}} \times 100$$

Studies with Fresh Human Serum Containing Rheumatoid Factor. The reaction mixture consisted of 0.5 ml of fresh human serum, 0.5 ml of γ-globulin, aggregated or nonaggregated and either reduced or nonreduced, and 1.0 ml of triethanolamine-buffered saline. A control tube containing fresh serum, triethanolamine-buffered saline, and bovine serum albumin at a concentration equal to the γ-globulin was included with each experiment. The tubes were incubated at 37° C for 60 minutes. The reaction was stopped by the addition of ice-cold triethanolamine- buffered saline. The test and control tubes were centrifuged in the cold at 2,000 rpm for 15 minutes, and residual total hemolytic complement activity was determined in the supernatants. The percentage of total complement fixed was calculated as:

$$\frac{C'H_{50}\text{ fixed by }\gamma\text{-globulin}}{C'H_{50}\text{ fixed by bovine serum albumin}} \times 100$$

Non reduced γ-globulin was studied in the aggregated and nonaggregated form. Solutions of γ-globulin (Cohn Fraction II) were made fresh in phosphate-buffered saline on the day of testing and adjusted to a concentration of 10 mg/ml. The protein solution was centrifuged at 35,000 rpm for 90 minutes in a Spinco model L2 ultracentrifuge, and passed through a 0.22 μ Millipore filter. This ultracentrifuged, Millipore-filtered preparation is referred to as nonaggregated, nonreduced γ-globulin. Aggregated, nonreduced γ-globulin is the same material heated at 63° C for 15 minutes.

Results

The results to be presented depend on the ability of aggregated, reduced γ-globulin to react with rheumatoid factor, but not to fix complement. Experiments demonstrating these two essential properties are shown in FIGURES 1 and 2. The precipitin curve obtained when increasing concentrations of aggregated, nonreduced γ-globulin are added to a serum containing a high titer of rheumatoid factor is shown in FIGURE 1. There is a slow rise in precipitable nitrogen, followed by a long flat zone that lacks a clear-cut equivalence or solubilization of the precipitate in the region of antigen excess. The curve obtained with aggregated, reduced γ-globulin differs in several respects. The total nitrogen precipitated is less, but there are well-defined zones of equivalence and antigen excess. Tests for rheumatoid factor in the supernatants showed no activity beyond the equivalence point. When rheumatoid serum was heated at 56° C for 30 minutes, or the reaction was performed in the presence of 0.01 M EDTA, there was a decrease in the amount of nitrogen precipitated with both the reduced and nonreduced, aggregated γ-globulin, but there was no significant change in the overall configuration of the two precipitin curves.

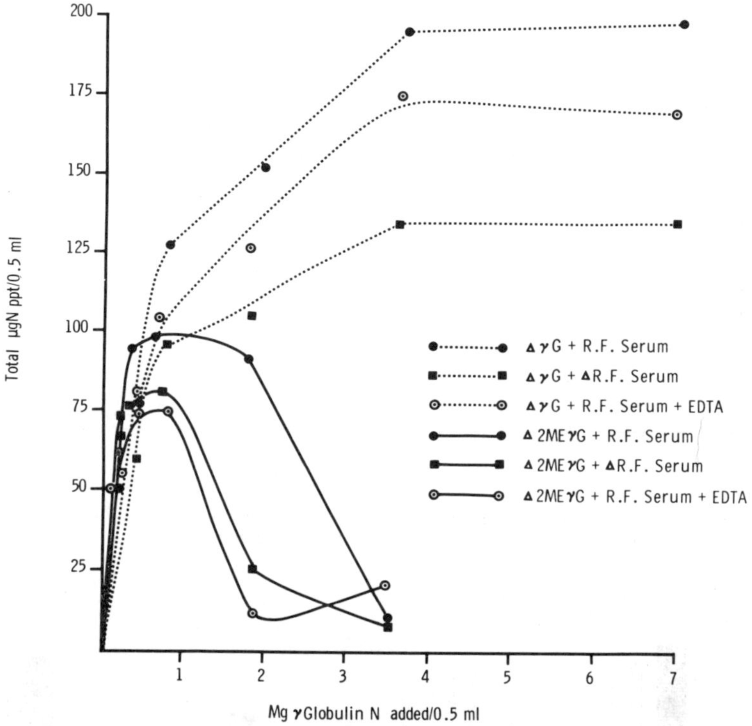

FIGURE 1. The effect of increasing concentrations of aggregated human γ-globulin (Δ γG) or aggregated, reduced human γ-globulin (Δ 2ME γG) on precipitable nitrogen (N) from 0.5 ml of serum containing rheumatoid factor (R.F.), and the influence of preheating or 0.01 M EDTA treatment.

A comparison of the complement-fixing ability of aggregated, nonreduced γ-globulin and aggregated, reduced γ-globulin is shown in FIGURE 2. As little as 100 μg of aggregated, nonreduced γ-globulin will fix 50% of the available guinea pig complement, while 10 mg of aggregated, reduced γ-globulin are unable to give a comparable degree of complement fixation. Similar results are obtained with fresh human serum as the complement source. Thus, reduced, aggregated γ-globulin combines with rheumatoid factor but does not by itself fix complement. Therefore, any complement fixation observed should come from the interaction of the reduced γ-globulin with rheumatoid factor.

Studies with Heat-Inactivated Human Serum Containing Rheumatoid Factor. The results of eight experiments analyzing complement fixation by the reaction of heat-inactivated rheumatoid factor serum with aggregated, reduced γ-globulin are summarized in FIGURE 3. Each experiment was performed with a serum of a different rheumatoid factor titer. Column I, in each instance, shows the residual complement after 60 minutes of incubation with only triethanolamine-buffered saline. Column II is the complement left after the reaction of serum containing rheumatoid factor and aggregated, reduced γ-globulin. Column III shows the residual complement with rheumatoid factor serum alone, and column IV the residual complement after reaction with only aggregated, reduced γ-globulin. The titer of rheumatoid factor for the individual sera is recorded beneath the

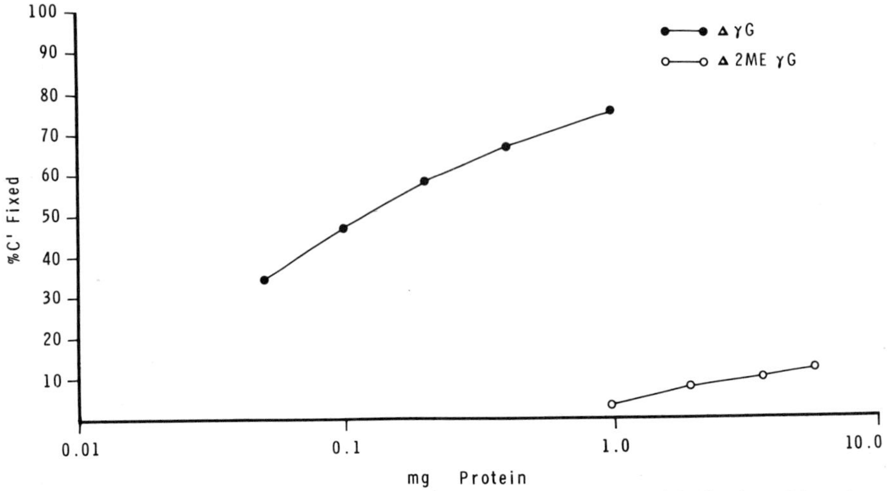

FIGURE 2. A comparison of the ability of aggregated human γ-globulin (Δ γG) and reduced, aggregated γ-globulin (Δ 2ME γG) to fix guinea pig complement.

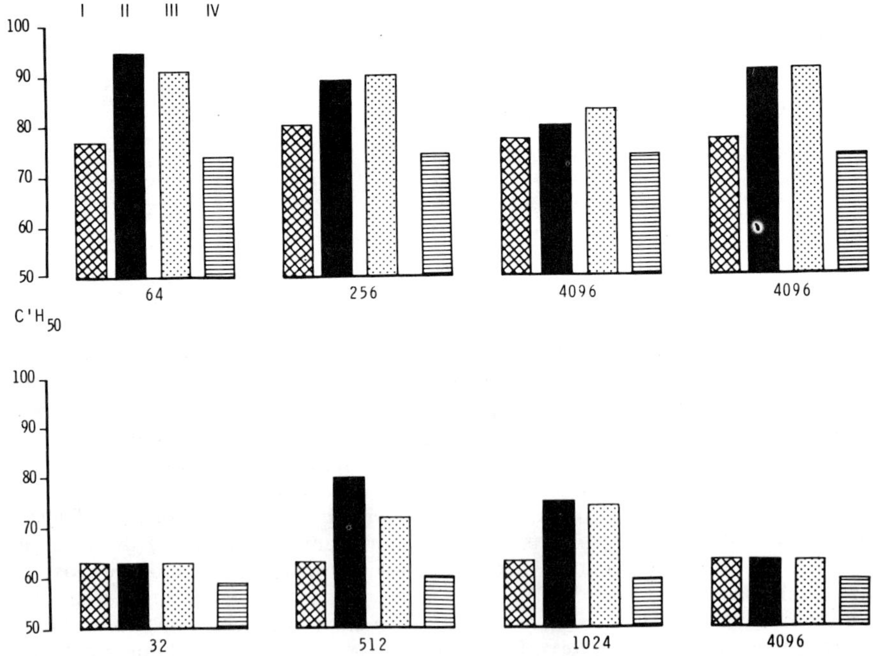

FIGURE 3. The residual guinea pig $C'H_{50}$ after the addition of reduced, aggregated γ-globulin to heat-inactivated serum containing rheumatoid factor. Reactants: complement alone (cross-hatched bar); complement, serum, and aggregated, reduced γ-globulin (solid bar); complement and serum (stippled bar); and complement and reduced γ-globulin (horizontally stripped bar). The number beneath each experiment is the reciprocal rheumatoid factor titer of the serum tested.

columns. There is no significant difference in the amount of residual complement in column III (rheumatoid factor serum plus complement) when compared with column II (rheumatoid factor serum and aggregated, reduced γ-globulin plus complement). Altogether, 18 sera with varying titers of rheumatoid factor were analyzed; no evidence for complement fixation could be demonstrated. An additional six sera were examined by comparing human complement with guinea pig complement; no complement fixation was noted in either case.

Studies with Preformed Complexes of Rheumatoid Factor and Reduced, Aggregated γ-Globulin. Complexes of rheumatoid factor and aggregated, reduced γ-globulin were incubated with fresh human serum at 37° C for two hours, or overnight at 4° C, and the residual complement was determined. Findings were compared with the fixation obtained with an equal concentration of aggregated, reduced γ-globulin alone. The results are shown in TABLE 1. At 4°C there was very little complement fixed by either the preformed complexes or the aggregated, reduced γ-globulin, but at 37° C the complex fixed 43% of the available complement. The complement fixation must be due to the complex, and not the reduced γ-globulin in the complex, for if all the protein in the complex were derived from aggregated, reduced γ-globulin, it would only fix 3% of the available complement. Neither the aggregated, reduced γ-globulin nor the complexes fix significant amounts of guinea pig complement, whether tested at 4° C or 37° C (TABLE 2). The effect of a change in concentration of the complexes on the amount of complement fixed is shown in FIGURE 4. Increasing the concentration of complex from 75 μg to 8.6 mg of protein resulted in increasing

TABLE 1

INCUBATION OF AGGREGATED, REDUCED γ-GLOBULIN AND RHEUMATOID FACTOR WITH HUMAN SERUM

Incubation Conditions	Reactants*	Residual $C'H_{50}$	% C' Fixed	β_{1C} Conversion
37° C, 2 hours	RF + ΔME FII	55	43	+
	ΔME FII	94	3	0
	Saline	97	—	0
4° C, 18 hours	RF + ΔME FII	107	0	0
	ΔME FII	95	8	0
	Saline	104	—	0

* RF = rheumatoid factor; ΔME FII = heat-aggregated, reduced γ-globulin (protein concentration, 3.0 mg/ml).

TABLE 2

INCUBATION OF AGGREGATED, REDUCED γ-GLOBULIN AND RHEUMATOID FACTOR WITH GUINEA PIG SERUM

Incubation Conditions	Reactants*	Residual $C'H_{50}$	% C' Fixed	β_{1C} Conversion
37° C, 2 hours	RF + ΔME FII	219	14	—
	ΔME FII	234	8	—
	Saline	255	—	—
4° C, 18 hours	RF + ΔME FII	212	9	—
	ΔME FII	203	13	—
	Saline	234	—	—

* RF = rheumatoid factor; ΔME FII = heat-aggregated, reduced γ-globulin (protein concentration, 3.0 mg/ml).

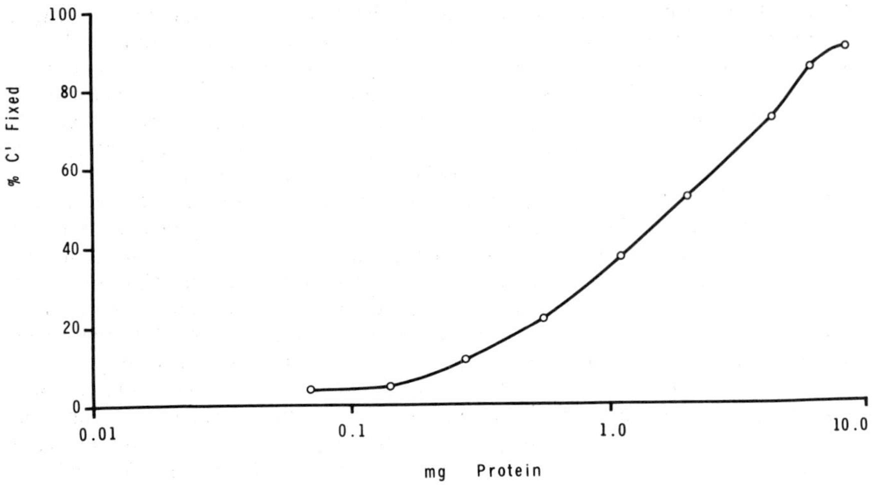

FIGURE 4. The effect of increasing concentrations of rheumatoid factor-reduced γ-globulin complexes on fixation of human complement. Preformed complexes were incubated with fresh human serum at 37° C for 120 minutes.

complement fixation; 2 mg of preformed complex fixed about 50% of the available complement, and 8 mg fixed more than 90%. Analysis of the second and third components of complement was performed to see if the rheumatoid factor-reduced γ-globulin complexes would fix complement in the conventional manner. The results are shown in TABLE 3. At a protein concentration of 75 μg, the rheumatoid factor-reduced γ-globulin complex fixed 35% of the total hemolytic complement and 33% of the available C′2, and reduced the immune-adherence titer by 50%. When the protein concentration was increased to 6.1 mg the preformed complexes fixed 95% of the total complement and 97% of the available C′2, reduced the immune-adherence titer to 13% of the value obtained with a similar concentration of aggregated, reduced γ-globulin.

Studies with Fresh Human Serum Containing Rheumatoid Factor. It was surprising that preformed complexes of rheumatoid factor and reduced, aggregated γ-globulin fixed human complement, while none was fixed by the addition of reduced, aggregated γ-globulin to heat-inactivated serum containing rheumatoid factor. Studies were done with serum that was not heated to determine if complement fixation occurred when the serum served both as the source of rheumatoid factor and hemolytic complement. Incubation of aggregated, reduced γ-globulin with a fresh serum containing a high titer of rheuma-

TABLE 3

FIXATION OF HUMAN COMPLEMENT COMPONENTS BY DIFFERENT CONCENTRATIONS OF RHEUMATOID FACTOR AND AGGREGATED, REDUCED γ-GLOBULIN

Reactants*	Protein (mg)	C′2	C′3	Total C′H_{50}
ΔME FII	0.75	160	1600	94
RF — ΔME FII	0.75	108	800	67
ΔME FII	6.1	300	1600	100
RF — ΔME FII	6.1	8	200	5

* RF = rheumatoid factor; ΔME FII = heat-aggregated, reduced γ-globulin.

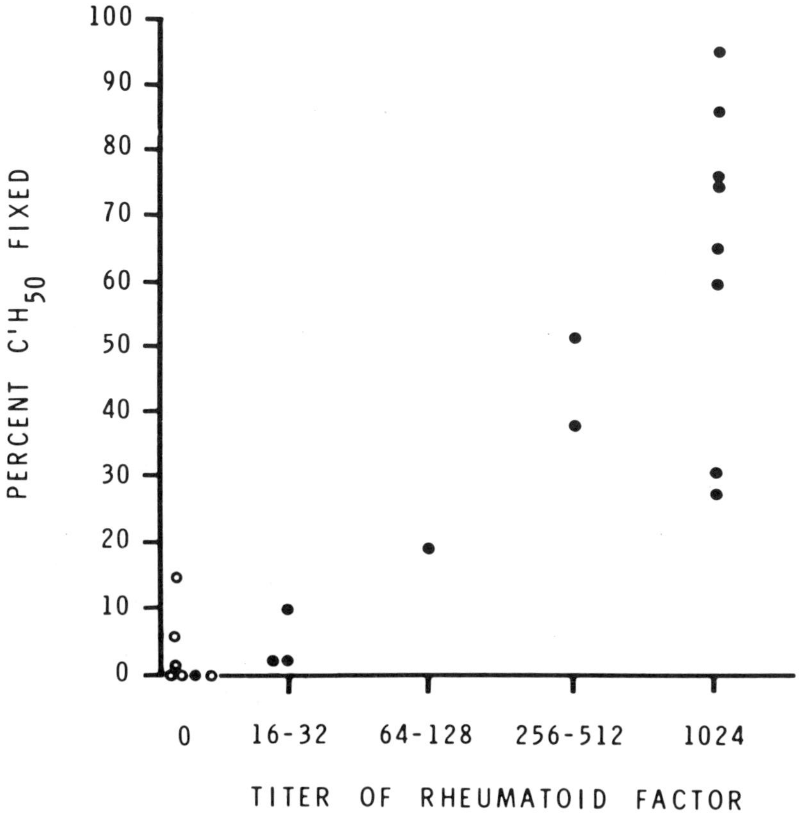

FIGURE 5. The percentage of total hemolytic complement fixed by the addition of reduced, aggregated γ-globulin to fresh serum containing rheumatoid factor. Open circles designate sera from normal subjects; closed circles represent sera from patients with rheumatoid arthritis.

toid factor resulted in the immunoelectrophoretic conversion of C′3 to C′3i. No conversion of C′3 was noted when aggregated, reduced γ-globulin was added to fresh serum containing no rheumatoid factor. This suggested that reduced, aggregated γ-globulin was reacting with a factor in rheumatoid serum to activate the third component of complement.

To investigate this reaction further, reduced, aggregated γ-globulin (10 mg/ml) was incubated with fresh sera of patients with rheumatoid arthritis. The residual hemolytic complement activity of the serum was measured. It was compared with the residual $C'H_{50}$ after similar treatment with bovine serum albumin (10 mg/ml). FIGURE 5 shows that the percentage of complement fixed by the reduced, aggregated γ-globulin was proportional to the titer of rheumatoid factor present in the serum. Little or no fixation was observed in fresh serum from normal subjects or rheumatoid patients with minimal amounts of rheumatoid factor. In contrast, the addition of reduced, aggregated γ-globulin to the serum of six of eight subjects with high titers of rheumatoid factor resulted in the fixation of more than 50% of their own complement.

Quantitative complement-fixation reactions were performed with the four rheumatoid sera that gave the greatest complement fixation. The results are shown in FIGURE 6. Increasing amounts of reduced, aggregated γ-globulin fixed a greater percentage of the available complement. Fixation of 50% of the complement occurred with 0.20, 0.33, 0.62, and 0.70 mg of reduced, aggregated γ-globulin. The efficiency of this complement-fixation reaction can be appreciated by the fact that 0.12 mg of nonreduced, aggregated γ-globulin is required to fix 50% of the complement in 0.5 ml of normal human serum (the average of seven experiments was 0.12 $\pm$ 0.02 mg). These studies showed that serum containing rheumatoid factor can fix autologous complement when reacted with reduced, aggregated γ-globulin. The complement fixation is probably accomplished by the rheumatoid factor; to date, however, experiments with isolated components of this system have not been successful.

Reduced γ-globulin is an artificial reagent; therefore, experiments were designed to test the ability of high-titer rheumatoid factor serum to fix complement with nonreduced γ-globulin. It was reasoned that if rheumatoid factor can fix complement, then the amount fixed in rheumatoid serum by a given concentration of γ-globulin should be greater than the amount fixed in normal serum by an identical concentration of γ-globulin. Thus, the amount of γ-globulin required to fix 50% of the available complement in rheumatoid sera should be less than the amount of γ-globulin needed to give 50% fixation in normal serum. The results of a representative experiment are depicted in FIGURE 7. The percentage of the total complement fixed by increasing concentrations of nonaggregated, nonreduced γ-globulin added to a high-titer rheumatoid serum and a normal serum

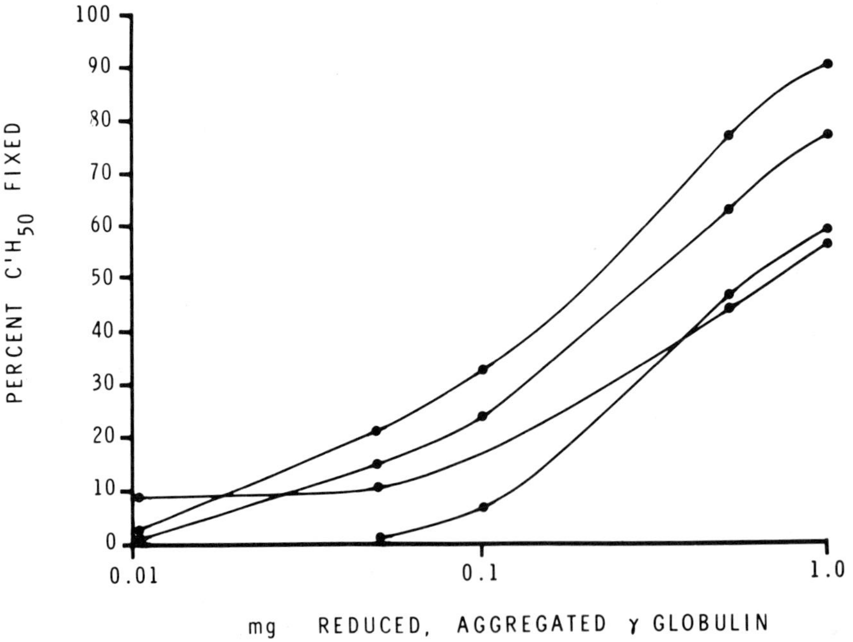

FIGURE 6. The relationship between the percentage of complement fixed in fresh human serum containing rheumatoid factor and the amount of added reduced, aggregated γ-globulin. Each curve designates an individual serum with a high titer of rheumatoid factor.

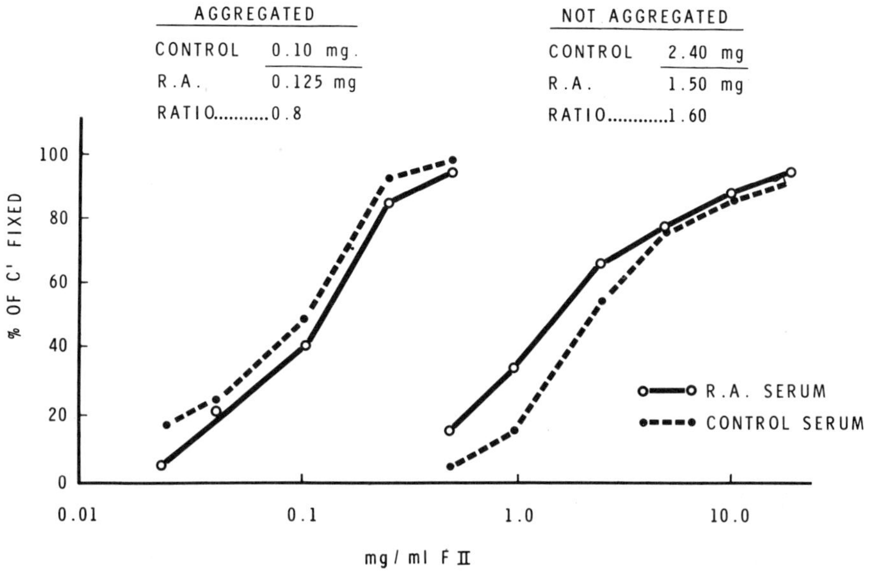

FIGURE 7. A comparison of the amounts of aggregated and nonaggregated γ-globulin needed to fix 50% of the complement in fresh normal and fresh rheumatoid serum.

is shown on the right-hand side of the figure; 2.40 mg of γ-globulin are required to fix 50% of the available complement in the normal serum, while the same percentage of fixation occurs in the rheumatoid serum with only 1.50 mg of γ-globulin. Therefore, 1.6 times more nonaggregated γ-globulin is necessary to fix 50% of the complement in normal serum than in rheumatoid serum. In five separate experiments comparing different rheumatoid and normal sera, this ratio ranged from 1.08 to 1.92, with an average of 1.45. Thus, less nonaggregated γ-globulin was required for 50% complement fixation in all rheumatoid sera studied. The results were just the opposite when heat-aggregated, nonreduced γ-globulin was studied. The curves on the left-hand side of FIGURE 7 compare the results obtained with the same normal and rheumatoid sera. Since the γ-globulin was aggregated, very little protein was required to give 50% fixation, but more was needed with the serum containing rheumatoid factor, 0.125 mg of aggregated γ-globulin with the rheumatoid serum, compared with 0.10 mg with the normal serum, for a ratio of 0.80. In experiments with five other high-titer rheumatoid factor-containing sera, the ratio varied from 0.49 to 0.83 with an average of 0.624.

DISCUSSION

The results of the studies with reduced, aggregated γ-globulin can be summarized as follows: Neither guinea pig or human complement is fixed when reduced, aggregated γ-globulin is added to heat-inactivated serum containing rheumatoid factor. Incubation of the same amount of reduced, aggregated γ-globulin with fresh serum containing rheumatoid factor results in good fixation of the complement in the serum. Preformed complexes of rheumatoid factor and reduced, aggregated γ-globulin fix human complement at 37° C but not at 4° C. Preformed complexes do not fix guinea pig complement at either temperature. These findings may not be as discordant as they first appear. The changes produced when human serum is heated to 56° C to destroy complement activity are probably important. γ-Globulin is susceptible to aggregation at temperatures above 37° C.[16] Thus, γ-globulin may be aggregated in the process of decomplementing rheumatoid serum. It would then be more likely to react with, or cover up, the complement-fixing sites on the rheumatoid factor molecule. The subsequent introduction of reduced, aggregated γ-globulin might not demonstrate complement fixation.

Human rheumatoid factor is a 19S antibody. Some other human 19S complement-fixing antibodies have shown a requirement for human complement and a reaction temperature of 37° C. Cunniff and Stollar reported that some rabbit and human 19S antibodies fix complement more efficiently at 37° C than at 4° C, which was never the case with 7S antibodies.[17] These results were obtained with guinea pig complement; the difference would be more exaggerated with human complement, since fixation of the first component of human complement to antigen-antibody complexes does not proceed will in the cold.[18] The absolute requirement for human complement and the inability to fix guinea pig complement are not without precedent. In a study of complement fixation by naturally occurring anti-A and anti-B antibodies, Ostgard and Orjasaeter[19] found a significantly higher frequency of positive results with human complement (43 of 54 samples) than with guinea pig complement. The immunoglobulin class of the anti-A and anti-B antibodies was not investigated, but the "naturally" occurring form is usually a macroglobulin.[20] Since γ-globulin does not normally exist in the reduced form, the relevance of these *in vitro* observations is of questionable significance for the patient with rheumatoid arthritis. Nevertheless, they do show that something in rheumatoid serum, most probably rheumatoid factor, has the capacity for fixing human complement.

The studies with nonreduced γ-globulin may have more biological and clinical significance. The observation that nonaggregated, nonreduced γ-globulin fixes complement in rheumatoid sera is of interest, but the designation "nonaggregated" γ-globulin is probably incorrect, since some denaturation undoubtedly occurs in the isolation process.[21] This mild denaturation is probably not unlike the changes in the γ-globulin molecule which result from its combination with antigen,[8] or which might be brought about by lysosomal proteases present in inflammatory effusions.[22] It has been shown that rheumatoid factor and γ-globulin exist *in vivo* as a complex,[20] but what evidence is there that complement fixation occurs in patients with these complexes? Vasculitis is common in rheumatoid arthritis, and complement fixation is required for the vascular lesion produced by antigen-antibody complexes.[23] The arteritis of rheumatoid arthritis is seen most often in patients with high titers of rheumatoid factor.[24] A group of patients has been described with mixed cryoglobulin complexes, consisting of IgM immunoglobulins with rheumatoid factor activity and IgG molecules. These patients usually have depressed serum complement levels, and frequently vasculitis and nephritis.[25] Hemolytic complement activity is depressed in the synovial effusions of patients with rheumatoid arthritis.[26-27] The low complement levels have been correlated with the presence of rheumatoid factor in the synovial fluid,[27] and in cytoplasmic inclusions of leukocytes from rheumatoid effusions.[28] Breakdown products of C′3 have been demonstrated in synovial fluids, and there is significant correlation with the presence of rheumatoid factor.[29]

The diminished complement fixation found when heat-aggregated γ-globulin is added to rheumatoid serum is like the protective effects noted previously.[1-5]

The relevance of this finding to the *in vivo* situation is questionable, however, for as the degree of denaturation of a protein increases, so does the rate at which it is removed from the circulation by the reticuloendothelial system.[30] This is also true in the articular cavity.[31] The ability of rheumatoid factor to enhance the clearance of soluble immune complexes may be a related phenomenon.[32]

Summary

Studies have been presented which analyze the complement-fixing ability of rheumatoid factor. These have been possible because reduced γ-globulin reacts with rheumatoid factor when heat aggregated, but does not, by itself, fix complement. Therefore, any complement fixation observed should result solely from the interaction of the aggregated, reduced γ-globulin with rheumatoid factor. Fresh serum from patients with rheumatoid arthritis can fix human complement when incubated at 37° C with reduced, aggregated γ-globulin. The complement fixation is proportional to the titer of rheumatoid factor in the serum. Preformed complexes of rheumatoid factor and aggregated, reduced γ-globulin also fix human complement, but they do not fix guinea pig complement.

The ability of high-titer rheumatoid factor serum to fix nonreduced γ-globulin was examined. When γ-globulin was heat aggregated, twice as much was required to fix 50% of the complement in fresh rheumatoid serum than in normal serum; conversely, rheumatoid factor serum fixed more complement when little or no aggregation was present. These studies were interpreted as showing that under appropriate conditions serum containing rheumatoid factor can give excellent complement fixation. The possible biological significance of these findings was also considered.

References

1. Bernhard, G. G., W. Cheng & D. W. Talmage. 1962. The reaction of rheumatoid factor and complement with gamma globulin coated latex. J. Immunol. **88:** 750.
2. Heimer, R., F. M. Levin, A. Primach, J. M. Corcos & C. Nosenzo. 1962. Inhibition of complement fixation by human serum. J. Immunol. **89:** 382.
3. Zvaifler, N. J. & K. J. Bloch. 1962. Rheumatoid factor: An inhibitor of the complement fixation reaction. Arthritis Rheum. **5:** 127.
4. Heimer, R., F. M. Levin & M. F. Kahn. 1963. Inhibition of complement fixation by human serum II. The activity of a gamma M_1 globulin and rheumatoid factor in complement fixation reactions. J. Immunol. **91:** 866.
5. Davis, J. S. & A. J. Bollet. 1964. Protection of a complement sensitive enzyme system by rheumatoid factor. J. Immunol. **92:** 139.
6. Wiedermann, G., P. A. Miescher & E. C. Franklin. 1963. Effect of mercaptoethanol on complement binding ability of human 7S gamma globulin. Proc. Soc. Exp. Biol. Med. **113:** 609.
7. Gough, W. W. & J. S. Davis. 1966. Effects of rheumatoid factor on complement levels *in vivo*. Arthritis Rheum. **9:** 555.
8. Ishizaka, K. 1963. Gamma globulin and molecular mechanisms in hypersensitivity reactions. Progr. Allergy **7:** 32.
9. Zvaifler, N. J. & P. Schur. 1968. Reactions of aggregated mercaptoethanol treated gamma globulin with rheumatoid factor: Precipitin and complement fixation studies. Arthritis Rheum. **11:** 523.
10. Bloch, K. J. & J. J. Bunim. 1959. Simple, rapid and diagnostic test for rheumatoid arthritis: Bentonite flocculation test. J.A.M.A. **169:** 307.
11. Barbaro, J. F. & E. L. Becker. 1962. Comparison of complement fixing potency of antiserum from various species. J. Infect. Dis. **111:** 175.
12. Austen, K. F. & F. Beer. 1964. Measurement of second component of human complement ($C'2^{hu}$) by its interaction with $EAC'1_a{}^{gp}$, 4^{gp} cells. J. Immunol. **92:** 946.
13. Nishioka, K. & W. D. Linscott. 1963. Components of guinea pig complement. I. Separation of a serum fraction essential for immune hemolysis and immune adherence. J. Exp. Med. **118:** 767.

14. SCHEIDEGGER, J. J. 1955. Une micromethode de l'immunoélectrophorèse. Int. Arch. Allerg. **7:** 103.
15. MARDINEY, M. R. & H. J. MULLER-EBERHARD. 1965. Mouse $\beta 1_c$-globulin: Production of antiserum and characterization in the complement reaction. J. Immunol. **94:** 877.
16. MARCUS, D. 1960. A study of the mechanism of the anticomplementary activity of γ-globulin. J. Immunol. **84:** 273.
17. CUNNIFF, R. V. & B. D. STOLLAR. 1968. Properties of 19S antibodies in complement fixation. I. Temperature dependence and role of antigen structure. J. Immunol. **100:** 7.
18. LEON, M. A. 1957. Kinetics of human complement. III. Intermediates in the reaction between human complement and sensitized cells. J. Immunol. **79:** 480.
19. OSTGARD, P. & H. ORJASAETER. 1962. Naturally occurring anti A and anti B and their ability to fix complement. Acta Path. Microbiol. Scand. **56:** 426.
20. KUNKEL, H. G. 1960. Macroglobulins and high molecular weight antibodies. *In* Plasma Proteins. F. W. Putnam, Ed. **I:** 279–307. Academic Press, Inc. New York, N. Y.
21. SINGER, J. & E. WITEBSKY. 1963. In a discussion of Experimental production of rheumatoid factor. Arthritis Rheum. **6:** 408.
22. WEISSMANN, G. 1966. Lysosomes and joint disease. Arthritis Rheum. **9:** 834.
23. WARD, P. A. & C. G. COCHRANE. 1965. Bound complement and immunologic injury of blood vessels. J. Exp. Med. **121:** 215.
24. SCHMID, F. R., N. S. COOPER, M. ZIFF & C. MCEWEN. 1961. Arteritis in rheumatoid arthritis. Amer. J. Med. **30:** 56.
25. MELTZER, M., E. C. FRANKLIN, K. ELIAS, R. T. MCCLUSKEY & N. COOPER. 1966. Cryoglobulinemia: A clinical and laboratory study. II. Cryoglobulins with rheumatoid factor activity. Amer. J. Med. **40:** 837.
26. PEKIN, T. J. & N. J. ZVAIFLER. 1964. Hemolytic complement in synovial fluid. J. Clin. Invest. **43:** 1372.
27. HEDBERG, H. 1967. Studies on synovial fluid in arthritis. Acta Med. Scand. (Suppl.) **479:** 5.
28. VAUGHAN, J. H., R. F. JACOX & P. NOELL. 1968. Relation of intracytoplasmic inclusions in joint fluid leukocytes to anti γG globulins. Arthritis Rheum. **11:** 135.
29. ZVAIFLER, N. J. 1969. Breakdown products of C'3 in human synovial fluids. J. Clin. Invest. **48:** 1532.
30. THORBECKE, G. J., P. H. MAURER & B. BENACERRAF. 1959. The affinity of the reticulo endothelial system for various modified proteins. Brit. J. Exp. Path. **41:** 190.
31. SLIWINSKI, A. J. & N. J. ZVAIFLER. 1969. The removal of aggregated and nonaggregated autologous gamma globulin from rheumatoid joints. Arthritis Rheum. In press.
32. LIGHTFOOT, R. W., R. E. DRUSIN & C. CHRISTIAN. 1969. The interaction of soluble immune complexes with rheumatoid factors. This monograph.

GENERAL DISCUSSION

DR. SCHMIDT (*Chicago, Ill.*): I'd like to comment on the effect of one variable in the system that we've been involved with, which may be of some interest in the paradoxical responses that have been reported for the action of rheumatoid factor in regard to whether or not it fixes or inhibits complement fixation. The variable that may be important here is one of those that are significant when one uses the red cell membrane as a site on which the reaction of fixation or rheumatoid factor binding takes place. This is the concentration of the IgG coat on the red cell. Our system consists of sheep red cells with rabbit IgG antibody in varying concentrations on the red cells. A constant amount of isolated rheumatoid factor is then added to such preparations. The resulting complement hemolysis is measured at the end of the incubation period.

In brief, the results indicate that when the concentration of the IgG coat is minimal, i.e., at a level of perhaps one-tenth or up to four-tenths the amount that would be optimal for fixation of complement by the IgG alone, the addition of rheumatoid factor to the system results in development of or augmentation of complement fixation. If one then adds increasing amounts of IgG coat, going from four-tenths of the optimal level to the full optimal level, then rheumatoid factor, which still adds to the coat – as can be determined with isotopically labeled rheumatoid factor—inhibits fixation. The fixation actually falls below that achieved by the IgG coat alone.

One thus has an explanation for the previously described results in which the rheumatoid factor was said to be competitive with complement, because most of those former studies were done with levels of IgG which were at the optimal range. Even at the range in which the IgG coat allows the rheumatoid factor to fix complement, the rheumatoid factor does not seem to possess an efficiency equal to an ordinary hemolytic IgM-antibody, but rather somewhat less. I got the impression from some of the results Dr. Zvaifler reported that he found approximately the same thing.

DR. ZVAIFLER: I think that what Dr. Schmidt is saying is essentially the same as what I referred to about nonaggregated and aggregated γ-globulin. We could, I suspect, spend a great amount of time discussing what is native γ-globulin vs what is denatured. I think Dr. Vaughan suggested in the symposium held ten years ago on rheumatoid factor that once the blood is drawn from the arm its γ-globulins are no longer native. Thus, when we speak of nonaggregated γ-globulin, certainly the material we use in the Cohn-fractionated human plasma has already undergone some changes that may be very analogous to the minimal coating Dr. Schmidt refers to, whereas aggregation that is produced by heating may be more comparable to the heavy coat he speaks of.

The efficiency of this system, I think, depends on a great number of variables. The preformed complexes obviously are not very efficient. But again we are confronted with the problem of how to make these preformed complexes and how to keep off complement components. We have used high-titer rheumatoid sera that were pooled and then heated. In the course of heat inactivating serum at 56° C, I am sure that, as Dr. Henney and many other people have shown, γ-globulins already have begun to be aggregated. Thus, many of the complement-fixing sites are probably tied up in the course of heat inactivation of complement. With preformed aggregates, we are only looking at a portion of the potential complement-fixing activity. I think in the completely autologous system this is much more analogous to γG complement fixation. We have no data on whether it is as good as one would expect from hemolytic 19S antibody.

DR. VAUGHAN: By making preformed aggregates, you had a reagent that was capable of fixing complement in normal human sera. Have you tried treatment of these preformed aggregates with 2-mercaptoethanol to determine whether the 19S component, which presumably is there, has anything to do with the complement-fixing activity?

DR. ZVAIFLER: Do you mean mercaptoethanol treatment before we make the complexes?

DR. VAUGHAN: No, make your preformed complexes and then treat with 2-mercaptoethanol.

DR. ZVAIFLER: No, we have not tried that.

DR. EPSTEIN: I'm not sure whether this is a semantic problem or not. You use the term complement fixation. To what is complement fixed? We are talking of the assay for complement after you have performed a certain procedure. If the soluble, preformed complexes can activate an enzyme system, e.g., esterase of entirely another pathway, these complexes may destroy complement components. We use the term complement fixation with cells, and we can demonstrate complement on the cells, but I wonder whether we are going to close some doors by using the term complement fixation.

As a second question, what direct evidence do you have that adding nonaggregated γ-globulin to perfectly normal serum does anything through rheumatoid factor? At a certain concentration of normal γ-globulin to normal serum, something abnormal happens. Do you draw the inference that this has something to do with the rheumatoid factor content of the normal serum?

DR. ZVAIFLER: No, this has to do with the fact that there is no such thing as nonaggregated γ-globulin. Some denaturation always occurs in any γ-globulin we work with. Therefore, it may take 5 mg of the substances to fix complement.

DR. EPSTEIN: Then you take the next step and assume that the element of aggregated γ-globulin is reacting with the rheumatoid factor content of the normal serum?

DR. ZVAIFLER: No, that's by itself. We are comparing it with the same γ-globulin added to rheumatoid serum to see if there is a difference, and all we can say is that there is a difference.

COMPLEMENT COMPONENTS IN SYNOVIAL FLUID: ACTIVATION AND FIXATION IN SEROPOSITIVE RHEUMATOID ARTHRITIS*

S. Ruddy, M.D.,† M. C. Britton, M.D.,‡ P. H. Schur, M.D., and K. F. Austen, M.D.

Department of Medicine
Harvard Medical School
Robert B. Brigham Hospital
Boston, Mass.

In 1964, Pekin and Zvaifler[1] observed that synovial fluids from patients with rheumatoid arthritis contained relatively less total hemolytic complement than did fluids from patients with other forms of arthritis. Hedberg[2] confirmed these findings and noted that the extent of this reduction in synovial-fluid complement activity was proportional to the titer of rheumatoid factor in the serum or synovial fluid. Vaughan and co-workers[3] also noted an association between reduced synovial-fluid complement activities and a positive serum test for rheumatoid factor. These latter workers found, in addition, that synovial fluids with relatively low complement activities contained, in their leukocytes, intracytoplasmic inclusions of γG- and γM-immunoglobulins and, in some cases, the third component of complement.

In the present study, the activities of individual components of the complement system have been measured in joint fluids from two groups of patients with rheumatoid arthritis, one seropositive and the other seronegative, and one group of patients with degenerative joint disease. Alterations in the levels of these complement components in the rheumatoid groups have been related to the intracytoplasmic deposition of complement proteins and immunoglobulins in synovial-fluid leukocytes.

The Complement Reaction Sequence

In order to appreciate the implications of the findings with respect to synovial-fluid complement, a brief review of the complement reaction mechanisms is required. The immune hemolytic sequence[4,5] depicted in FIGURE 1 uses sheep erythrocytes (E) as the target cell, but similar reactions have been demonstrated for other cell systems and for soluble antigen-antibody complexes. Antibody (A) combines with antigens on the surfaces of the E, and, as a result, the A is altered in such a way as to become capable of initiating the events of the complement sequence. Similar alterations in immunoglobulins can result from physical treatment such as heating.[6]

C1, the first component of complement, consists of three subunits: C1q, C1r, and C1s.[7] The C1q subunit carries the binding site of C1, and the union of C1 with the immunoglobulin results in the appearance of enzymatic activity on the C1s portion of the C1 molecule. The complex of erythrocyte, antibody, and activated C1 ($C\bar{1}$) is shown in FIGURE 1 as $EAC\bar{1}$. $C\bar{1}$ is susceptible to the $C\bar{1}$-

* Supported by grants nos. AI-07722, AM-11414, AM-12051, and AM-05577 from the National Institutes of Health, United States Public Health Service, a grant from the Massachusetts Chapter of the Arthritis Foundation, and a grant from the New England Peabody Home for Children.

† Investigator, Howard Hughes Medical Institute.

‡ Clinical Trainee supported by training grant no. AM-05076 from the National Institutes of Health, United States Public Health Service.

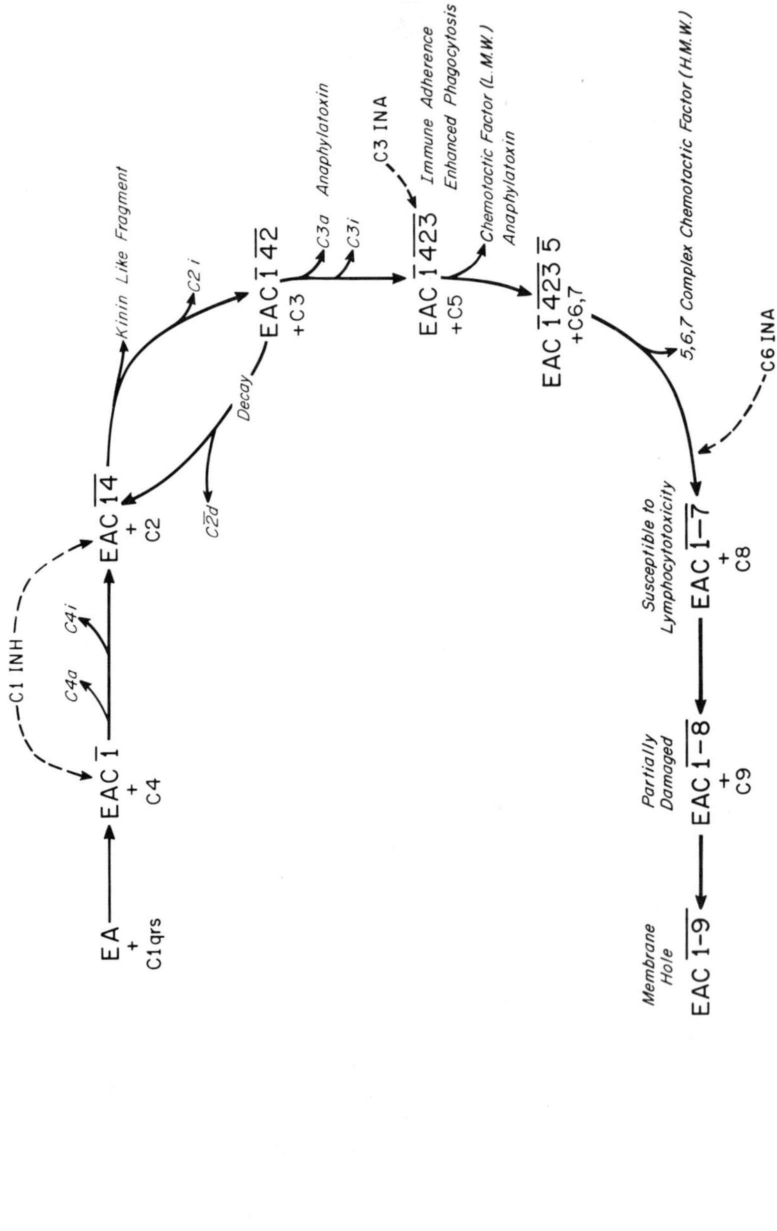

FIGURE 1. The reactions of the complement system.

inhibitor ($C\overline{1}INH$), a polyspecific α_2 neuraminoglycoprotein[8] that combines stoichiometrically with activated $C\overline{1}$ and blocks its activity.

The action of $C\overline{1}$ on C4 cleaves a small fragment from the C4[9]; the larger portion of the C4 molecule is either bound to the cell surface, generating the intermediate $EAC\overline{14}$, or remains free in the fluid phase as the inactive product, C4i. The reaction of $C\overline{1}$ with C4 greatly increases the capacity of C1 to act on C2.[10] The latter component is also cleaved, and the larger fragment is bound to the cell, generating the $EAC\overline{142}$ intermediate. A kinin-like permeability factor may be released at this step.[11] $EAC\overline{142}$ cells are unstable and rapidly decay to the $EAC\overline{14}$ state, liberating the decay product $C\overline{2}d$.[12]

The action of $C\overline{1}$ on C4 and C2 generates from these components a new enzymatic activity, C3-convertase.[13] This enzyme cleaves C3 into at least two pieces, one of which is anaphylatoxin, a small peptide with histamine-releasing capabilities.[14] The larger fragment of C3 is either bound to the cell surface or remains free in the fluid phase as C3i. Immune complexes to which C3 has been bound participate in the immune-adherence phenomenon and experience enhanced phagocytosis by polymorphonuclear leukocytes.[15] These biological effects of the cell-bound C3 fragment are reversed by the C3-inactivator (C3INA), an enzyme in normal serum.[16] The remaining steps in the sequence result in the production of two chemotactic factors for polymorphonuclear leukocytes,[17,18] cells that are susceptible to lymphocytotoxic reactions[19] and, ultimately, lysis and death of the target cells.

It is important to note that the total hemolytic complement determination (CH_{50}) measures the interaction of all nine components and the three control steps of the complement sequence in terms of the end product, immune hemolysis. For purposes of this presentation, the following points also deserve emphasis: the C1 molecule can be quantitatively bound to the immune complex, with a resulting diminuition in the fluid-phase activity of this component; the activation of C1 is manifested by the destruction of C4 and C2, its two natural substrates, or by the binding of these components to the immune complex; and levels of C3, the substrate of C3-convertase, can provide information about the generation of this enzyme.

Materials and Methods

Subjects for study were chosen from patients at the Robert B. Brigham Hospital chiefly on the basis of availability for biopsy and for the collection of synovial fluid. There were 53 patients with rheumatoid arthritis who had a positive serum or euglobulin latex fixation test[20] for rheumatoid factor, and 30 patients with rheumatoid arthritis and a negative latex test. The high proportion of seronegative rheumatoid arthritis patients reflects a deliberate attempt to obtain such patients for study. Of these 83 patients, 80 had "classical" or "definite" and three had "probable" rheumatoid arthritis according to the Arthritis and Rheumatism Association criteria.[21] In addition, 21 patients with degenerative joint disease were also studied. Biopsies were obtained from 86 of the 104 patients and were, in all cases, consistent with the diagnosis.

Synovial fluid was usually obtained from the knee joint, allowed to clot briefly at room temperature, centrifuged, aliquoted, and frozen at $-70°$ C. A portion of the synovial fluid for immunofluorescent study was collected in 0.01 M disodium ethylenediaminetetraacetate. The cells from this fluid were washed four times in 0.01 M phosphate-buffered saline (pH 7.5) containing 1% human albumin. They were resuspended in this same buffer, smeared on siliconized microscope slides, dried, fixed in alcohol, and stored at $-20°$ C.

Total hemolytic complement (CH_{50}) was measured by a modification of the Kent-Fife technique.[22] The technique of Hanauer and Christian[23] was used for the radial immunodiffusion measurement of C1q protein; the techniques for the measurement of C3 and C4 protein have been previously described.[24] Complement component activities were measured on a sample of 33 fluids, with effective molecule titrations according to techniques previously described for C1,[25] C4,[26] C2,[27] and C3.[16]

Synovial-fluid leukocytes were stained for inclusions of γM, γA, γG and the four subgroups of γG with fluorescein-conjugated antisera prepared against the respective immunoglobulins. Cells were also stained for deposits of C1q, C4, and C3 with fluorescein-conjugated specific antisera to these complement components, purified by previously described techniques.[16,26,28] In all cases, the immunofluorescence was specifically inhibited by the appropriate purified antigen. For each synovial fluid and for each antiserum stain, at least 200 cells were examined and graded with respect to the percentage of cells staining for intracytoplasmic inclusions with the specific antiserum.

Results

The synovial-fluid activities of total hemolytic complement, C1, C4, C2, and C3 are given for each of the three groups of patients in TABLE 1. Results are expressed as units of activity per gram of protein contained in the synovial fluid. The means and standard error of this mean are shown for each category of patients. The synovial-fluid CH_{50} activities of the seronegative rheumatoid arthritis group were not significantly different from those of the patients with degenerative joint disease. The synovial fluid CH_{50} levels of the seropositive rheumatoid arthritis patients were significantly lower than those of either of the other two groups.

The mean synovial-fluid C1 activity was 7,300 units/g of protein in the degenerative joint disease group, and 10,000 units/g in the seronegative rheumatoid arthritis group. The mean C1 activity in the seropositive rheumatoid arthritis group was only moderately reduced, but six of the 17 fluids in that group had levels below 1,500 units/g. The activities of C4 and C2, the two natural substrates of $C\bar{1}$, paralleled each other. Compared with the degenerative joint disease group, the seropositive rheumatoid arthritis synovial fluids contained markedly lower activities of C4 and C2, while the seronegative rheumatoid arthritis fluids contained only moderately lower activities. The mean C4 activity was 7,800

TABLE 1

ACTIVITIES OF TOTAL HEMOLYTIC COMPLEMENT AND OF INDIVIDUAL COMPLEMENT COMPONENTS IN SYNOVIAL FLUID

Measurement	No. of Determinations	Activity (units/gram of synovial fluid protein)*		
		RA-pos	RA-neg	DJD
CH_{50}	104	11.6 ± 1.0	27.7 ± 1.3	24.3 ± 1.5
C1	33	5,100 ± 1,200	10,100 ± 2,000	7,300 ± 1,100
C4	33	700 ± 200	4,300 ± 500	7,800 ± 1,100
C2	33	25.4 ± 3.8	94.3 ± 19.3	128.9 ± 31.0
C3	33	3,900 ± 1,000	8,900 ± 800	6,800 ± 1,100

* Mean ± standard error of mean. RA-pos = seropositive rheumatoid arthritis patients; RA-neg = seronegative rheumatoid arthritis patients; DJD = degenerative joint disease patients.

TABLE 2

INTRACYOTPLASMIC INCLUSIONS OF COMPLEMENT PROTEIN*

Patient Group†	Complement Components		
	C1q	C4	C3
RA-pos	20/27	23/27	14/30
RA-neg	8/13	5/13	2/14
DJD	0/6	0/6	0/6

* Number of specimens with >10% of cells staining out of the total number examined.
† RA-pos = seropositive rheumatoid arthritis; RA-neg = seronegative rheumatoid arthritis; DJD = degenerative joint disease.

units/g for the degenerative joint disease group, 4,300 units/g for the seronegative rheumatoid arthritis group, and 700 units/g for the seropositive rheumatoid arthritis group. For C2, the corresponding mean values were 128.9, 94.3, and 25.4 units/g, respectively.

The activity of the third component was significantly depressed in the fluids form the seropositive rheumatoid arthritis patients, with a mean value of 3,900 units/g. Fluids form the seronegative rheumatoid arthritis patients did not differ from those of the degenerative joint disease patients with respect to C3 activity. Diminutions in the activities of C3 and C4 were paralleled by reductions in the protein concentrations of these components, as measured by radial immunodiffusion. The overall correlation coefficient for C4 activity and C4 protein concentration was 0.79, and for C3 the corresponding coefficient was 0.69. Since C4i or C3i in the joint fluid would have been measured as C4 or C3 protein on radial immunodiffusion but not as activity in the hemolytic assays, the correlation between these two determinations implies that variable amounts of the hemolytically inactive products were not present in the joint fluids.

The low component activities in the seropositive rheumatoid arthritis group might indicate either intraarticular inactivation or impaired influx of these components into the joint space. The results of immunofluorescent studies favor the former alternative: Deposits of complement proteins were found in intracytoplasmic inclusions in synovial-fluid leukocytes, and the intensity of this deposition was correlated with the reductions in the levels of these components in the surrounding joint fluid. TABLE 2 shows the results of staining for C1q, C4, and C3. Leukocytes from a given fluid were scored as positive if more than 10% of the cells exhibited specific immunofluorescence. None of the six specimens from the degenerative joint disease group stained positively for any complement proteins. Twenty of 27 preparations from seropositive rheumatoid arthritis patients had more than 10% of cells staining for C1q, as did eight of 13 preparations from seronegative rheumatoid arthritis patients. Among the cell preparations from seropositive rheumatoid arthritis patients, 23 of 27 exhibited specific immunofluorescence for C4, as did five of 13 preparations from seronegative rheumatoid arthritis patients. For C3, the proportion of preparations that stained positively was lower: 14 of 30 in the seropositive rheumatoid arthritis group and two of 14 in the seronegative rheumatoid arthritis group stained for this component.

Depletion of a complement protein from the joint fluid was associated with the deposition of this same protein in the leukocytes contained in that fluid. As the C4 protein level decreased, the percentage of cells staining for C4 protein increased. Most of the specimens with low C4 concentrations in the joint fluid and a high percentage of the cells containing C4 inclusions were from seropositive rheumatoid arthritis patients. A similar inverse relationship between fluid concentration and leukocyte inclusions was observed for C3, but was not observed for C1q.

TABLE 3 gives the results of staining for immunoglobulins in the synovial-fluid leukocytes. No positive reactions were observed among the seven specimens from patients with degenerative joint diseases. A high proportion of positive reactions for immunoglobulin inclusions was seen in the seropositive rheumatoid arthritis group, while only an occasional specimen from a seronegative rheumatoid arthritis patient was positive. Synovial-fluid levels of complement protein were also related to γG- and γM-immunoglobulin deposition, the specimens with the lowest concentrations of complement proteins having the highest percentage of cells staining for γG and γM. This relationship was not observed when the cells were stained for γA. Stains for the subgroups of γG revealed that if the cells of a given fluid contained any of the four subgroups, all were usually present. It is noteworthy, however, that two seronegative rheumatoid arthritis patients with relatively high levels of C4 and C2 stained exclusively for γG_2 and γG_4, subgroups that have been reported to fix complement poorly, if at all.[29]

TABLE 3

INTRACYTOPLASMIC INCLUSIONS OF IMMUNOGLOBULINS*

	Immunoglobulin Class		
Patient Group†	γG	γA	γM
RA-pos	28/31	16/31	25/31
RA-neg	2/13	2/14	1/14
DJD	0/7	0/7	0/7

* Number of specimens with $>10\%$ of cells staining out of the total number examined.

† RA-pos = seropositive rheumatoid arthritis; RA-neg = seronegative rheumatoid arthritis; DJD = degenerative joint disease.

Discussion

The total hemolytic complement activity of the synovial fluids from the seropositive rheumatoid arthritis patients was approximately one-half that of the fluids from either the seronegative rheumatoid arthritis or the degenerative joint disease patients. In the seropositive rheumatoid arthritis group, these low CH_{50} levels were associated with variable reductions in C1 activity, marked depressions of C4 and C2 activities, and moderate depressions of C3 activity (TABLE 1). These alterations in component levels are consistent with intraarticular activation of C1, as originally postulated by Fostiropoulos and his colleagues.[30] This activation can be inferred from the marked and parallel reductions of C4 and C2, the natural substrates of $C\overline{1}$.

Evidence from the component analyses suggests also that this activation of C1 is immunological in origin. The very low C1 activities observed in six of the 17 fluids from seropositive rheumatoid arthritis patients are consistent with binding to an immune complex rather than with activation by a nonimmunological mechanism. The absence of reduced C1 activities in some of these fluids may relate to the known ability of $C\overline{1}$ to dissociate from immune complexes at physiological ionic strength.[31] The reductions in C3 activities suggest the generation of significant amounts of C3-convertase, a process that is more efficiently completed by solid-state activation, such as occurs on an immune complex, than by the random fluid-phase action of $C\overline{1}$ on C4 and C2.

The immunofluorescent studies on synovial-fluid leukocytes reveal that the deposition of complement and immunoglobulin proteins occurs predominantly in those joints in which complement activation is evident from fluid-phase reductions of C4 and C2 activities. Presumably, complexes of immunoglobulins and complement protein are phagocytosed by the synovial-fluid leukocytes. Since the third component is known to enhance phagocytosis,[15] it is not surprising that the intracellular deposition of C3 and C4 is most intense in those joints in which complement activation is occurring. The inverse relationship between synovial-fluid levels of C4 and C3 and the frequency of intracellular inclusions of these complement proteins and immunoglobulins γM and γG are consistent with this view. A similar inverse relationship between CH_{50} activity and C3 deposition was suspected by Vaughan and co-workers,[3] but the number of cell preparations stained for C3 was too small to permit a firm conclusion in this regard. It is noteworthy that the synovial fluids from latex-negative patients with rheumatoid arthritis did contain reduced levels of C4 and C2 activities as compared with the fluids from the patients with degenerative joint diseases. The fluids from the seronegative rheumatoid arthritis patients occasionally contained demonstrable deposits of immunoglobulins and complement protein. These findings are consistent with the view that synovial fluids from both seronegative and seropositive rheumatoid arthritis patients share the abnormality which leads to activation of C1. Either the rheumatoid factor in the seropositive fluids reflects a greater underlying abnormality or the factor itself augments the derangement of the complement system.

Data concerning the effect of anti-γ-globulin antibodies on the complement system are in apparent conflict. Gough and Davis have demonstrated that rheumatoid factor protects against the complement-lowering effects of intraperitoneal injections of aggregated γ-globulin[32] in the rat. In addition *in vitro* studies have also demonstrated the ability of rheumatoid factor to interfere with complement fixation or activation.[33,34] By contrast, recent studies by Zvaifler and Schur[35] reveal that rheumatoid factor can enhance the complement-fixing properties of reduced and alkylated heat-aggregated γG-globulin. The diverse behavior of rheumatoid factor-containing sera with respect to complement fixation may relate to the antigen-antibody ratios used in individual experiments, or to the presence of other inhibitory substances in heat-inactivated sera employed as a source of rheumatoid factor.[36]

The evidence for the intense immunological activation of the complement system in the joint fluid of seropositive rheumatoid arthritis patients and for the lesser activation in fluids from seronegative patients does not offer direct insight into the eliciting event. Nevertheless, these findings can perhaps be related to other recent observations. Evidence that synovial fluid from patients with rheumatoid arthritis contains immune complexes consisting of γG and 7S anti-γG has recently been obtained by Winchester and co-workers.[37] They have associated the finding of this material with reductions in the synovial-fluid CH_{50}. Furthermore, Ziff and his coworkers have observed that the addition of rheumatoid factor to synovial fluid from patients with seronegative arthritis markedly promotes the intracellular deposition of C3.[38] Whether this finding reflects the interaction of 19S rheumatoid factor with γG-anti-γG complexes or with an altered form of γG itself is unknown. The various pathways by which complement activation could occur in rheumatoid arthritis and the possible augmenting effect of 19S rheumatoid factor are indicated schematically in FIGURE 2. This scheme leaves completely unanswered the question of the mechanism by which altered

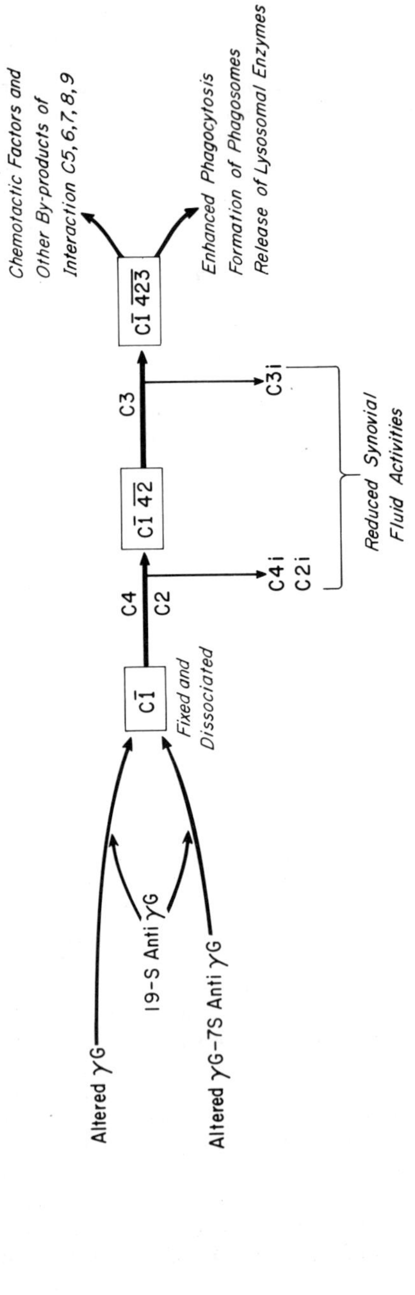

FIGURE 2. Possible pathways by which complement activation occurs in rheumatoid arthritis, and biological consequences of this activation.

γG appears so as to initiate the formation of anti-γ-globulins and to participate in the intraarticular activation of the complement system.

Acknowledgment

We are grateful for the assistance of Miss Mary Graves, Miss Margaret Monroe, Miss Sally Newell, and Mrs. Ann Platt Walker.

References

1. PEKIN, T. J. & N. J. ZVAIFLER. 1964. Hemolytic complement in synovial fluid. J. Clin. Invest. **43:** 1372.
2. HEDBERG, H. 1967. Studies on synovial fluid in arthritis. Acta Med. Scand. (Suppl.) **479**.
3. VAUGHAN, J. H., E. V. BARNETT, M. V. SOBEL & R. F. JACOX. 1968. Intracytoplasmic inclusions of immunoglobulins in rheumatoid arthritis and other diseases. Arthritis Rheum. **9:** 127.
4. NELSON, R. A., J. JENSEN, I. GIGLI & R. TAMURA. 1966. Methods for the separation, purification, and measurements of nine components of hemolytic complement in guinea pig serum. Immunochemistry **3:** 111.
5. MÜLLER-EBERHARD, H. J. 1968. Chemistry and reaction mechanisms of the complement system. Adv. Immunol. **8:** 1.
6. CHRISTIAN, C. L. 1960. Studies of aggregated γ-globulin. J. Immunol. **84:** 112.
7. LEPOW, I. H., G. B. NAFF, E. W. TODD, J. PENSKY & C. F. HINZ. 1961. Chromatographic resolution of the first component of human complement into three activities. J. Exp. Med. **117:** 983.
8. PENSKY, J. & H. G. SCHWICK. 1969. Human serum inhibitor of C′1 esterase. Identity with α2-neuraminoglycoprotein. Science **163:** 698.
9. PATRICK, R. A. & I. H. LEPOW. 1969. Fragmentation of the fourth component of human complement by $\overline{C1}$s. Fed. Proc. **28:** 817 (Abstr.).
10. GIGLI, I. & K. F. AUSTEN. 1969. Fluid phase destruction of $C2^{hu}$ by $C\overline{1}^{hu}$. I. Its enhancement and inhibition by homologous and heterologous C4. J. Exp. Med. **129:** 679.
11. DONALDSON, V. H., O. D. RATNOFF, M. R. KLEMPERER & F. S. ROSEN. 1968. Studies on a peptide from hereditary angioneurotic edema plasma with permeability factor and kinin activity. J. Immunol. **101:** 818 (Abstr.).
12. MILLER, J. A. & M. M. MAYER. 1968. On the cleavage of C′2 by C′1a: Immunological and physical comparisons of $C'2a^{d}$ and C′2a/i. Proc. Soc. Exp. Biol. Med. **129:** 127.
13. MÜLLER-EBERHARD, H. J., M. J. POLLEY & M. A. CALCOTT. 1967. Formation and functional significance of a molecular complex derived from the second and the fourth components of human complement. J. Exp. Med. **125:** 359.
14. COCHRANE, C. G. & H. J. MÜLLER-EBERHARD. 1968. The derivation of two distinct anaphylatoxin activities from the third and fifth components of human complement. J. Exp. Med. **122:** 99.
15. GIGLI, I. & R. A. NELSON. 1968. Complement dependent immune phagocytosis. Exp. Cell Res. **51:** 45.
16. RUDDY, S. & K. F. AUSTEN. 1969. C3 inactivator of man. I. Hemolytic measurement by the inactivation of cell-bound C3. J. Immunol. **102:** 533.
17. WARD, P. A., C. G. COCHRANE & H. J. MÜLLER-EBERHARD. 1966. Further studies on the chemotactic factor of complement and its formation *in vivo*. Immunology **11:** 141.
18. WARD, P. A. & L. J. NEWMAN. 1969. A neutrophil chemotactic factor from human C5. J. Immunol. **102:** 93.
19. PERLMANN, P., H. PERLMANN, H. J. MÜLLER-EBERHARD & J. A. MANNI. 1969. Cytotoxic effects of leukocytes triggered by complement bound to target cells. Science **163:** 937.
20. HALL, A. P., A. D. MEDNIS & T. B. BAYLES. 1958. Latex agglutination and inhibition reactions: Clinical experience in diagnosis of rheumatoid arthritis. New Eng. J. Med. **258:** 731.
21. ROPES, M., G. A. BENNETT, S. COBB, R. F. JACOX & R. A. JESSAR. 1958. Revision of diagnostic criteria for rheumatoid arthritis. Arthritis Rheum. **2:** 16.
22. KENT, J. F. & E. H. FIFE. 1963. Precise standardization of reagents for complement fixation. Amer. J. Trop. Med. Hyg. **12:** 103.
23. HANAUER, L. B. & C. H. CHRISTIAN. 1967. Clinical studies of hemolytic complement and the 11S component. Amer. J. Med. **42:** 882.

24. RUDDY, S., C. B. CARPENTER, K. F. AUSTEN & H. J. MÜLLER-EBERHARD. 1968. Complement component levels in hereditary angioedema and isolated C2 deficiency in man. *In* Mechanisms of Inflammation Induced by Immune Reactions, Fifth International Immunopathology Symposium. P. A. Miescher and P. Grabar, Eds. : 231–251. Benno Schwabe & Co. Basel, Switzerland.
25. BORSOS, T. & H. J. RAPP. 1963. Chromatographic separation of the first component of complement and its assay on a molecular basis. J. Immunol. **91**: 851.
26. RUDDY, S. & K. F. AUSTEN. 1967. Stiochiometric measurement of the activity of the fourth component of complement (C′4) in whole human serum. J. Immunol. **99**: 1162.
27. BORSOS, T. & H. J. RAPP. 1967. Immune hemolysis. A simplified method for the preparation of EAC′4 with guinea pig or human complement. J. Immunol. **99**: 263.
28. MÜLLER-EBERHARD, H. J. & H. G. KUNKEL. 1961. Isolation of a thermolabile serum protein which precipitates γ-globulin aggregates and participates in immune hemolysis. Proc. Soc. Exp. Biol. Med. **106**: 291.
29. ISHIZAKA, T., K. ISHIZAKA, S. SALMON & H. FUDENBERG. 1967. Biologic activities of aggregated γ-globulin. VIII. Aggregated immunoglobulins of different classes. J. Immunol. **99**: 82.
30. FOSTIROPOULOS, G., K. F. AUSTEN & K. J. BLOCH. 1965. Total hemolytic complement (CH50) and second component of complement (C2): Activity in serum and synovial fluid. Arthritis Rheum. **8**: 219.
31. RAPP, H. J. & T. BORSOS. 1963. The effects of low ionic strength on immune hemolysis. J. Immunol. **91**: 826.
32. GOUGH, W. W. & J. S. DAVIS. 1966. Effects of rheumatoid factor on complement levels *in vivo*. Arthritis Rheum. **9**: 555.
33. ZVAIFLER, N. J. & K. J. BLOCH. 1962. Rheumatoid factor: An inhibitor of the complement fixation reaction. Arthritis Rheum. **5**: 127.
34. HEIMER, R., F. M. LEVIN & M. F. KAHN. 1963. Inhibition of complement fixation by human serum. II. The activity of γ1M globulin and rheumatoid factor in complement fixation. J. Immunol. **91**: 866.
35. ZVAIFLER, N. J. & P. H. SCHUR. 1968. Reactions of aggregated mercaptoethanol treated gammaglobulin with rheumatoid factor: Precipitin and complement fixation studies. Arthritis Rheum. **11**: 523.
36. KEMPF, R. A., I. GIGLI & K. F. AUSTEN. 1969. Inhibition of the lytic effect of guinea pig complement by rabbit complement. J. Immunol. **102**: 795.
37. WINCHESTER, R., V. AGNELLO & H. G. KUNKEL. 1969. The joint-fluid γG globulin complexes and their relationship to intraarticular complement diminution. This monograph.
38. HURD, E. R., J. LOSPALLUTO & M. ZIFF. Studies on the formation of leukocyte inclusions *in vivo* and *in vitro*. Arthritis Rheum. In press.

General Discussion

DR. ZVAIFLER: I don't think the people who have not worked in this area can appreciate how hard Dr. Ruddy and his co-workers have worked to load the system against themselves by using degenerative joint disease as a control. In point of fact, if they had used as a control diseases in which comparable degrees of inflammation occur, i.e., nonrheumatoid inflammatory joint diseases, I'm sure the differences they showed would be much greater. In degenerative joint disease, there are less cells and there is less protein ingress into the joint. Thus, the changes they have shown, which are distinct from degenerative joint disease, would be even more exaggerated with other inflammatory infusions.

The material I presented with Dr. Peter Ward a year ago in Atlantic City showing the trimolecular complex of C5, 6, 7 in joint fluids, mainly from patients with rheumatoid arthritis, suggests also that complement activation goes on beyond the third component step. And I suspect that if we were to measure all the way to the end, we'd show all of the complement sequence involved.

DR. RUDDY: We think it probably does proceed further along the line than merely to C3 and plan on determinations of C9 in a relatively short period of time.

DR. EPSTEIN: Dr. Ruddy, what is the very best way to collect synovial fluid so that you don't use up complement, don't let the leukocytes ingest complement components during clotting, and don't activate the kinin or any other plasmin or enzyme-active system? You passed over that. In our lab, we let the fluid clot briefly at room temperature.

DR. RUDDY: As a collector of synovial fluids, Dr. Epstein, I think you probably know that there is no good answer to your question. I defer the collection of specimens for kinin to Dr. Austen or to you. In regard to collecting for complement, all I can say is that we collected the specimens as described and we do not consider that there were any alterations that occurred after the drawing of the specimen.

DR. VAUGHAN: May I ask about the patients who were seronegative and had inclusions? I gather that you had the same experience that we did, that fewer cells were involved when there were inclusions in the seronegative patients, and perhaps there were fewer inclusions per cell. Did you also have the experience that γM was rarely if ever seen in these patients? What proportion of patients who were seronegative actually did show inclusions?

DR. RUDDY: Among our seronegative patients, one out of 14 stained for IgM among the seropositive patients, 25 out of 31 stained. I would say, therefore, that in general our experience was similar to yours. The seronegative patients who did stain for IgG were the ones that I mentioned who showed subgroup-specific staining for γG_2 in one case and for γG_2 and γG_4 in another case.

DR. VAUGHAN: Have you seen in your investigation of joint fluid some patients that were seropositive in the face of a negative peripheral blood serum? This has been talked about; we haven't seen it, but perhaps you have.

DR. RUDDY: Yes, on rare occasions we have seen such patients, but they are distinctly unusual.

DR. HANNESTAD: Are the changes that you observe in the synovial fluid from seropositive patients caused by true immune complexes or by nonspecificially aggregated γG? I think this would be very difficult to determine because the seronegative patients probably have less severe joint inflammation. Incidentally, are you aware of control studies in which they have taken cells from pus, intensively inflammed regions other than joints, and studied these cells for inclusions of IgG, M, A, and complement components to see if such inclusions contain the same type of changes as you find in these synovial fluid cells?

DR. RUDDY: To answer the first question, the changes that we have observed in complement component activities are compatible with the activation of the complement system either by an altered immunoglobulin or by specific immune complexes. The point, I think, is that the system is immunological in the sense that it proceeds in the orderly and sequential fashion in which one would expect component alterations to occur. I think Dr. Schur should answer the question about staining for pus cells.

DR. SCHUR: One pleural fluid was examined from a patient with rheumatoid arthritis, and we found the same type of inclusion body.

DR. CATHCART: I think I can add to that. By means of immunofluorescent techniques in studying pus we have found inclusions that contain complement, IgG, and nucleoprotein, but not IgM.

DR. RUDDY: This was C3 that you published.

DR. CATHCART: Yes.

DR. KUNKEL: Was the complement down in the pleural fluid along with these inclusion bodies?

Dr. Schur: Yes, it was undetectable by whole hemolytic complement, and the β_{1C}, β_{1E}, and C1q by radial diffusion were barely detectable. I don't think it's possible to get normal pleura fluid. Do you?

Dr. Barnett: We looked as synovial fluid prior to synovectomy of the knee, and then six months later. The complement levels consistently rise six months later. So for what it's worth, there are apparent local factors that can be altered by synovectomy.

Dr. Hannestad: That doesn't surprise me. When you do a synovectomy, you are removing the inflammed territory, so obviously you would expect the complement to rise. I don't think that this really tells us anything about the basic problem here. Is it nonspecifically aggregated or is it immune complexes present in these aggregates?

RHEUMATOID FACTOR AND KININ GENERATION*

Wallace V. Epstein, M.D., Margaret Tan, M. S.,
and Kenneth L. Melmon, M.D.

Rheumatic Disease Group and Division of Clinical Pharmacology
Department of Medicine, University of California School of Medicine
San Francisco, Calif.

It is evident from individual case presentations and from retrospective studies that the synovitis characteristic of peripheral rheumatoid arthritis bears some meaningful association with the presence of high concentrations of circulating rheumatoid factors. Most vexing to those who would attempt to show a close correlation between inflammation and the presence of rheumatoid factor is the unmistakable synovitis in seronegative rheumatoid arthritics, both young and old, and the noninflammatory nature of some strongly seropositive conditions. Examination of the mediators of inflammation is required to bridge the gap between the presence or absence of detectable rheumatoid factor and sustained inflammation.

Many of the substances that generate and regulate the inflammatory process are derived from cells such as mast cells, from tissue and circulating leukocytes, from cell fragments such as platelets, and in some instances from organ parenchymal cells, as in pancreatic tissue. Of greatest interest to this presentation are those inflammatory mediators that derive entirely from soluble blood proteins.

The coagulation system, complement system, and the kinin system impinge on one another at a number of points. Much evidence has been presented emphasizing the involvement and utilization of complement components in the plasma and synovial fluid of patients with inflammatory arthritis. The generation of the short-lived group of linear polypeptides collectively termed kinins depends upon the activation of a series of protein precursors, depicted in FIGURE 1. The α_2-globulin, kininogen, is acted upon by one or more esterolytic enzymes designated active kallikrein. Peptides of the kinin group are split from the parent kininogen, and a variety of events associated with inflammation can then result. The kinins, in turn, are destroyed by kininases found in plasma leukocytes, and tissue parenchymal cells. Particular interest is focused on the key role occupied by the inactive precursor of esterolytic kallikrein and of Hageman Factor. The inhibitor of C′1 esterase and the naturally occurring plasma kallikrein inhibitors may be identical or closely related substances. The association of Hageman Factor with the kinin system as well as the coagulation system further asserts the interrelationship of these several elements that contribute to inflammation. The many sources and high efficiency of cellular and plasma kininases give the kinins a half-life measured in seconds.

Evidence involving the kinin system in the inflammatory process of rheumatoid arthritis derives from observations on the presence of Hageman Factor, kininogen, and granulocytes in rheumatoid synovial fluid, as well as the presence of kininogen and kinin in several forms of inflammatory synovitis. Melchiorri in 1963[1] noted increased kinin and kinin precursors in the synovial fluid of patients with rheumatoid arthritis. Jenson and co-workers in 1965[2] measured the urinary excretion of kinins and found these decreased in rheumatoid arthritics com-

* Supported in part by United States Public Health Service grants nos. AM–1229, HE–09964 and GM-16496, as well as School of Medicine and Academic Senate Research Funds and the Northern California chapter of the Arthritis Foundation.

pared with a control population. Briseid and his colleagues in 1966[3] found normal plasma kininogen concentrations in rheumatoid arthritics but low plasma kininase concentrations. More recently, Melmon and his associates in 1967[4] measured increased concentrations of kinins in the synovial fluid obtained from persons with several forms of synovitis and noted that the intraarticular injection of synthetic bradykinin in dogs caused an experimental synovitis.

In attempting to evaluate these observations one must first consider the nature of the biological assay for bradykinin. The biological test system consists of the contraction of a uterine muscle strip from an estrogen-treated rat in a bath containing an antihistaminic drug, an anticholinergic drug, and an antiserotonin drug. Contraction under these circumstances is regarded as a specific test for the kinin content of the test solution. A refinement involves the capacity of carboxypeptidase to destroy the muscle-contracting capacity; this further characterizes the test solution as kinin-like. Additional characterization is possible, based upon chromatographic procedures as well as the definitive structural identification of the polypeptides.

In addition to the intrinsic uncertainty of any biological assay, there is the problem of assembling the materials to be studied. The ease with which kinin can be generated in plasma makes collection of the plasma substrate a singularly difficult undertaking. Change of temperature, saline dilution, or contact with glass, or the presence of any particulate matter, pH change, or the presence of foreign chemicals is sufficient to initiate the enzymatic steps that lead to kinin production. Therefore, the steps in manipulation always involve a balance of kinin generation and kinin destruction. Truly, this is a field that deserves a specific immunoassay, and Dr. Austen and his group as well as others are moving rapidly in that direction. However, the problem of substrate collection as well as the specificity of the activating systems will remain even after the "nasty bit of tissue on a piece of string," to quote Dr. Brocklehurst, has been eliminated. The activation of the bradykinin system by antigen-antibody complexes has been suggested by the work of Movat, who identified kinin activity after the addition of antigen-antibody precipitates to guinea pig serum.[5] Dr. Movat traces the origin of his own work back to Friedburger's studies in 1910

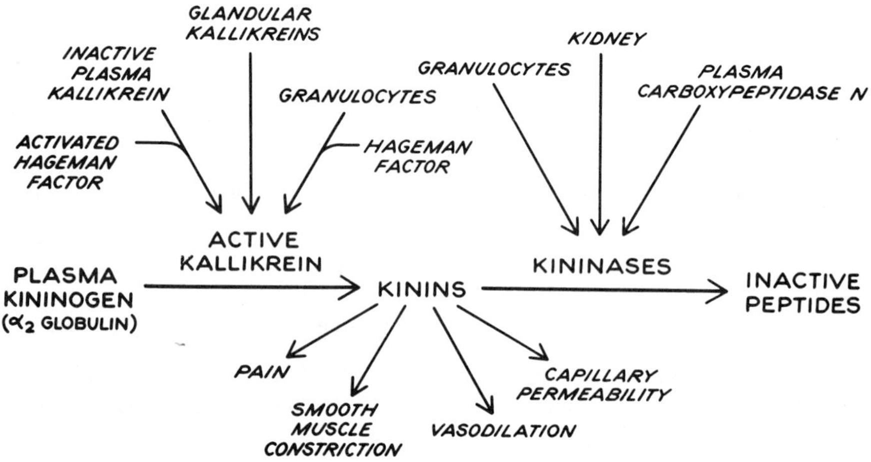

FIGURE 1. Activators and inactivators of the kininogen-kinin system.

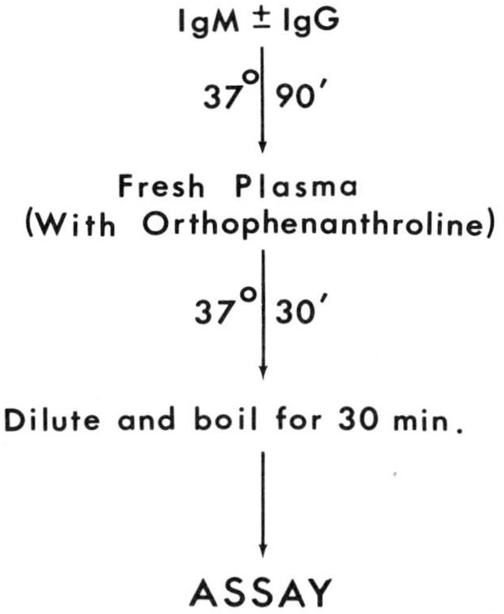

FIGURE 2. Scheme for the release and direct assay of kinin.

on the activation of guinea pig serum by antigen-antibody precipitates with complement-fixing capability.[14] It was the failure of antihistaminics to entirely suppress enhanced vascular permeability that led him to identify kinin-like activity in such activated serum. The enhancement of this activity by kininase inhibitors and the failure of antihistaminics to prevent guinea pig ileum contraction as well as the induced fall of blood pressure produced by such serum provided further indirect supportive evidence that kinin had been generated. Rather than attempting to generate kinin activity in serum by particulate antigen-antibody precipitates, we have used combinations of human IgG and IgM rheumatoid factor added to freshly obtained normal human plasma in the presence of a kininase inhibitor. A likely site for antigen-antibody activation of the system is at the point of conversion of inactive to active Hageman factor, while another potential site of activity is the point of conversion of inactive kallikrein to active kallikrein; evidence dealing with these two possible points of activity will be presented. Activation of plasma kallikreins alone has proven capable of converting from 30–50% of the available substrate plasma kininogen,[6] and this would be the largest quantity of kinin generation that one might seek in the action of soluble antigen-antibody complexes. We have used citrated human plasma as our substrate material and have taken great care to centrifuge all protein solutions free of particulate matter. Indeed, the two technical problems of how to handle substrate plasma and how to keep reagents particle free have provided us with a continuous challenge. There is, in fact, no clear evidence in the literature bearing on the ability of soluble isolated serum proteins free of kinin, activated kallikrein, or activated Hageman factor to initiate those steps resulting in kinin release.

The procedure used for the direct assay of kinin is shown in FIGURE 2. The IgM-rich fraction of selected sera, with or without the addition of normal human IgG-globulin, is added to freshly drawn citrated plasma in the presence of *o*-phenanthroline. Following incubation of this combination, the plasma is diluted and boiled for 30 minutes, and then the material assayed by the biological test system. The IgG used in these studies is either Cohn Fraction II or the IgG-globulin obtained from normal human serum by Sephadex G-200 chromatography combined with DEAE-exchange chromatography. IgG solutions that have been heated for 15 minutes at 63° C are designated as aggregated or heated γ-globulin. These, as well as all other solutions, are centrifuged immediately prior to use to remove any particulate matter. The IgM-rich fractions of serum are obtained by steps shown in FIGURE 3. These are isolated from the euglobulin fractions obtained by passage of sera through a Sephadex G-25 column equilibrated at low ionic strength. The pseudoglobulin fractions are first removed, and then the euglobulin fractions are obtained by passage of high-ionic strength buffer. The euglobulin fractions subjected to DEAE chromatography yield IgM-rich fractions.[7] The rheumatoid factor titers of the original serum and the isolated IgM fractions are measured by the FII tanned cell hemagglutination technique[8] with doubling dilutions beginning at a concentration of the isolated fraction of 0.2 mg of protein per milliliter of test solution. We have found it most desirable to perform the biological assay on the same day on which the kinin is generated. We follow standard procedures in the biological assay,[9] using a 10-ml chamber; DeJalon's strip bath, containing atropine sulfate (10^{-6} g/ml); and mepyramine maleate (10^{-7} g/ml). The temperature of the bath was 23°–25°, and we have based our standardization upon the ability of 2 ng of synthetic bradykinin to cause a contraction of 8–9 cm. Those familiar with biological assay systems will appreciate our reluctance to ascribe quantitative values in this direct assay of kinin activity.

The controls used in this direct assay of kinin are shown in FIGURE 4. The addition of 2 ng of synthetic bradykinin results in a contraction of the uterine strip of 8–9 cm. The normal plasma exposed only to plastic surfaces does not generate sufficient kinin to result in a detectable contraction, while the same plasma exposed to a glass surface generates kinin-like activity sufficient to cause the contraction shown at the third point.

Following these control points is shown the behavior of the strip following the sequential addition of two IgM-rich fractions obtained from sera of patients with rheumatoid arthritis. These two IgM fractions appeared to be similar upon immunoelectrophoretic analysis. Both had approximately the same strongly positive reaction for the presence of rheumatoid factor by hemagglutination, but

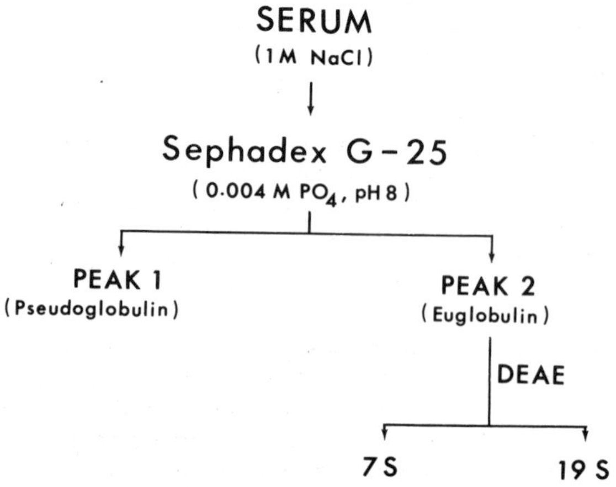

FIGURE 3. Steps used to isolate the 19S IgM-rich fraction of serum.

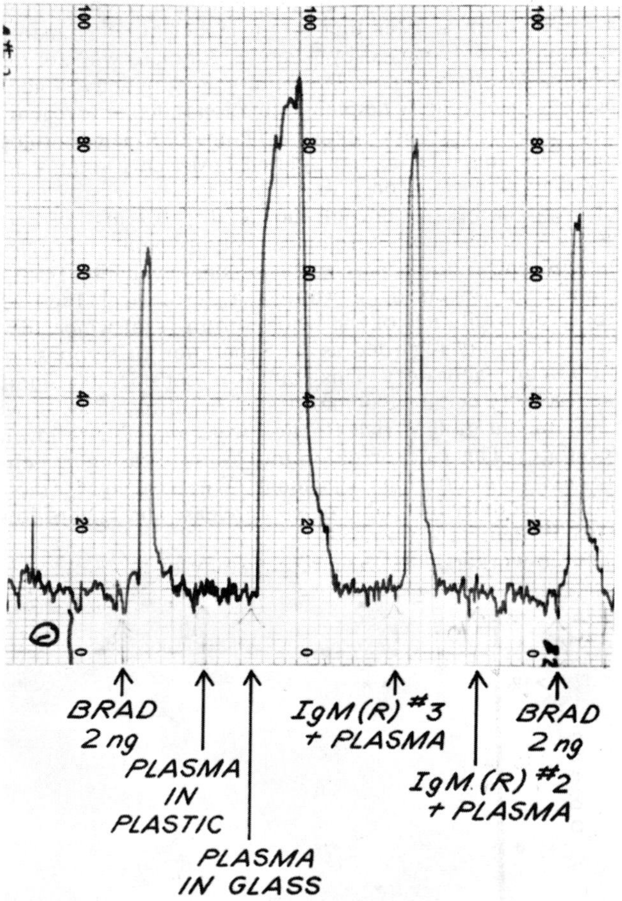

FIGURE 4. Contractions of uterine muscle strip following addition of synthetic bradykinin or IgM-rich fractions of serum. Plasma controls are included.

one of them, IgM (R) #3, on contact with plasma caused the release of uterine-contracting activity while the other, IgM (R) #2, failed to do so. The final contraction shown in FIGURE 4 was produced by reference synthetic bradykinin. The material or materials released in plasma by glass exposure, by the addition of IgM-rich fractions, or by complexes of IgG-and IgM-rich globulin caused rat uterine muscle contraction in the presence of atropine and mepyramine. This activity was destroyed by carboxypeptidase and by chymotrypsin. None of these activities could be produced in plasma which was deficient in Hageman factor, nor could this activity be produced by any of the foregoing methods when the kallikrein inhibitor-soybean trypsin inhibitor was added although it could be produced in the presence of ovomucoid. All of these findings constitute reasonable characterization of kinin as the agent responsible for the uterine contraction shown.

In general, it was possible to categorize individual IgM-rich fractions as positive or negative in respect to kinin-generating ability since contractions were either less than 1 cm or greater than 6 cm in height. Presumably, very small quantities of kinin were destroyed by whatever kininase was not blocked by the *o*-phenanthroline. Attempts to correlate kinin-releasing activity and the rheumatoid factor activity measured by hemmaglutination failed to reveal an unequivocal association of kinin-releasing activity with rheumatoid factor serological activity. FIGURE 5 shows the $\log_2$ titer of the isolated IgM-rich fractions and their categorization for kinin-releasing (positive) or non-kinin-releasing (negative) activity. In all of these studies, a concentration of 0.1–0.2 mg/ml of the IgM-rich fraction was used to test both serological activity and kinin-releasing ability. This protein concentration was selected as one available from all isolation procedures and one which demonstrated a serological titer approximately equivalent to a 1:100 dilution of the whole serum from which the fraction was derived. This is generally regarded as the separation of seropositive from seronegative serum in our laboratory. This point is of considerable significance, since kinin-releasing activity could be demonstrated in all instances in which concentrations of 1–2 mg/ml of IgM-rich fraction were available following chromatographics procedures. This categorization into kinin-releasing or non-kinin-releasing is, therefore, concentration dependent. We have IgM fractions of high rheumatoid factor activity incapable of kinin release and IgM of low rheumatoid activity capable of definite kinin release.

Colman and co-workers,[10] in their recent study of the nature of serum kalli-

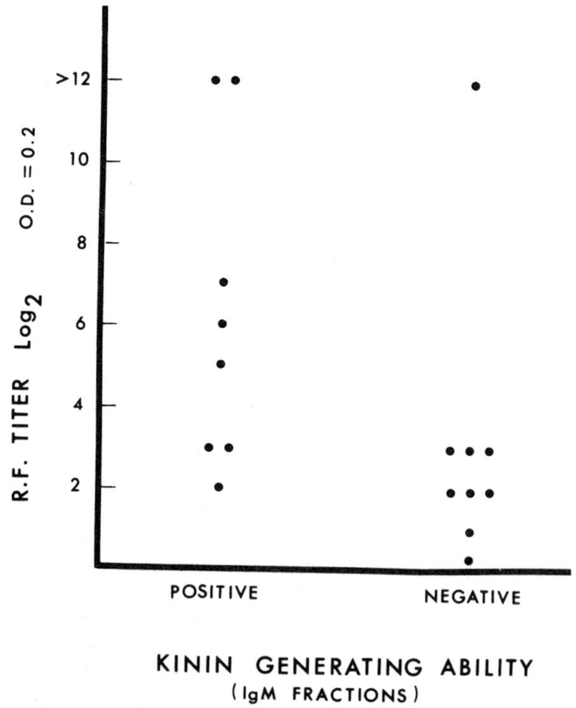

FIGURE 5. Relation of $\log_2$ rheumatoid factor titer of IgM fractions to kinin-releasing ability.

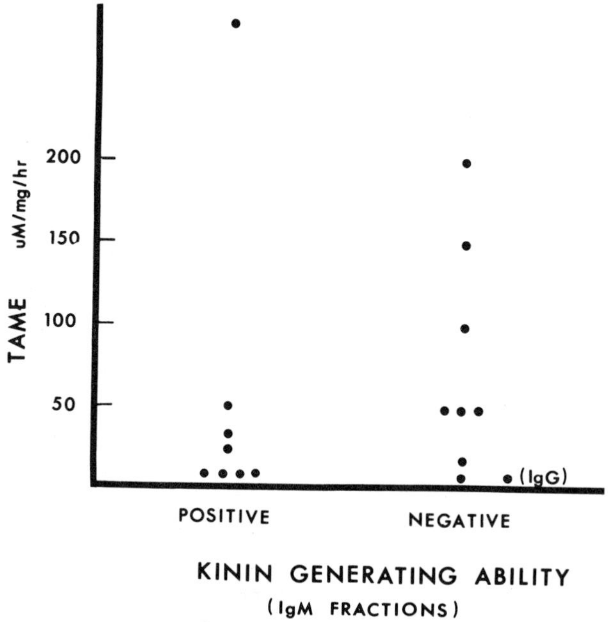

FIGURE 6. Relation of esterolytic capability (TAME assay) to kinin-releasing ability of IgM-rich fractions and normal IgG.

krein, used chromatographic steps for the isolation of kallikrein. They found a molecular weight of approximately 160,000 for their kallikrein II, which migrated as a fast γ-globulin. Robert[11] has recently described TAME esterolytic activity in highly purified human IgG. In order to examine whether we might be studying active kallikrein in these IgM-rich fractions, we subjected these fractions to the TAME enzyme assay: The ability of kallikrein to hydrolyze the synthetic arginine ester tosylargininemethyl ester (TAME) was used to examine the esterase capability of our IgM-rich fractions.

FIGURE 6 shows a comparison of kinin-generating ability with TAME-hydrolyzing ability. No correlation of TAME-hydrolyzing ability and kinin-generating ability was found. The inability of the IgM-rich fraction to generate bradykinin in Hageman factor-deficient plasma also made it unlikely that preformed active kallikrein in the IgM fraction was responsible for kinin generation. There remains the possibility, however, that enzyme systems not detectable by the TAME assay could contribute to the generation of kinin from kininogen.

In contrast to the activity of IgM-rich fractions of serum, serum itself in con-

TABLE 1

KININ GENERATING ABILITY OF WHOLE SERUM*

Rheumatoid Factor Activity of Serum	Kinin Generation (no. of sera)	
	Positive	Negative
Positive	1	12
Negative	0	10

* Serum dilution, 1:100.

centrations that provided approximately the same rheumatoid factor activity as the IgM fractions almost uniformly failed to cause kinin generation. As shown in TABLE 1, only one of thirteen sera strongly positive for rheumatoid factor activity caused kinin release in fresh normal plasma while none of ten sera free of rheumatoid factor activity caused kinin release. These sera were tested at 1:100 dilutions.

Since our major interest was the ability of the soluble complex of IgG and IgM to cause kinin generation, an explanation was sought for the variable capability of isolated IgM by the addition of IgG to those IgM fractions incapable of bradykinin release. FIGURE 7 shows test results with 0.5 mg of normal human IgG, which produced an insignificant contraction when added to fresh plasma, and with 0.02 mg of an isolated IgM-rich fraction, which produced no detectable release of kinin activity. The combination of the two prior to addition to normal plasma caused the release of kinin activity. Doubling the concentration of the

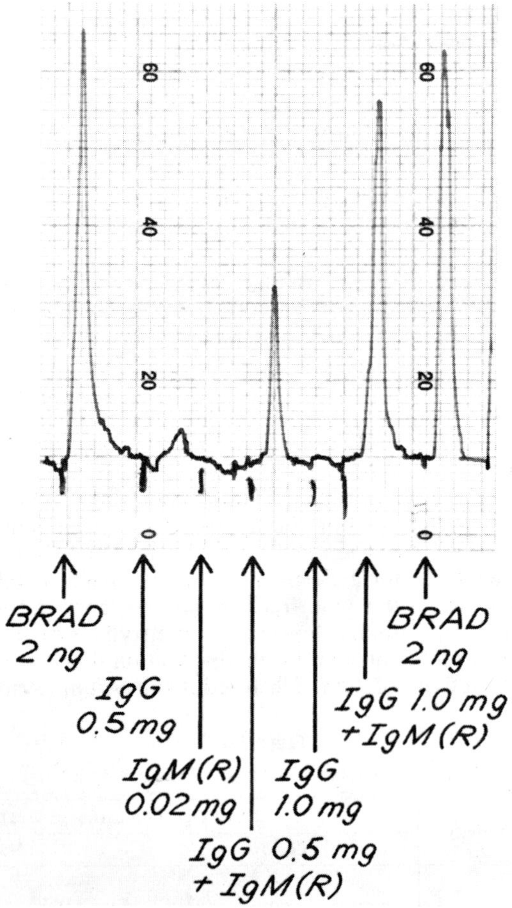

FIGURE 7. Contractions of uterine muscle strip produced by the addition of IgG plus IgM to normal plasma.

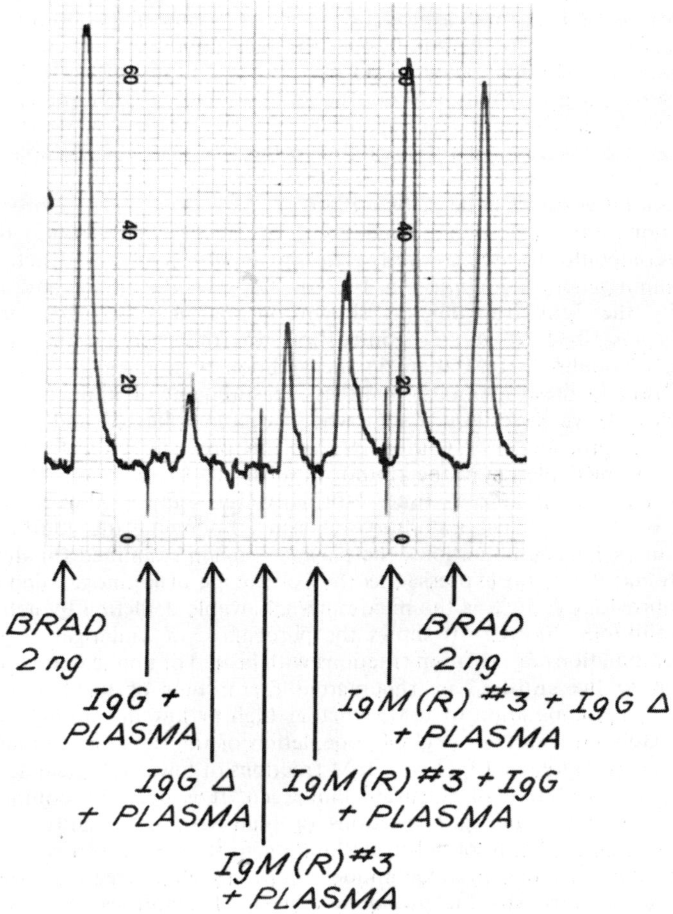

FIGURE 8. Comparison of IgG and heated IgG added to IgM before addition of such combinations to normal plasma.

IgG protein (1.0 mg/ml) did not cause kinin generation, but the addition of the higher concentration of IgG to IgM caused further evidence of kinin release. The reference contractions to synthetic bradykinin are shown at the beginning and end of the strip in FIGURE 7. The capacity to "turn on" inactive samples of IgM by adding IgG has been limited to those IgM fractions that showed rheumatoid factor activity, whether obtained from the serum of normal individuals or from those with peripheral rheumatoid arthritis. We have examined the tubes containing the combination of IgG-globulin and IgM-rich fractions after incubation for 90 minutes at 37° C and found no gross visual evidence of particulate matter. This ability of IgG to induce kinin-generating ability in an IgM-rich fraction is our strongest, albeit, indirect evidence that it is actually the anti-IgG rheumatoid factor activity that we are measuring in the IgM fractions. This result implies that those IgM fractions which generate kinin without the addition of IgG-globulin may already contain such biologically active complexes. Nothing in our isolation procedure precludes the presence of such complexes in the IgM-rich fractions. A comparison of IgG- and heated IgG-globulin is shown in FIGURE 8. Slight activity was produced by the addition of the IgG-globulin to plasma. None was demonstrated on adding heated IgG-globulin to plasma. The IgM fraction selected showed some activity without the addition of IgG-globulin. The addition of IgG-globulin to the IgM fraction produced little change, while the addition of the heated or aggregated IgG-globulin to the IgM led to what appears to be an increased amount of kinin release. Although we have continued to avoid the use of quantitative terms in describing these results, TABLE 2 shows three different IgM fractions and suggests a greater ability of heated IgG-globulin than non-heated IgG-globulin to induce kinin-releasing activity in an IgM fraction. There was no kinin-generating ability in IgG or heated IgG alone, and negligible activity by the IgM fractions, as shown on uterine strips standardized as previously described. A greater contraction was observed on the addition of heated IgG-globulin to IgM than on the addition of nonheated IgG.

In addition to these methods of direct measurement of kinin released from normal plasma, we have used a somewhat more complicated and less sensitive indirect assay procedure[12,13] (FIGURE 9). In this procedure, the fresh plasma is examined for the depletion of the kininogen substrate. Fresh plasma is assayed for its kininogen content at zero time. Normally, this ranges between 4,000 and 6,000 ng of kininogen per milliliter of plasma. Following the addition of IgG and IgM in various combinations, the plasma is again examined for the residual kininogen and the result expressed as the percentage of kininogen depletion. As indicated previously, 50% is the maximum achievable depletion by activation of plasma kallikrein. FIGURE 10 shows the percentage of kininogen depletion of various combinations of IgM-rich fractions with heated or nonheated IgG-globulin in relation to the anti-IgG or rheumatoid factor titer of the individual IgM fractions. The combination of IgM, whether high or low in serological activity, with IgG-globulin results in negligible depletion of the substrate kininogen. The combination of aggregated IgG with IgM fractions of low serological activity also produces little depletion of substrate kininogen. It is only the combination of heated IgG-globulin and IgM fractions of high serological activity that produces significant depletion of substrate kininogen. In comparison with our direct assay procedure, this depletion technique requires much greater kininogen utilization, which explains why the production of small quantities of bradykinin by IgM protein alone could not be detected by this method, although it was detected in the direct assay procedure. This method confirms the specificity of the complex formed by the combination of aggregated IgG with IgM, and suggests

TABLE 2

COMPARATIVE EFFECT OF HEATED AND NONHEATED IGG-GLOBULIN ON THE INDUCTION OF KININ-RELEASING ACTIVITY IN IGM FRACTIONS

IgM Fraction No.	Kinin-Generating Ability*		
	IgM	IgM + IgG	IgM + △ IgG
1	0	4	7
2	1	3	9
3	1	2	8

* Measured in centimeters of contraction of a uterine strip. Reference standard, produced by 2 ng of bradykinin, 8–9 cm; positive reaction, >6 cm; IgG and heated (Δ) IgG produced contractions of 0 cm, i.e., no effect.

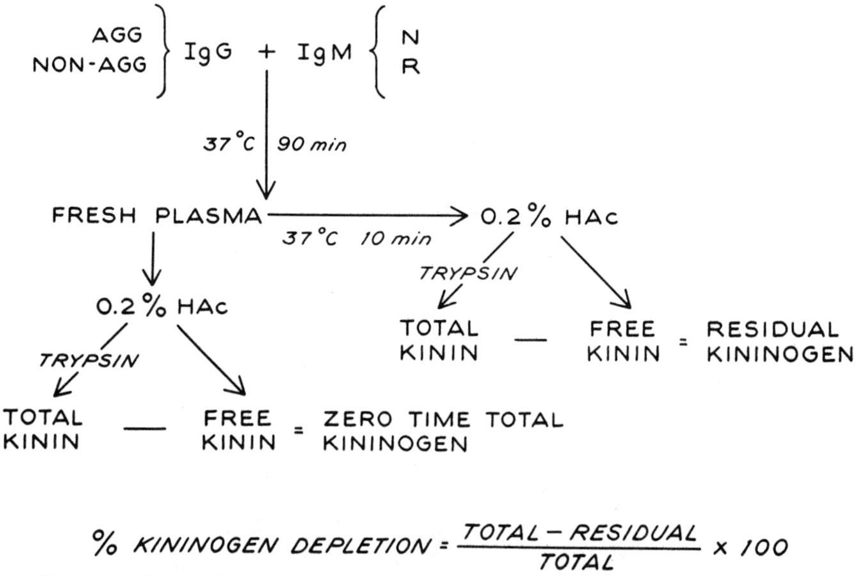

FIGURE 9. Scheme for the release of kinin and measurement of kininogen depletion.

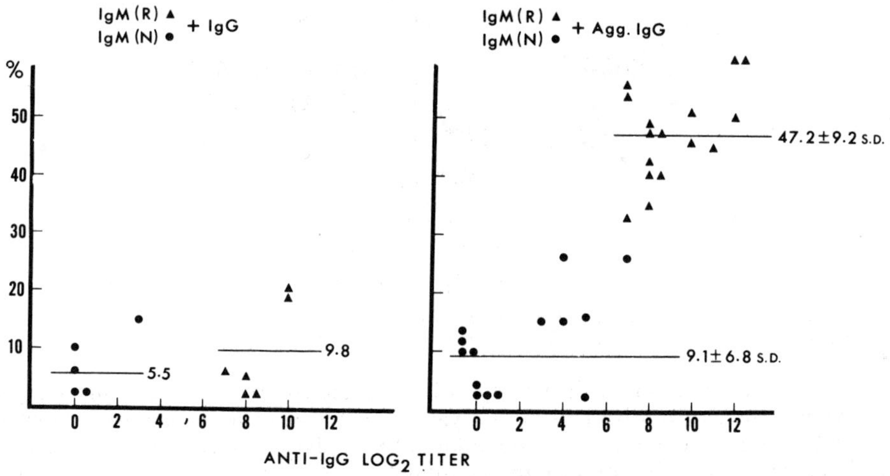

FIGURE 10. Percentage of kininogen depletion caused by the addition of combinations of heated or nonheated IgG and different IgM fractions to normal plasma.

greater activity of seropositive IgM fractions than seronegative fractions with aggregated IgG.

We have begun to examine body fluids other than serum from patients with rheumatoid arthritis. Inflammatory synovial fluids contain both fibrin and leukocytes which are capable of initiating kinin formation as well as serving as a source, together with plasma, of the kininases. There is clearly much in the handling and storing of synovial as well as pleural fluid that will determine

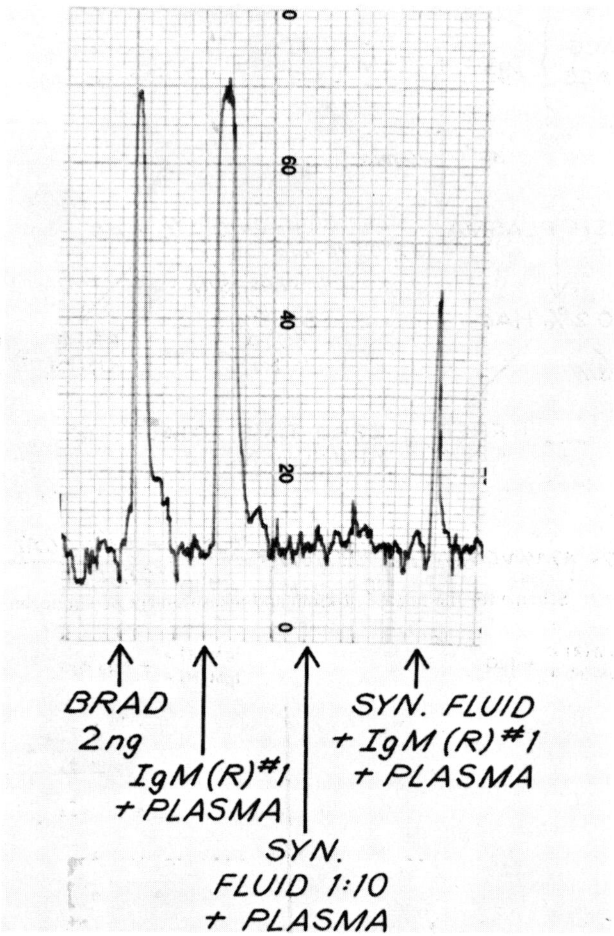

FIGURE 11. Demonstration of kininase activity of synovial fluid when added to an IgM capable of causing kinin release from plasma. Reaction time was 30 minutes.

whether kinin or kininase activity will be detected. We have examined eight synovial fluids from patients with a variety of forms of inflammatory synovitis, and in none of these have we found kinin-like activity as measured by the direct biological assay. In contrast to the studies of Melmon and co-workers,[4] this synovial fluid was not obtained by techniques that would destroy kininase activity. The addition of these synovial fluids to fresh normal plasma has not caused generation of bradykinin. One synovial fluid was found to have kininase-like activity, as shown in FIGURE 11. In this instance, the ability of synovial fluid added to an IgM fraction capable of causing kinin release resulted in diminished kinin activity. The combination of this synovial fluid with synthetic bradykinin abolished the muscle-contracting ability of the bradykinin. A pleural fluid from a strongly seropositive rheumatoid arthritic was found to contain both aggregated IgG-globulin, based upon precipitate formation with rheumatoid factor, and kininase activity sufficient to destroy 50,000 ng of synthetic bradykinin with

1 ml of pleural fluid in 30 minutes. Synovial and pleural fluid is now being collected with attention to those details that might influence kinin generation and the activity of kininase enzymes.

Summary

The soluble complex formed by the combination of aggregated normal human IgG with some IgM-rich fractions of serum results in the release of a kinin-like activity when normal human plasma is used as the substrate material. The strongest evidence suggesting that the kinin-releasing ability is directly correlated with anti-IgG activity is the ability of IgG protein, especially heated IgG, to enable IgM-globulin to show kinin-releasing activity. The direct assay detects a kinin-releasing capability in some IgM fractions alone, while the less-sensitive kininogen-depletion method demonstrates this activity only with the combination of aggregated IgG-globulin and IgM fractions of high rheumatoid factor activity. Various tests of kinin specificity indicate that bradykinin or a closely related substance is released from normal plasma under these circumstances; no correlation was found between esterolytic activity of the IgM fraction and its ability to release kinin. Free kinin has not been detected in samples of stored synovial fluid studied, but kininase activity has been detected in both synovial fluid and in pleural fluid from patients with rheumatoid arthritis.

References

1. Melchiorri, P. 1963. Occurrence of bradykinin in the synovia of subjects affected with rheumatoid arthritis. *In* Bradykinin and Its Precursors. F. Sicuteri, Ed. : 65. Centro Editionale Publicario Italiano. Rome, Italy.
2. Jensen, K. B., S. F. Rinvik & O. K. Dyrud. 1965. Excretion of urinary kinins in rheumatoid arthritis. Acta Pharmacol. Toxicol. **23:** 231.
3. Breseid, K., O. K. Dyrud & S. F. Rinvik. 1966. Determination of plasma kininogen, plasma kininase and erythrocyte kininase in men with rheumatoid arthritis. Acta Pharmacol. Toxicol. **24:** 179.
4. Melmon, K. L., M. E. Webster, S. E. Goldfinger & J. E. Seegmiller. 1967. The presence of a kinin in inflammatory synovial effusion from arthritides of varying etiologies. Arthritis Rheum. **10:** 13.
5. Movat, H. Z. 1967. Activation of the kinin system by antigen-antibody complexes. *In* Symposium on Vaso-Active Peptides. Proc. Third Int. Pharmacol. Congr., Sao Paulo, 1966. M. Rocha e Silva, Ed. : 177–188. Pergammon Press. Oxford, England.
6. Vogt, W. 1966. Demonstration of the presence of two separate kinin-forming systems in human and other plasma. *In* Hypotensive Peptides. Proc. Int. Symp., 1965. E. Erdös, N. Bach, I. Sicuteri & A. F. Wilde, Eds. : 185–192. Springer-Verlag. New York, N. Y.
7. Epstein, W. V. & M. Tan. 1962. Gamma globulin interactions in the sera of two patients with rheumatoid arthritis studied by gel filtration. J. Lab. Clin. Med. **60**(1): 125–137.
8. Heller, G., A. S. Jacobson, M. H. Kolodny & W. H. Kammerer. 1954. The hemagglutination test for rheumatoid arthritis. II. The influence of human plasma fraction II (gamma globulin) on the reaction. J. Immunol. **72:** 66.
9. Erdös, E. G. 1966. Hypotensive peptides: bradykinin, kallidin and eledoisin. Advances Pharmacol. **4:** 1–90.
10. Colman, R. W., L. Mattler & S. Sherry. 1969. Studies on the prekallikrein (kallikreinogen)–kallikrein enzyme system of human plasma. I. Isolation and purification of plasma kallikreins. J. Clin. Invest. **48:** 11.
11. Robert, B. 1968. Origine des activities esterolytiques et proteolytiques des preparations de gamma-globulines de differentes especes. Ann. Inst. Pasteur (Paris) **115:** 813–825.
12. Diniz, C. R. & I. F. Carvalho. 1963. A micromethod for determination of bradykininogen under several conditions. Ann. N. Y. Acad. Sci. **104:** 77–89.
13. Epstein, W. V., K. L. Melmon, M. Tan & J. Stoff. 1968. Kinin generation by human IgG-rheumatoid factor complex. J. Clin. Invest. **47:** 30a–31a.
14. Friedberger, E. 1910. Weitere Unterschungen über Erweisanaphylaxie. 1. Das Anaphylaxiegift. Z. Immunitätsforsch. **4:** 636–689.

General Discussion

DR. MACKENZIE: Aren't the fractions produced out of the G-25 column euglobulins? If so, these in themselves will contain γG.

DR. EPSTEIN: But then they are passed through DEAE.

DR. MACKENZIE: Even so, you still may get some fast-moving γG in your γM preparations. Could this explain some of your differences in your kinin generation?

DR. EPSTEIN: Yes, I think so.

DR. RUDDY: Did you examine your IgM-rich fractions for other esterase activity besides that with TAME? The solubility characteristics and the performance on DEAE of C1, for example, would probably make this material also wind up in the IgM-rich fraction. It might be interesting to look at acetyltyrosinemethyl ester.

DR. EPSTEIN: Would it not show activity on TAME substrate assay?

DR. RUDDY: I think acetyltyrosinemethyl ester would probably be more sensitive.

DR. EPSTEIN: We now have two other studies in progress. I really modeled this experiment after the kallikrein study of Dr. Sherry.

DR. COLEMAN: Some of your data indicated that the positive and negative kinin-like activities were not related to the titer of rheumatoid factor activity, but most demonstrated a strong relationship. Can you clarify this discrepancy?

DR. EPSTEIN: First, a direct assay of kinin release is a more sensitive assay and demonstrates the release of kinin activity from material having a wide spectrum of serological activities. It would be preferable to use quantitative techniques, such as the immunological assay for kinin, in order to establish meaningful correlations, rather than positive or negative assays. In our experiments, no very clear relationship was apparent.

With the less-sensitive technique, which requires depletion of 30% or more of the total kininogen substrate, activity was found in IgM that was high in serological rheumatoid factor activity, and when heated rather than unheated γG was used. Thus, the difference in relation to rheumatoid activity is not clear in the more-sensitive direct assay, but it is in the less-sensitive utilization assay.

DR. AUSTEN: We have been working with the radioimmunoassay of the known nonapeptide bradykinin. The problems, even with the specific immunological assay, are similar to those that Dr. Epstein has mentioned. The major problem, which is only now being resolved, is, how does one process a biological fluid so as to get a true assessment of the endogenous bradykinin value? We took advantage of an intrinsically labeled bradykinin preparation that has carbon-14 in the two prolines. We found, to our distress, that all existing methods of processing biological fluids resulted in about 90% inactivation, including use of the inhibitors of the radiolabeled bradykinin. Therefore, a new approach for obtaining meaningful values of free kinin is required. I think this explains, in part, why you have had such difficulty and why you have not obtained good correlations with your kinin assay. In all likelihood, your second method, evaluation of kinonogen depletion, although blunter in some ways, is at least less affected by the inactivation of any kinin that exists in the joint space.

DR. EPSTEIN: I'm aware of the use of the Hageman factor-stabilizing material together with EDTA. With trypsin as the assay material, we still find the normal range of available kinin that we obtain with our usual method of handling the fluids. Do you regard that as an adequate description of the preservation of the kininogen substrate?

DR. AUSTEN: No, and for a very good reason. You have to use intrinsically labeled bradykinin, and you have to measure the bradykinin present. If your intrinsically labeled bradykinin disappeared and you still obtained a normal native level, then obviously there was some generation. All of the existing methods for harvesting are still susceptible to a combination of destruction of the known nonapeptide and introduction of new nonapeptide; therefore, you look at some combination thereof. The only way of appreciating this problem is to use intrinsically radiolabeled material, and I don't think anybody has really solved the problem of looking at endogenous levels. That is why I said that I would consider your second approach as more reliable.

EXPERIMENTAL ARTHRITIS IN MAN AND RABBIT DEPENDENT UPON SERUM ANTI-IMMUNOGLOBULIN FACTORS*

Arnold J. Rawson, M.D., Sc.D., Joseph Lee Hollander, M.D.,
Francisco P. Quismorio, M.D., and Neva M. Abelson, M.D.

Departments of Pathology and Medicine
University of Pennsylvania School of Medicine
Philadelphia, Pa.

Experimental Arthritis Based upon Exogenous Antigen and Antibody

Several investigators have established that the intraarticular injection of an antigen into a previously hyperimmunized animal results in an arthritis which exhibits many of the histological features of rheumatoid arthritis in man.[1-4] As far back as 1933, Klinge[1] hyperimmunized rabbits by repeated subcutaneous injection of horse serum, and elicited arthritis by a single intraarticular injection of this material after a high-antibody titer had been achieved. More recently, rabbits have been hyperimmunized by intracutaneous injections of human or rabbit fibrin in Freund's adjuvant, and, after demonstration of delayed hypersensitivity to these materials, arthritis has been elicited by an intraarticular injection of the antigen.[2]

That the reaction was dependent upon local factors and not upon circulating antibody per se was demonstrated by the intraarticular injection into a normal rabbit of freshly prepared complexes of antigen and rabbit antibody in the presence of complement.[3] This procedure resulted in an arthritis that was similar in histological appearance to those produced by the previously described methods. In the early phase, after a single injection, there was evidence of synovial cell injury with exudation of polymorphonuclear leukocytes into the synovial fluid. Following repeated injections, proliferation of synovial cells occurred, and in chronic lesions there was villous change with nodules of lymphocytes and plasma cells. The exudate cells contained cytoplasmic granules in which IgG was demonstrable.

Recent studies of the Arthus reaction by a number of investigators have provided much information relevant to the studies described. It has been clearly shown that activation of the complement system by immune complexes results in chemotaxis of polymorphonuclear leukocytes,[5] and that the release of lysosomal enzymes from the granules of these cells is capable of inducing synovial proliferation as well as the other inflammatory changes noted.[6]

Experimental Arthritis Dependent upon Autologous Antigen and Autoantibody

Most normal rabbits have a spontaneously occurring 7S autoantibody called homoreactant.[7] This combines specifically with the Fab fragment of rabbit IgG, but not with the intact molecule. The intraarticular injection of autologous or pooled rabbit Fab fragment into a rabbit with homoreactant regularly elicits an arthritis similar in appearance and sequence of events to the arthritis elicited by exogenous antigen.[8] The injection of Fab fragment into the joint of a rabbit lacking homoreactant produces no lesion, nor does any lesion result from the intraarticular injection of autologous or pooled intact rabbit IgG, even in the presence of homoreactant.

*Supported in part by grant no. GM–6218 from the National Institutes of Health, United States Public Health Service.

The arthritis elicited by the injection of Fab fragment into the joint of a rabbit having serum homoreactant can be detected within 24 hours by evidence of synovial cell injury and exudation of polymorphonuclear leukocytes into the joint fluid. These cells have cytoplasmic granules within which IgG can be demonstrated. With repeated intraarticular injections of Fab fragment, the histological appearance within two weeks consists of synovial cell proliferation and fibrous organization of fibrin exudates. Continued injections result in early villous proliferation and accumulations of lymphocytes and plasma cells.

The repeated intraarticular injection of Fab fragment into a rabbit whose serum lacks homoreactant stimulates rising titers of serum homoreactant, first detectable one to two weeks after the initial injection. Although no immediate lesion is found in the injected joint, acute exudative changes first make their appearance about two weeks after the initial injection, at about the time that the autoantibody can be detected in the serum. Thereafter, subsequent chronic changes appear with continued injections. In the subsequent consideration of rheumatoid arthritis, the importance of the establishment of a hypersensitive state by the intraarticular route will be discussed. Also of interest in this connection is the ease with which the intraarticular introduction of an autologous IgG fragment, administered without adjuvants, gives rise to autoantibody.

Under the conditions described, the synovial lesions persist and progress only if antigen is continually supplied to the joint. An injection schedule of three times weekly suffices. If injection of antigen is discontinued, the lesion regresses. In addition, it was found that a minimum amount of antigen was required in order to elicit arthritis. In the case of Fab fragment, this was about 0.5 mg of protein; when 0.1 mg was given, no lesion appeared.

Rheumatoid Factor as an Autoantibody to IgG

Rheumatoid factor has been shown to be produced abundantly by the lymphoid and plasma cells of the synovial membrane of joints involved by rheumatoid arthritis.[9,10] It has the physicochemical characteristics of an antibody of the IgM class, although minor components having characteristics of other antibody classes may be present.[11] Although rheumatoid factor reacts with several mammalian γ-globulins, its primary specificity appears to be directed toward human IgG.[12] It reacts best with denatured human IgG, and the degree of the reaction seems to depend upon the extent of the denaturation.[13]

Many rheumatoid factors exhibit isospecificity, although autospecificity may also be demonstrated.[14] The technique of separating rheumatoid factor from complexes existing in serum facilitates the demonstration of its autospecificity by freeing it from substances that tend to inhibit its combination.[15] Studies utilizing fragments of IgG as antigens indicate that the major specificity of rheumatoid factor appears to be directed toward the Fc fragment.[16,17] A minor degree of specificity may be directed toward the Fab fragment[17] and pepsin-digested fragments.[18,19] The Fc fragment appears to contain antigenic loci Gm(a), Gm(x), and Gm(b), whereas Gm(f) and Gm(z) seem to be on the Fd portion of the Fab fragment.[20,21]

Experimental Arthritis Dependent upon Rheumatoid Factor and IgG

Since spontaneous rheumatoid arthritis is apparently limited to man, it was necessary to conduct experiments in human volunteers. In the initial experiments,[22] 2–4 ml of autologous whole serum was injected into the quiescent knees of six rheumatoid patients. In three instances, the injected serum had previously been heated to 63° C for ten minutes. In no instance was there any reaction in the injected joint.

In order to exclude activity of inhibitory substances, IgG was separated from serum by chromatography on diethylaminoethyl cellulose, and the quiescent knee joints of each of five rheumatoid patients received autologous isolated IgG. Four of the five responded within two hours with an acute arthritis characterized by pain, effusion, and leukocytic exudate. The cytoplasm of these cells contained granules within which both IgG and IgM were demonstrated. Initially, the amount of injected IgG was somewhat larger, but it soon became evident that a consistent response could be evoked by 3 mg. The standard rabbit test showed no evidence of pyrogens in the IgG preparations used.

When autologous IgG in similar dosage was introduced into the knees of four patients with osteoarthritis and one without arthritis, no inflammatory response was evoked. These early experiments seemed to indicate that rheumatoid arthritics were capable of responding to an autoantigen with an acute inflammatory reaction; thus, it was of interest to determine whether the response was related to the antigen or to a special degree of reactivity on the part of the rheumatoid arthritic.

To investigate this point, five rheumatoid patients each received an injection of 3 mg of IgG obtained from a normal donor. Four of the five showed no response, and in one patient only a very mild inflammatory reaction appeared. It is noteworthy that one of the test subjects had previously exhibited a severe inflammatory response to autologous IgG, but no reaction was elicited by IgG from a normal donor. This seemed to indicate that the inflammatory response of rheumatoid arthritics was indeed a reaction to an autoantigen associated with IgG. The one rheumatoid arthritic who did not respond to autologous IgG was discovered to have a negative serum latex test at the time of the experiment even though it had previously been positive. This suggested the possibility that antibody was not available to initiate a reaction even though antigen had been introduced into the joint.

The part played by Gm types was studied in an attempt to define further the nature of the autoantigen. With the cooperation of Dr. H. H. Fudenberg,[23] all donors and recipients were typed for Gm(a), Gm(b), Gm(f), Gm(x), and Gm(z). When autologous IgG was injected into one knee of a rheumatoid patient, and IgG from another rheumatoid arthritic was injected into the other knee, essentially similar inflammatory responses were elicited in the two knees if there were Gm groups in common between donor and recipient. In each of seven patients tested, this proved to be the case, and in an additional two trials run without autologous IgG controls, a significant inflammatory response was elicited by matched Gm types. By contrast, two subjects receiving IgG from rheumatoid donors who differed from the recipients with respect to all five Gm groups tested developed no inflammatory response. One additional subject, who had only Gm(b) in common with the donor, developed a very mild reaction detectable only by changes in the joint fluid.

If Gm loci themselves are the autoantigens responsible for the inflammatory reaction, it would be expected that IgG from normal donors might elicit a synovial reaction in rheumatoid recipients if the donors and recipients were matched with respect to Gm groups. To test this possibility, ten rheumatoid patients received IgG from normal donors sharing two or three Gm groups with the recipients. Only one of the recipients developed an inflammatory response, and this was a very mild one. Although these experiments suggest that the autoantigen which elicits the synovial inflammation observed in these experimental subjects bears some relation to the Gm type of the IgG molecule, the Gm locus itself does not seem to be the autoantigen. If it were, it would be expected that IgG from a properly matched normal donor would provoke a reaction.

In view of the finding that rheumatoid factor appears to be directed principally against the Fc fragment of human IgG, it seemed worthwhile to observe the effect of injecting this fragment into the quiescent joint of a rheumatoid patient. An experiment was conducted[24] with a normal donor having Gm(b) and Gm(f) in common with a rheumatoid recipient. Four antigens were prepared from the donor material: IgG, Fc and Fab fragments prepared by papain digestion, and $F(ab')_2$ prepared by pepsin digestion. The Fc was given in 1.0-mg dosage, and the remaining materials in a dosage of 3.0 mg each. Neither the IgG nor the $F(ab')_2$ elicited any inflammatory response in the recipient's knees. The Fc fragment evoked a severe response, however, and the Fab fragment produced a moderate reaction.

In view of these results, we proceeded to study additional subjects for their response to IgG fragments.[25] Five additional rheumatoid recipients were given Fc fragment, from a normal donor in three instances and from a rheumatoid donor in two. The antigen was given in dosage ranging from 0.1 to 1.0 mg. In each case, a definite inflammatory reaction was observed. The two rheumatoid recipients who received Fc fragment from rheumatoid patients also received Fab fragment from the same donor in the opposite knee. In one case, in which the Fab fragment was given in 0.1-mg dosage, no reaction was observed. Another patient, who received 3.0 mg of Fab, had a moderate reaction. These findings suggest that the autoantigens involved in this form of experimental arthritis may be associated with the Fc fragment, and possibly to a lesser extent with the Fab fragment, and that they may be exposed to a greater degree in IgG from a rheumatoid arthritic than that from a normal subject. The interpretation of the results is uncertain, however, since the injected IgG fragments were not tested for pyrogens.

Relevance of Experimental Arthritis to Rheumatoid Arthritis

The foregoing experiments indicate that, in either rabbit or man, an arthritis may be produced by the introduction of an antigen derived from autologous material into the joint of a subject who has a corresponding autoantibody. If rheumatoid factor is the autoantibody concerned in the pathogenesis of rheumatoid arthritis by a mechanism of this type, the identity of the presumed antigen must be considered. Since rheumatoid factor is an antibody directed primarily against certain antigenic groupings of human IgG, it would seem logical that an altered form of IgG might be found in the active joints of rheumatoid arthritics. Evidence of the presence of such material has recently been reported.[26]

There is little information on how altered IgG might find its way into a joint apart from the larger question of how IgG might be altered to become an autoantigen. It has been proposed that antibody IgG might become an autoantigen following combination with infectious agents, bacterial or viral; clinical as well as experimental observations have been cited to support this thesis.[27] Of interest in this connection is the recent observation that lysosomal proteases of human synovial origin are capable of splitting human IgG to produce fragments which react with antisera to Fc and Fab and with rheumatoid factors.[28]

It is also possible that IgG may become an autoantigen in consequence of some intrinsic abnormality of IgG peculiar to rheumatoid arthritics. The experiments described indicate a definite difference between IgG from a rheumatoid arthritic and that from a normal subject with respect to their ability to induce acute arthritis. Although there is little additional definite support for this idea, one interesting observation has had some bearing on this point: Normal subjects of blood group O respond to an injection of group A or B substance by making abundant antibody of IgG type. Rheumatoid subjects of blood group O, by contrast, are capable of making only a very limited amount of isohemagglutinin of IgG type.[29] This might possibly be explained by minor anomalies of tertiary structure in some of the IgG molecules of rheumatoid arthritics. Such structural change might expose hidden antigenic determinants such as the one recently shown to be exposed on the Fc portion of the heavy chain by various forms of aggregation.[30]

The experiments concerned with the injection of Fab fragment into rabbit joints indicate that autoantibody may be stimulated by the presence of autoantigen in a joint cavity. The demonstration of synovial lymphoid cells as a major source of rheumatoid factor in rheumatoid arthritis is compatible with a hypothesis of sensitization by an intraarticular autoantigen.

References

1. KLINGE, F. 1933. Der Rheumatismus: Die experimentelle serumhyperergie. Ergebn. Allg. Path. **27:** 245.
2. GLYNN, L. E. 1965. Arthropathy in man and animals. Proc. Roy. Soc. Med. **58:** 365.
3. RAWSON, A. J. & T. P. TORRALBA. 1967. Induction of proliferative synovitis in rabbits by intra-articular injection of immune complexes. Arthritis Rheum. **10:** 44.
4. WILLKENS, R. F., R. V. ANDERSON & B. C. GILLILAND. 1968. Response of sensitized rabbits to intra-articular gamma globulin. Arthritis Rheum. **11:** 418.
5. WARD, P. A. & C. G. COCHRANE. 1965. Bound complement and immunologic injury of blood vessels. J. Exp. Med. **121:** 215.
6. WEISSMANN, G., I. SPILBERG & K. KRAKAUER. 1969. Arthritis induced in rabbits by lysates of granulocyte lysosomes. Arthritis Rheum. **12:** 103.
7. MANDY, W. J. & L. C. KORMEIER. 1966. Homoreactant: A naturally occurring autoantibody in rabbits. Science **154:** 651.
8. RAWSON, A. J., F. P. QUISMORIO & N. M. ABELSON. 1969. The induction of synovitis in the normal rabbit with Fab. Amer. J. Path. **54:** 95.
9. MELLORS, R. C., A. NOWOSLAWSKI & L. KORNGOLD. 1961. Rheumatoid arthritis and the cellular origin of rheumatoid factors. Amer. J. Path. **39:** 533.
10. BONOMO, L., A. TURSI & U. GILLARDI. 1968. Distribution of antigamma globulin factors in the synovial membrane and other tissues in different diseases. Ann. Rheum. Dis. **27:** 122.
11. SCHROHENLOHER, R. E. 1966. Characterization of the γ-globulin complexes present in certain sera having high titers of anti-γ-globulin activity. J. Clin. Invest. **45:** 501.
12. BUTLER, JR., V. P. & J. H. VAUGHAN. 1965. The reaction of rheumatoid factor with animal gamma globulins: quantitative considerations. Immunology **8:** 144.
13. HENNEY, C. S. & D. R. STANWORTH. 1965. The reactivity of rhumatoid factor with human gamma G globulin. Immunology **9:** 139.
14. BANDILLA, K. K. & F. C. MCDUFFIE. 1969. Reactivity of rheumatoid factor with autologous IgG antibodies. Arthritis Rheum. **12:** 74.
15. ALLEN, J. C. & H. G. KUNKEL. 1966. Hidden rheumatoid factors with specificity for native-γ-globulins. Arthritis Rheum. **9:** 758.
16. HARBOE, M., B. RAU & K. AHO. 1965. Properties of various anti-γ-globulin factors in human sera. J. Exp. Med. **121:** 503.
17. GOODMAN, J. W. 1961. Reaction of rheumatoid sera with fragments of papain-digested rabbit gamma globulin. Proc. Soc. Exp. Biol. Med. **106:** 822.
18. NATVIG, J. B. 1966. Heterogenicity of anti-γ-globulin factors detected by pepsin-digested human G-globulin. Acta Path. Microbiol. Scand. **66:** 369.
19. SCHOENFELD, L. S. & W. V. EPSTEIN. 1965. Macroglobulin rheumatoid factors directed toward buried antigenic sites of human γ-globulins. Vox Sang. **10:** 482.

20. STEINBERG, A. G. & S. H. POLMAR. 1965. The relation of the S and F fragments and the H and L chains of gamma globulin to the Gm groups. Vox Sang. **10:** 369.
21. LITWIN, S. D. & H. G. KUNKEL. 1966. A gamma-globulin genetic factor related to Gm(a) but localized to a different portion of the same heavy chains. Nature **210:** 866.
22. RESTIFO, R. A., A. J. LUSSIER, A. J. RAWSON, J. H. ROCKEY & J. L. HOLLANDER. 1965. Studies on the pathogenesis of rheumatoid joint inflammation. III. The experimental production of arthritis by the intra-articular injection of purified 7S gamma globulin. Ann. Intern. Med. **62:** 285.
23. HOLLANDER, J. L., H. H. FUDENBERG, A. J. RAWSON, N. M. ABELSON & T. P. TORRALBA. 1966. Further studies on the pathogenesis of rheumatoid joint inflammation. Arthritis Rheum. **9:** 675.
24. OWEN, E., F. P. QUISMORIO, A. J. RAWSON, N. M. ABELSON & J. L. HOLLANDER. 1967. Induction of synovitis in rheumatoids by fragments of IgG. Abst., IV Pan Amer. Congr. Rheum., E29, I26. Excerpta Med. Int. Congr. Ser. **143.**
25. QUISMORIO, F. P., E. OWEN, A. J. RAWSON, N. M. ABELSON & J. L. HOLLANDER. 1968. Synovitis from injected IgG fragments in rheumatoid patients. Arthritis Rheum. **11:** 113 (Abstr.).
26. HANNESTAD, K. 1967. Presence of aggregated gamma-G-globulin in certain rheumatoid synovial effusions. Clin. Exp. Immunol. **2:** 511.
27. HOLLANDER, J. L., E. M. BROWN, JR., R. A. JESSAR, K. HUMMELER & W. HENLE. 1962. Studies on relationship of virus infections to early or acute rheumatoid arthritis. AIR (Arch. Interam. Rheum.) **5**(2)**:** 137.
28. FEHR, K., J. LOSPALLUTO & M. ZIFF. 1968. Exposure of hidden antigenic sites in human IgG after digestion by lysosomal proteases. Arthritis Rheum. **11:** 822 (Abstr.).
29. RAWSON, A. J., N. M. ABELSON & D. J. MCCARTY. 1961. The isohemagglutinin partition in rheumatoid arthritis. Arthritis Rheum. **4:** 463.
30. HENNEY, C. S. & K. ISHIZAKA. 1968. Antigenic determinants specific for aggregated γG-globulins. J. Immunol. **100:** 718.

General Discussion

DR. CATHCART: Did you use patients without rheumatoid arthritis but with rheumatoid factor in the serum as controls for your γ-globulin injection studies?

DR. RAWSON: We have not studied nonrheumatoids with rheumatoid factor. We have been unable to obtain permission for such studies.

DR. WALLER: I noted that you gave Fab fragments to rabbits with homoreactant. I presume the specificity that you obtained was to the papain-digested fragments. Was this controlled by using Fab fragments digested with pepsin? The specificity is entirely different, depending upon which enzyme is used for hydrolysis.

DR. RAWSON: We did not study the pepsin-digested fragment. We followed the methods described by Mandy, who was the original worker with the homoreactant.

DR. WALLER: The same study was done in man, and the same rule holds. These antibodies in man are called agglutinators, and they are quite specific for the type of enzymatic hydrolysis used for the γG-globulin. In the instances in which you administered the Fab fragment, how did the titers vary in your recipients? Our experience has been that individuals can have high titers of agglutinator to the pepsin-hydrolyzed fragment and low titers to the papain-digested fragment, and vice versa. Thus, you have a built-in control in man in many instances. Did you notice any difference between the two pepsin fragments that depended upon their titers of agglutinator?

DR. RAWSON: We only studied titers to these fragments in rabbits, not in human beings.

DR. VAUGHAN: You reported on studies with Fc fragment from normal γG-globulin and Fc fragment from rheumatoid γG-globulin. Did you have enough data from these two different sources to know whether or not they behaved differently when injected into patients with rheumatoid arthritis? You have reported that whole γG seemed to make a difference, depending on the source. Did the Fc fragment?

DR. RAWSON: We are not entirely satisfied with the Fc fragment studies, for the reason I mentioned. We also have a rather small series, three sera from normal sources and two from rheumatoid sources. However, it was our impression that the Fc fragment from rheumatoid sources gave a much more severe reaction than did the Fc fragment from normal sources.

DR. VAUGHAN: Are you satisfied that any residual papain in the preparation plays no role?

DR. RAWSON: Yes. We studied these preparations for residual papain by a number of methods, including Ouchterlony assay using antipapain antibody.

THE JOINT-FLUID γG-GLOBULIN COMPLEXES AND THEIR RELATIONSHIP TO INTRAARTICULAR COMPLEMENT DIMINUTION*

R. J. Winchester, M.D., V. Agnello, M.D., and H. G. Kunkel, M.D.
The Rockefeller University, New York, N. Y.

Accumulating evidence implicates local immune reactions in the pathogenesis of rheumatoid arthritis. Early studies by Pekin and Zvaifler[1,2] and Hedberg[3] have described the disproportionate lowering of total hemolytic complement in certain joint fluids obtained from patients with rheumatoid arthritis. Additional studies on the concomitant depression of various complement components in these fluids indicated that intraarticular fixation and activation of complement was most probably responsible for this complement depletion.[4,5] Although immune complexes or their equivalents were held likely to be the initiating agents of complement activation, no evidence of directly measurable complexes associated with the occurrence of complement depletion was advanced.

A characteristic feature of the serum and joint fluid from patients with rheumatoid arthritis is the presence of different types of γ-globulin complexes visible on ultracentrifugation. Investigations primarily in the serum demonstrated that these complexes are based on the anti-γ-globulin specificity of mainly either γM or γG rheumatoid factors. The property of 7S γG rheumatoid factor, that of being an antibody to γG-globulin molecules similar to itself, results in the formation of various immune complexes sedimenting intermediate between 7S and 19S, and occasionally in heavier zones.[6] There was, however, no certain pathogenic role demonstrated for these complexes.

Recently, Hannestad redirected attention to the γ-globulin complexes in the joint fluid of patients with rheumatoid arthritis with his description of high-molecular weight components precipitable from certain joint fluid by the addition of rheumatoid sera or γM rheumatoid factor.[7] Subsequent studies demonstrated that the complexes were composed of γG-globulin and were not found in inflammatory arthritis other than rheumatoid arthritis. It was further observed that their occurrence was associated with the presence of a continuum of γ-globulin sedimenting in the intermediate and in some cases heavier than 19S regions upon ultracentrifugation.[8] Complexes obtained from the regions between 7S and 12–14S did not precipitate with γM rheumatoid factor but united with the rheumatoid factor, thus inhibiting its agglutinating ability. Heavier γ-globulin complexes gave direct precipitin reactions with γM rheumatoid factor.

Results and Discussion

The joint fluid from rheumatoid arthritis patient Cr., upon analytic ultracentrifugation, exhibits a continuum of components not present in similar concentration in the serum (FIGURE 1); 1.2 mg/ml of components sedimenting in a region heavier than 19S are present in the joint fluid but are not detectable in the serum in similar concentration. Between the 7S and 19S regions, the joint fluid has 5.1 mg and the serum 2.6 mg of component per milliliter. The 7S peaks are 11 and 13 mg, respectively. These complexes are found principally in the

* This investigation was supported by United States Public Health Service grant no. AM-04761.

euglobulin fraction, and the complexes of this fraction are dissociable to 7S γ-globulin.

Joint fluids such as Cr., containing abundant γ-globulin complexes, gave the precipitin reactions with γM rheumatoid factor described by Hannestad, whereas those with small amounts of complexes or none gave no precipitin band. A precipitin reaction carried out on an ouchterlony plate is depicted in FIGURE 2.

The phenomenon of precipitin permits the complexes to be isolated and further characterized. Following the addition at equivalence of purified γM rheumatoid factor[9] to 4 ml of joint fluid Ea., the precipitate was harvested, washed, and dissociated in 0.1M acetate buffer at pH 4.0. Gel filtration was performed in a Sephadex G-200 column equilibrated with the same buffer. The effluent diagram is shown in FIGURE 3. The γ-globulin complexes were dissociated to 150,000-molecular weight γG. Testing of fractions by the FII latex reagent or heat-

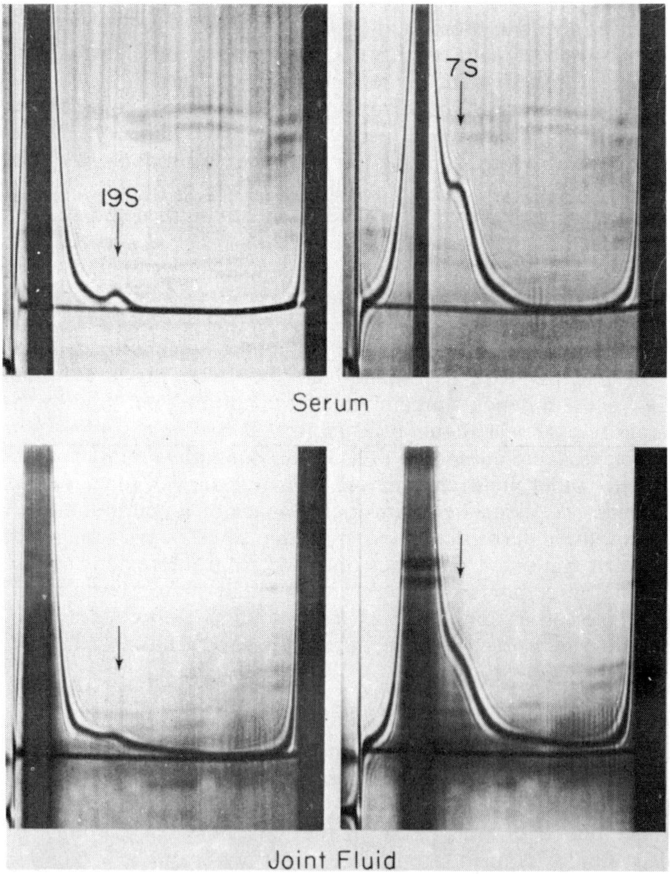

FIGURE 1. Analytic ultracentrifugation of serum and joint fluid from patient Cr. (52,640 rpm at 20° C). The left-hand frames were taken at 32 minutes, and the 19S component is indicated. The right-hand frames were taken at 96 minutes, and the 7S peak is indicated. A spectrum of components is present in the joint fluid, heavier than 7S, at concentrations greater than in the serum.

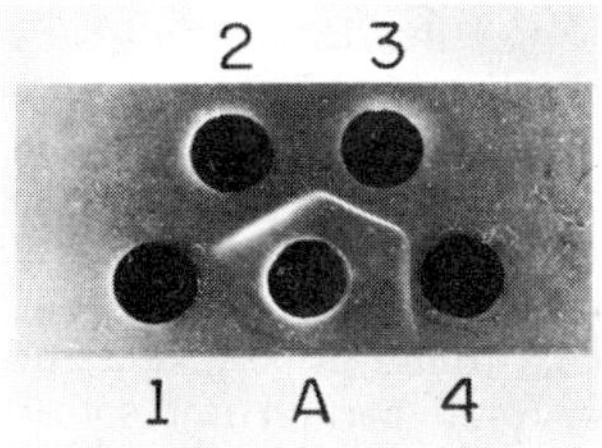

FIGURE 2. Precipitation reaction with purified γM rheumatoid factor. The central well, A, contains purified γM rheumatoid factor; wells 3 and 4, aggregated γ-globulin at 0.1 and 0.05 mg/ml, ml, respectively; well 1, joint fluid Mo., without γ-globulin complexes; and well 2, fluid from patient Lo., with abundant γ-globulin complexes. A precipitin band is present with aggregated γ-globulin and joint fluid Lo. No reaction is seen with joint fluid Mo.

aggregated γ-globulin according to methods of Schrohenloher[10] revealed the presence of rheumatoid factor activity in the 150,000-molecular weight fraction as well as in the void-volume fractions that contained the added γM rheumatoid factor. From this and other experiments it was inferred that 7S γG rheumatoid factor was a constituent of the high-molecular weight γ-globulin complex. Accordingly, the question arose whether 7S γG rheumatoid factor could under certain circumstances form complexes large enough to be precipitated by γM rheumatoid factor.

Two of 15 cases of hyperglobulinemic purpura, a disease containing complexes of 7S γG rheumatoid factor in the serum,[6] gave precipitin reactions with γM rheumatoid factor. Analytic ultracentrifugal analysis of serum Da., which gave the most abundant precipitate with γM rheumatoid factor, is shown in FIGURE 4. A sloping continuum of components sedimenting in regions appreciably heavier than 19S is present. Analysis of this serum on density gradient under nondissociating conditions is shown in FIGURE 5. γ-globulin complexes are demonstrable in fractions heavier than 7S both by their property of inhibiting the agglutination by rheumatoid factor and by their precipitation with γM rheumatoid factor. The

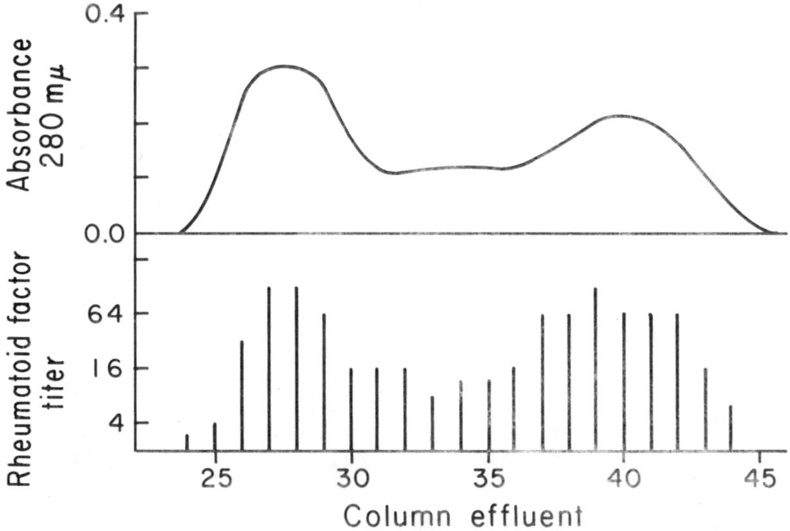

FIGURE 3. Resolution of dissociated γM rheumatoid factor precipitate of γG-globulin complexes. (*Top*) Effluent concentration of protein. (*Bottom*) Results of testing fractions for FII latex-agglutinating activity. The first peak is the excluded volume and contains the added γM rheumatoid factor. The second peak overlies a 150,000-molecular weight marker occurring in tube 40.

precipitation was apparent in the heavier fractions. From the 7S region to the bottom fractions of the gradient, β-mercaptoethanol-resistant, FII latex-agglutinating activity was present, indicating the presence of 7S γG rheumatoid factor activity. This was confirmed by the presence of reactivity with aggregated γ-globulin. Thus, certain sera, with γ-globulin complexes based on 7S γG rheumatoid factor, can precipitate with added γM rheumatoid factor. However, in rheumatoid arthritis the various complexes of γ-globulin found in both sera and joint fluids are not fully characterized, and there are still certain unresolved differences between the complexes in the two locations.

In the course of investigations on γG complexes, a relationship was encountered in various joint fluids between the occurrence of abundant complexes and diminished complement. TABLE 1 shows the average total hemolytic complement levels as a function of the quantity of γ-globulin complex. The eight fluids from rheumatoid arthritis patients with more than 6 mg of precipitate per gram had complement levels of less than 3.4 $C'H_{50}$ units/100 mg. Conversely, fluids from rheumatoid arthritis patients with less than 1 mg of complex had average complement levels of 23 $C'H_{50}$ units/100 mg, within the same range as control fluids from various inflammatory and degenerative arthritides. FIGURE 6 shows the relationship between the quantity of γ-globulin complex and the complement level. The average levels of two components of the complement system, C′1q and β_{1A}, are shown in TABLE 1. These were similarly diminished in

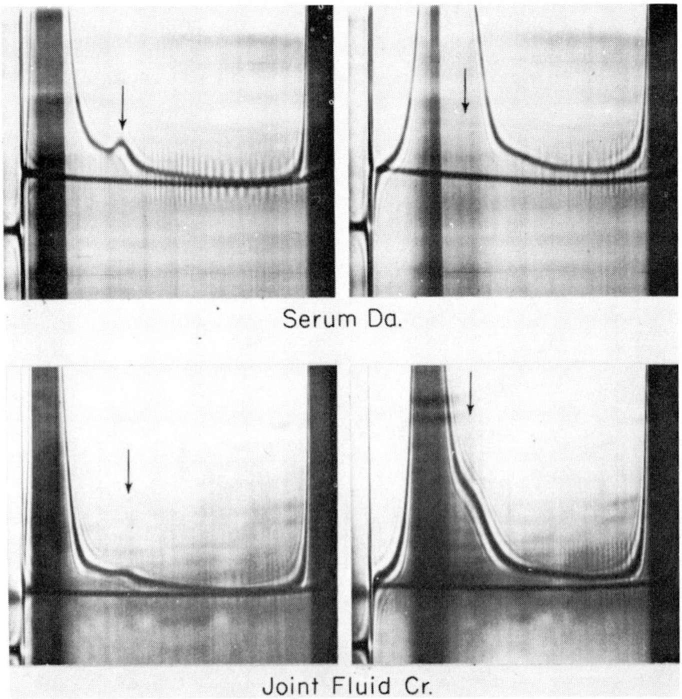

FIGURE 4. Analytic ultracentrifugation of serum Da. and joint fluid Cr. Centrifugation and frame time are the same as in FIGURE 1. A continuum of complexes is present in serum Da. similar to that present in joint fluid Cr.

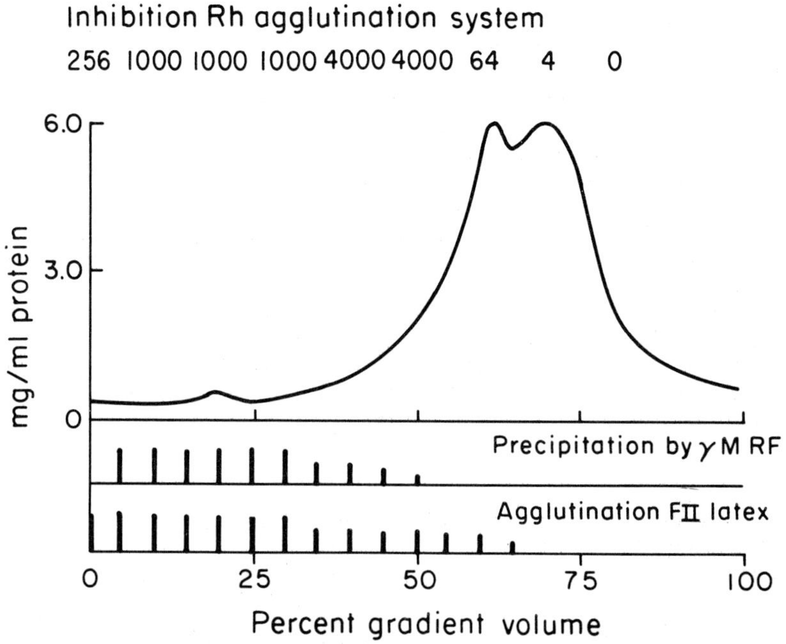

FIGURE 5. Density-gradient analysis of hyperglobulinemic purpura serum. Sucrose-density gradient of serum Da. in phosphate-buffered saline, (pH 7.2). A 19S marker is at 25% and a 7S marker at 60% of the gradient volume. Protein concentration content of fractions is as indicated. The reciprocal of inhibition titer measures the quantity of γ-globulin complexes as does precipitation with added γM rheumatoid factor (RF). The mercaptoethanol-resistant agglutination of FII-coated latex is indicated in the lower section.

TABLE 1

COMPARISON OF THE QUANTITY OF γ-GLOBULIN COMPLEX WITH THE LEVEL OF HEMOLYTIC COMPLEMENT AND TWO COMPLEMENT COMPONENTS

γ-Globulin Complex* (mg/g)	Complement Level† (C′H_{50} units/100 mg)	C′1q† (mg/g)	β_{1A}† (mg/g)
>6 (8)	0.8 (0– 3.4)†	1.3 (.7–2.5)†	3.2 (1.8– 8.2)†
1–6 (5)	15 (11–20)	2.8 (2.0–3.6)	6.8 (3.6– 8.8)
<1 (5)	23 (19–31)	2.8 (1.9–3.1)	7.2 (3.4–11.1)
0‡ (8)	26 (15–39)	3.0 (2.1–4.5)	8.7 (4.7–11.0)

* Numbers in parentheses indicate the number of fluids in each group.
† Mean value and range.
‡ Control fluids.

proportion to the amount of γ-globulin complex present, although there was more individual variation present than with total hemolytic complement.

The association of the diminution of C′1q with the occurrence of γ-globulin complexes suggests that the γ-globulin complexes themselves may be capable of fixing C′1q. The decrease in β_{1A} levels indicates that activation of the complement system followed fixation of C′1q. In view of this correlation, it was decided to investigate whether the joint fluids containing the γ-globulin complexes were capable of interacting with the complement system *in vitro*. Two methods were employed to evaluate this: precipitation with isolated C′1q, which indicates the presence of immune complexes with the ability to fix this subcomponent,[11] and assessment of an anticomplementary effect, which indicates subsequent activation. When normal serum was used as the complement source and incubation was carried out at 4° C, only three fluids showed an anticomplementary effect, and these were from the group of seven joint fluids with abundant γ-globulin complexes, markedly depressed hemolytic complement, and undetectable C′1q. However, an anticomplementary effect was manifest in an additional five fluids when rheumatoid serum was employed as the complement source and incubation was performed at 37° C. All joint fluids manifesting an anticomplementary effect under these conditions had moderate to abundant γ-globulin complexes. All joint fluids exhibiting an anticomplementary effect with rheumatoid serum gave direct precipitation reactions with C′1q. FIGURE 7 depicts the precipitin reaction. This precipitation represented a second method for the isolation of the complexes. This procedure also gave evidence for 7S γG rheumatoid factor as a dominant constituent of the complexes.

Conclusion and Summary

A relationship was encountered between the amount of γ-globulin complexes and the diminution of total hemolytic activity in joint fluid. The depression in levels of C′1q and β_{1A} were generally correlated with the quantity of γ-globulin

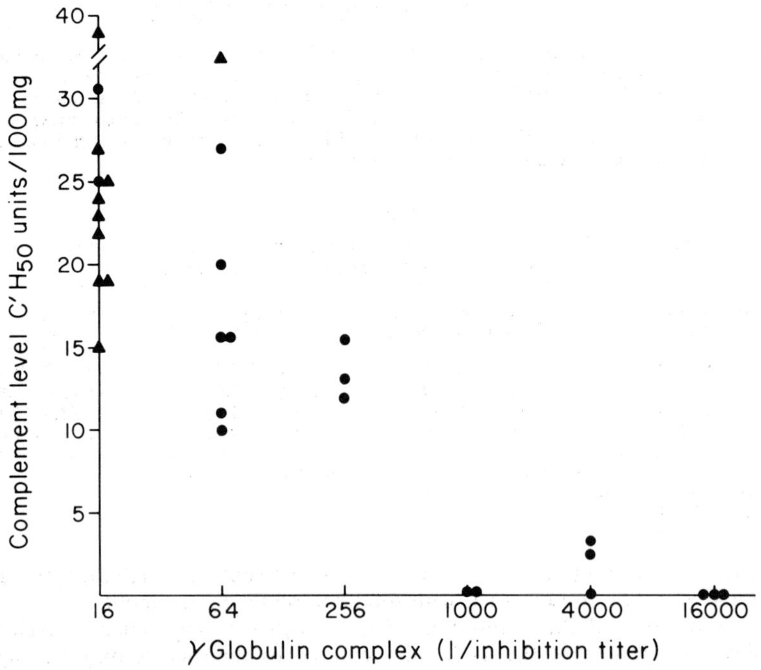

FIGURE 6. Relationship of the quantity of γ-globulin complex to hemolytic complement level. The ordinate expresses the total hemolytic complement $C'H_{50}$ units/100 mg of joint fluid protein. The abscissa expresses the quantity of γ-globulin complex measured by the inhibition of the agglutination of Ripley coated erythrocytes by a high-titer rheumatoid serum. Control fluids are indicated by triangles.

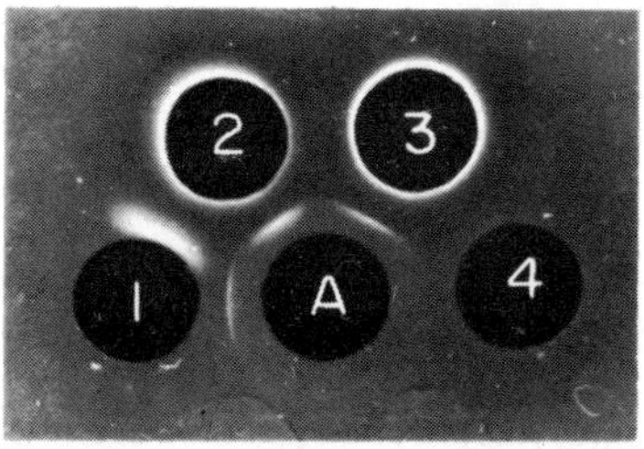

FIGURE 7. Direct precipitation reaction with C′1q. The C′1q (well A) gives precipitin bands with aggregated γ-globulin (well 1) and joint fluids Lo. (well 2) and Ea. (well 3), both of which contain γ-globulin complexes. No precipitin band is given by joint fluid Mo., which does not contain complexes (well 4).

complex, suggesting that the complement diminution in these instances was due to fixation and activation of the complement system by the γ-globulin complexes. Additional evidence for the interaction of these fluids with the complement system was obtained. Fluids with abundant complexes manifested an anticomplementary effect accentuated by 19S rheumatoid factor and formed direct precipitates with C′1q. Isolation of the complexes was accomplished by precipitation with 19S rheumatoid factor or C′1q. The 7S γG rheumatoid factor has been identified as a major constituent of the complexes. The central implication in the present study is that γG-globulin complexes containing 7S γG rheumatoid factor are responsible for the intraarticular activation of the complement system, and thereby may initiate immune injury.

References

1. PEKIN, T. J. & N. J. ZVAIFLER. 1962. Measurement of hemolytic complement in synovial fluids. Arthritis Rheum. **5:** 314.
2. PEKIN, T. J. & N. J. ZVAIFLER. 1964. Hemolytic complement in synovial fluid. J. Clin. Invest. **43:** 1372.
3. HEDBERG, H. 1963. Studies on the depressed hemolytic complement activity of synovial fluid in adult rheumatoid arthritis. Acta Rheum. Scand. **9:** 165.
4. ZVAIFLER, N. J. & T. J. PEKIN. 1963. Complement components in synovial fluids. Clin. Res. **11:** 180.
5. FOSTIROPOULOS, G., K. F. AUSTEN & K. J. BLOCH. 1965. Total hemolytic complement (CH_{50}) and second component of complement ($C'2^{hu}$) activity in serum and synovial fluid. Arthritis Rheum. **8:** 219.
6. KUNKEL, H. G., H. J. MÜLLER-EBERHARD, H. H. FUDENBERG & T. B. TOMASI. 1961. Gamma globulin complexes in rheumatoid arthritis and certain other conditions. J. Clin. Invest. **40:** 117.
7. HANNESTAD, K. 1967. Presence of aggregated γ globulin in certain rheumatoid synovial effusions. Clin. Exp. Immunol. **2:** 511.
8. WINCHESTER, R. J. & H. G. KUNKEL. 1968. High molecular weight complexes involving γ globulin in joint fluids from rheumatoid arthritis patients. Arthritis Rheum. **11:** 849 (Abstr.).
9. SCHROHENLOHER, R. E., H. G. KUNKEL & T. B. TOMASI. 1964. Activity of dissociated and reassociated 19S anti-γ-globulins. J. Exp. Med. **120:** 215.
10. SCHROHENLOHER, R. E. 1966. Characterization of the γ globulin complexes present in certain sera having high titers of anti γ globulin activity. J. Clin. Invest. **45:** 501.
11. AGNELLO, V., R. I. CARR, D. KOFFLER & H. G. KUNKEL. 1969. Gel diffusion reactions of C′lq with aggregated γ globulin, DNA and various anionic substances. Fed. Proc. **28:** 2447 (Abstr.).

General Discussion

DR. HANNESTAD: Your precipitin curve between rheumatoid factor and the γG-anti-γG complexes from the hyperglobulinemic purpura sera shows very strong inhibition in antigen excess. When I performed quantitative precipitation of joint fluids containing γG aggregates, I did not observe inhibition in antigen excess. Have you observed similar inhibition in antigen excess during quantitative precipitation with joint fluids containing γG aggregates?

DR. WINCHESTER: Yes, we have. In most instances, we find inhibition when we use the joint fluids in antigen excess.

DR. HANNESTAD: From the analytical ultracentrifuge appearance of this particular serum, did you have the impression that the complexes were smaller than in the joint fluids? I wonder whether the inhibition that was so strong with the serum could be explained by rather small complexes, whereas the lesser degree of inhibition in joint fluids could be explained by larger complexes. Possibly there are other explanations for this difference in inhibition.

DR. WINCHESTER: I think we are seeing inhibition by 7S γ-globulin of precipitation of relatively small aggregates or complexes. These complexes should not be viewed in the same context as those created from γ-globulin by incubation at 63° C for ten minutes, which are 50–100S.

DR. VAUGHAN: Does the 20% of complex which has not dissociated in acid respond to mercaptoethanol? Can you dissociate it, for instance, with 0.1 or 0.2 M 2-mercaptoethanol?

DR. WINCHESTER: Recent experiments have been carried out on highly purified complexes minimally contaminated with γM rheumatoid factor. Here acid dissociation of the γG complex was essentially complete.

DR. AUSTEN: How does your complement data correlate with the content of rheumatoid factor? You show a nice correlation with your complex.

DR. WINCHESTER: All of the joint fluids with low complement levels came from patients who were seropositive. It was, however, of interest to encounter one fluid with zero complement activity and abundant complexes; yet by various means γM rheumatoid factor was barely detectable in the serum, and not evident in the joint fluid.

DR. SCHMIDT: You drew certain parallels between the γG complexes in people with hypergammaglobulinemic purpura and those seen in the joint fluids of people with rheumatoid arthritis. I understand that in the joint fluids the complexes are readily precipitable by adding γM rheumatoid factor. In the serum of the patients with purpura, however, only two of 15 apparently were precipitable by γM rheumatoid factor. Is any information as to why this happened?

DR. WINCHESTER: I can only speculate on that. It may reflect the fact that the affinity of the 7S γG rheumatoid factor in these two patients differed from that of the other 13.

DR. VAUGHAN: I gather your thought, if not proof at the moment, is that the complexes that you are dealing with are simply γG-anti-γG complexes without being necessarily abnormal γG molecules, in the sense of some denaturation process having involved the γG-globulin molecule. In other words, the complex is related to γG-anti-γG activity rather than some other type of polymerization of γG. Is this correct?

DR. WINCHESTER: That interpretation is most consistent with the data that we have. I think it goes beyond our data in the joint fluid, however, to conclude at this time that all the complexes are so formed. We have not obtained evidence to suggest that other varieties of polymerization are operating.

DR. VAUGHAN: Dr. Hannestad, have you any information to suggest otherwise?

DR. HANNESTAD: I have one synovial fluid in which the complexes were not completely dissociable in acid, down to pH 3.7. When I went down to pH 2.6, I got some evidence of denaturation by the low pH alone. I wonder whether, in addition to γG-anti-γG complexes there is another factor making these complexes larger, and why they don't completely dissociate at pH 3.0. Is it because of a very high affinity or is it because of an added denaturation of these complexes? I would think that, if they were simply immune complexes, one should see complete dissociation of the complexes.

DR. VAUGHAN: You didn't have any of the 19S rheumatoid factor involved in yours?

DR. HANNESTAD: No, it was γG. It went to the bottom in the regular sucrose gradient, and at 20,000 rpm it still went to the bottom. Thus, we must be dealing with extremely large complexes. They were not completely dissociated, which means to me that there must be something else than just pure antibody-antigen, or γG-anti-γG.

DR. ZVAIFLER: Dr. Slowensky in our laboratory has done some studies that have a bearing on the thoughts about γG. By means of radioisotope dilution techniques, he has shown that 10–25% of all the γ-globulin in a single rheumatoid joint is produced locally. Since we know the half-life of γ-globulin in the joint and can estimate the size of the effusions, we calculate that as much as 50 mg of γ-globulin protein are made in a single knee joint in a day. Thus, I think there is ample opportunity for the kinds of reaction that Dr. Winchester and Dr. Hannestad have been talking about to take place.

SUMMARY

John H. Vaughan, M.D.
Department of Medicine
University of Rochester School of Medicine and Dentistry
Rochester, N. Y.

Epidemiological Considerations

The incidence of anti-γ-globulins in the sera of individuals in the general population is about 1–5%. As noted by Drs. Cathcart and O'Sullivan, as well as by others, only about 20–25% of these seropositive persons have what may be diagnosed as rheumatoid arthritis. If you study those persons in the general population who have the highest titers of seropositivity, however, the likelihood goes up to 60–70% that they will have rheumatoid arthritis.

As has been reported, there is some tendency for persons without joint disease but who are seropositive to exhibit rheumatoid arthritis later on. The numbers of patients involved in this conversion from a clinically negative state to a clinically positive state are very few, and whether this apparent tendency is borne out over long periods I don't know; even if we consider the data of Ball and Lawrence on the same subject, it seems to me we have precious little evidence to support this point. It remains a fact that many persons in the general population are seropositive but do not have rheumatoid arthritis.

Some of this seropositivity may be attributed to the fact that anti-γ-globulins accompany diseases other than rheumatoid arthritis. What disease states are these? They include the chronic infectious diseases. We believe this is the result of chronic immunization and supposed alterations of the configuration of, or metabolism of, γG-globulin molecules that have combined with antigen. Subacute bacterial endocarditis is a good example of such a disease, as are tuberculosis, leishmaniasis, trypanosomiasis, and leprosy. In infectious mononucleosis, a type of anti-γG-globulin that looks much like rheumatoid factor is produced. Thus, chronic infections can explain at least some of the seropositivity in the general population that is not attributable rheumatoid arthritis.

Aging is recognized as a process that tends to be accompanied by the production of anti-γ-globulins. This may mean a succession of acute or chronic infections, but nobody really knows. We also recognize that patients who have received organ transplants tend to develop anti-γ-globulins. Needless to say, this particular means of developing anti-γ-globulins will not affect our statistics on the general population to a significant degree, but it emphasizes that there are possibly many types of immunization other than ordinary infection that can result in anti-γ-globulins. Hypergammaglobulinemic purpura, Sjögren's syndrome, cryptogenic cirrhosis, and idiopathic pulmonary fibrosis are further examples. All these together cannot, however, account for much of the seropositivity in the general population, and Dr. Cathcart has told us that he does not detect any disease in most of the seropositive individuals in his population who do not have rheumatoid arthritis. Most of these normal persons who are seropositive will, of course, be persons with low titers of anti-γ-globulins.

These facts serve to emphasize the extent to which the presence of anti-γ-globulins cannot be equated simply to the presence of rheumatoid arthritis. A point is equally well made from the opposite direction. If you examine the general population for rheumatoid arthritis, 75% of persons with the disease, using the Ball and Lawrence criteria for diagnosis, do not have positive serology. If you use Dr. Cathcart's criteria, 60% with disease do not have positive serology. Thus, there is, in the general population, a very large group of persons who are seronegative but by current diagnostic criteria must nevertheless be said to have possible or probable rheumatoid arthritis.

Relation of Serology to Patterns of Arthritis

Dr. Ansell reported that juvenile arthritis patients with anti-γ-globulins present a clinical picture that resembles the adult form of the disease. Patients with seronegative juvenile rheumatoid arthritis often develop something that looks more like ankylosing spondylitis.

In adult-onset rheumatoid arthritis, those who have anti-γ-globulins generally exhibit more severe disease. Deposits of complexes occur in the tissues, and there is a lowering of the complement component titers in the fluid, corresponding to fixation of complement components during the deposition. This may be the reason why seropositive disease is more severe than is seronegative disease.

We must question whether seronegative and seropositive rheumatoid arthritis are different diseases. This question is presented not only by the general population studies, but also by the study of arthritic patients themselves. Obviously, the question is hard to answer. Further understanding of the bases for the development of precipitates between the joint fluids of patients with seronegative rheumatoid arthritis and isolated rheumatoid factors from seropositive patients, such as have been reported by Dr. Winchester and his colleagues and by Dr. Hannestad, may provide a solution.

Pathogenetic Considerations

Are rheumatoid factor complexes important in pathogenesis of the disease? Dr. Rawson and his co-workers have reported the production of arthritis both in the experimental animal and in man by the intraarticular injection of γG-globulins or their subunits. Their studies suggest that development of the arthritis depends upon presence of anti-γG-globulins in the injected individual. We have heard that in seropositive rheumatoid arthritis, rheumatoid factor complexes are deposited in the tissues, complement components are also present in the desposits, and there are lowered complement titers in the joint fluids. In patients with complicating peripheral vasculitis, the serum anti-γ-globulin levels are higher, and the serum complement titers lower compared with those without vaculitis. All of these observations provide "guilt by association," and to my way of thinking strong evidence of guilt. Obviously, the anti-γ-globulins in rheumatoid arthritis may be a secondary development in the disease. It is a reasonable assumption, that seronegative and seropositive rheumatoid arthritis are fundamentally identical, but complicated in the case of the seropositivity by the presence of the γ-globulin complexes.

Specificities

Rheumatoid factors precipitate better with aggregated forms of γG-globulin. Dr. Henney's data suggest to him that the rheumatoid anti-γG-globulins are primarily directed to a denatured form of γG globulin. In ultracentrifugation, however, completely unaggregated γG globulin will react with 19S anti-γG-globulin to give perfectly good 22S complexes. This has been used as an argument that anti-γ-globulin (at least the 19S variety) will react with perfectly normal γG-globulin configurations.

The dilemma present by these seemingly contradictory results remains unresolved because of two facts: (1) we do not have clear data to indicate that greater precipitability with aggregated γG is not related simply to a greater "valence" for the γG-globulin due to its physical aggregation; and (2) we have no real assurance that γG-globulins which are unaggregated are entirely free of denaturation.

All of the subclasses of γG-globulins can be found in the inclusion bodies in joint-fluid leukocytes. Ultracentrifugation data indicate that each of the subclasses of myeloma proteins may react with isolated rheumatoid factors, although γG_3 has been thought to be less reactive than the others. These findings suggest a contradiction with the experiments that Dr. Rawson and his associates have described on the need of similarity between the Gm subtypes of the injected γ-globulin and those of the patient if the injection is to elicit arthritis. This is not a direct contradiction, however, and it is possible that rheumatoid factors may exhibit activities *in vitro* that are not important *in vivo*.

Dr. Hannestad has made the interesting suggestion that the anti-γ-globulin activity of the rheumatoid factor is really a cross-reaction. He finds precipitation between DNP or TNP conjugates of hemocyanin and rheumatoid factors. He finds the same with DNA. It has been brought out that the materials that he has worked with are prone to react nonspecifically with γ-globulins. Dr. Hannestad is aware of this and has tried to guard against it. Possibly, we can ignore this technical question and ask whether the anti-γ-globulins of the rheumatoid factors really might be derived by way of immunization with an agent such as DNA. It is difficult to imagine that DNA has in it all the different configurations that are represented on the γ-globulins of the various animal species with which rheumatoid factors react, as well as the configurations represented in the various Gm specificities that have been recognized among the rheumatoid factors. These specificities argue overwhelmingly in favor of the idea that rheumatoid factors are truly and primarily anti-γ-globulin in nature.

In studies of the rheumatoid factors with Fc fragments and comparison with the anti-γ-globulins that can be elicited in the rabbit, Drs. Cerottini and Grey have emphasized the low avidity exhibited by the rheumatoid factors. This low avidity may be important as a mechanism for allowing these complexes to persist in the circulations of patients rather than to be swept out by the reticuloendothelial system. Further support for the true antibody nature of the 19S anti-γ-globulins is provided by the evidence for a valence of 10 for a 19S rheumatoid factor in the studies reported by Drs. Chavin and Franklin.

Biological Phenomena

Sera from patients with rheumatoid arthritis exhibit several interesting biological properties. There is some factor in these sera that releases histamine from guinea pig lung. This activity is associated with γG-globulins that separate in Sephadex with components $\geqq$ 19S. There is some reason from the data of Dr. Broder and his associates to believe that the activity may not be due to the rheumatoid factors. I believe, however, that this needs more exploration. We now have *in vitro* evidence that rheumatoid factor can fix complement of human origin; the work of both Dr. Zvaifler and Dr. Schmidt indicates this. This presents an important *in vitro* parallel to the evidence of depletion of joint-fluid complement components and their deposition in tissues with rheumatoid factor complexes. Rheumatoid factors also are capable of kininogen consumption, presumably with kinin formation.

These are activities that would contribute to inflammation. Rheumatoid factors may also exhibit activities that could play quite different roles in the body economy. For instance, inhibition or potentiation of opsonic activity of the antibodies from subacute bacterial endocarditis sera may be seen, the direction of the effect depending upon the particular conditions of the experiment. Rheumatoid factors may inhibit complement fixation, if the anti-γ-globulins are used in the right proportion to the other reactants. As Dr. John Davis in Charlottesville has argued, maybe some of these blocking or enhancing activities reflect a protective value for rheumatoid factors. Effects of rheumatoid factors on lymphocyte transformation and in the inhibition of formation of anti-γG-reactive lymphocytes suggest that rheumatoid factors may have yet other roles in immunological homeostasis. These are important questions raised by persons who visualize that the rheumatoid factors were not created by Nature simply to contribute to rheumatoid arthritis; thus, they must have some more useful role in the body's normal physiology.

Future Considerations

What are some of the things we need to see developed in the next two, three, or four years? A further careful delineation of the biological potentials of the various classes and subclasses of the rheumatoid factors is surely needed. What of the complement-fixing ability of the 7S as compared with the 19S anti-γG-globulins? Certainly the 19S fraction fixes complement very inefficiently, as Dr. Schmidt noted. Perhaps the 7S fraction with anti-γG-globulin is more potent in this respect. We don't know; we don't have quantitative data on this subject yet. We also might speculate about the relative efficiencies of the various classes and subclasses of anti-γG-globulins in respect to all the other biological activities that have been designated for rheumatoid arthritis sera.

We ought to think about how to construct ways to determine whether there are some anti-γ-globulins being produced by patients with rheumatoid arthritis which are taken up by the reticuloendothelial system and other phagocytic activities as fast as they get into the fluids, because of their high avidity, so that they never accumulate. This question implies that we may all be looking at the wrong thing. Obviously, we study what we can get out of the blood. Are there types of anti-γ-globulins, or other complexes, which have very short lifetimes in the circulation and which are, therefore, never seen in our test-tube experiments? Possibly, *in vivo* labeling techniques can be used to obtain data describing rates of production of γ-globulins and to determine whether there is a portion of very newly made γG-globulin, for instance, which disappears almost as rapidly as it is made.

Finally, as always, a continued effort should be made toward finding a viral or other microbial agent, if there is one, involved in rheumatoid factor production. A most intriguing possibility in this realm was presented in the experiments described by Hannestad and Winchester and his colleagues. Will some foreign material be found among the aggregated γ-globulins they described in the joint fluids they studied? If not, what more can we discover about the nature of the aggregated γG-globulin itself? Hopefully, another conference five years from now will see answers to all of these questions.

Printed in the United States of America